Biosimilars in Europe

Biosimilars in Europe

Editors

Arnold G. Vulto
Steven Simoens
Isabelle Huys

MDPI • Basel • Beijing • Wuhan • Barcelona • Belgrade • Manchester • Tokyo • Cluj • Tianjin

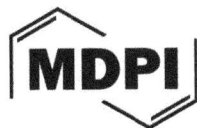

Editors
Arnold G. Vulto
Hospital Pharmacy
Erasmus University Medical Centre
Rotterdam
Netherlands

Steven Simoens
Department of Pharmaceutical and Pharmacological Sciences
KU Leuven
Leuven
Belgium

Isabelle Huys
Department of Pharmaceutical and Pharmacological Sciences
KU Leuven
Leuven
Belgium

Editorial Office
MDPI
St. Alban-Anlage 66
4052 Basel, Switzerland

This is a reprint of articles from the Special Issue published online in the open access journal *Pharmaceuticals* (ISSN 1424-8247) (available at: www.mdpi.com/journal/pharmaceuticals/special_issues/biosimilars_Europe).

For citation purposes, cite each article independently as indicated on the article page online and as indicated below:

LastName, A.A.; LastName, B.B.; LastName, C.C. Article Title. *Journal Name* **Year**, *Volume Number*, Page Range.

ISBN 978-3-0365-6575-0 (Hbk)
ISBN 978-3-0365-6574-3 (PDF)

© 2023 by the authors. Articles in this book are Open Access and distributed under the Creative Commons Attribution (CC BY) license, which allows users to download, copy and build upon published articles, as long as the author and publisher are properly credited, which ensures maximum dissemination and a wider impact of our publications.

The book as a whole is distributed by MDPI under the terms and conditions of the Creative Commons license CC BY-NC-ND.

Contents

About the Editors vii

Steven Simoens and Isabelle Huys
Emerging Insights into European Markets of Biologics, Including Biosimilars
Reprinted from: *Pharmaceuticals* 2022, 15, 615, doi:10.3390/ph15050615 1

Manuel García-Goñi, Isabel Río-Álvarez, David Carcedo and Alba Villacampa
Budget Impact Analysis of Biosimilar Products in Spain in the Period 2009–2019
Reprinted from: *Pharmaceuticals* 2021, 14, 348, doi:10.3390/ph14040348 5

Konstantin Tachkov, Zornitsa Mitkova, Vladimira Boyadzieva and Guenka Petrova
Did the Introduction of Biosimilars Influence Their Prices and Utilization? The Case of Biologic Disease Modifying Antirheumatic Drugs (bDMARD) in Bulgaria
Reprinted from: *Pharmaceuticals* 2021, 14, 64, doi:10.3390/ph14010064 21

Steven Simoens, Arnold G. Vulto and Pieter Dylst
Simulating Costs of Intravenous Biosimilar Trastuzumab vs. Subcutaneous Reference Trastuzumab in Adjuvant HER2-Positive Breast Cancer: A Belgian Case Study
Reprinted from: *Pharmaceuticals* 2021, 14, 450, doi:10.3390/ph14050450 31

Evelien Moorkens, Teresa Barcina Lacosta, Arnold G. Vulto, Martin Schulz, Gabriele Gradl and Salka Enners et al.
Learnings from Regional Market Dynamics of Originator and Biosimilar Infliximab and Etanercept in Germany
Reprinted from: *Pharmaceuticals* 2020, 13, 324, doi:10.3390/ph13100324 39

Félix Lobo and Isabel Río-Álvarez
Barriers to Biosimilar Prescribing Incentives in the Context of Clinical Governance in Spain
Reprinted from: *Pharmaceuticals* 2021, 14, 283, doi:10.3390/ph14030283 59

Philippe Van Wilder
The Off-Patent Biological Market in Belgium: Is the Health System Creating a Hurdle to Fair Market Competition?
Reprinted from: *Pharmaceuticals* 2021, 14, 352, doi:10.3390/ph14040352 75

Liese Barbier, Steven Simoens, Caroline Soontjens, Barbara Claus, Arnold G. Vulto and Isabelle Huys
Off-Patent Biologicals and Biosimilars Tendering in Europe—A Proposal towards More Sustainable Practices
Reprinted from: *Pharmaceuticals* 2021, 14, 499, doi:10.3390/ph14060499 81

Arnold G. Vulto, Jackie Vanderpuye-Orgle, Martin van der Graaff, Steven R. A. Simoens, Lorenzo Dagna and Richard Macaulay et al.
Sustainability of Biosimilars in Europe: A Delphi Panel Consensus with Systematic Literature Review
Reprinted from: *Pharmaceuticals* 2020, 13, 400, doi:10.3390/ph13110400 109

Beverly Ingram, Rebecca S. Lumsden, Adriana Radosavljevic and Christine Kobryn
Analysis of the Regulatory Science Applied to a Single Portfolio of Eight Biosimilar Product Approvals by Four Key Regulatory Authorities
Reprinted from: *Pharmaceuticals* 2021, 14, 306, doi:10.3390/ph14040306 127

Ali M. Alsamil, Thijs J. Giezen, Toine C. Egberts, Hubert G. Leufkens and Helga Gardarsdottir
Type and Extent of Information on (Potentially Critical) Quality Attributes Described in European Public Assessment Reports for Adalimumab Biosimilars
Reprinted from: *Pharmaceuticals* **2021**, *14*, 189, doi:10.3390/ph14030189 . . . . **143**

Yannick Vandenplas, Steven Simoens, Philippe Van Wilder, Arnold G. Vulto and Isabelle Huys
Informing Patients about Biosimilar Medicines: The Role of European Patient Associations
Reprinted from: *Pharmaceuticals* **2021**, *14*, 117, doi:10.3390/ph14020117 . . . . **157**

About the Editors

Arnold G. Vulto

Arnold Vulto is Emeritus Professor at the Erasmus Medical Center in Rotterdam and Visiting Professor at KU Leuven. He is a hospital pharmacist and pharmacologist. In 2008, he was one of the co-founders of the Generics & Biosimilar Initiative and the GaBI Journal. In 2013, he was one of the founders of the Dutch Initiative Group on Biosimilars.

Steven Simoens

Steven Simoens is a senior full professor of health economics at KU Leuven. His research interests focus on health economic aspects of medicinal products. Steven has carried out numerous cost(-of-illness) analyses, economic evaluations and budget impact analyses of medicinal products. He has also worked extensively in the area of policy relating to market access of medicinal products, with a particular interest in oncology medicinal products, orphan medicinal products, advanced therapy medicinal products, antibiotics, vaccines, generics and biosimilars.

Isabelle Huys

Isabelle Huys is full professor at KU Leuven and specialises in intellectual property rights and regulatory sciences. Her research interests focus on legal and regulatory strategies for medicine development, with the aim to promote access to medicines, (human) biological samples and related therapies/diagnostics, as certain therapies remain underdeveloped and, hence, unavailable for patients due to legal or regulatory barriers.

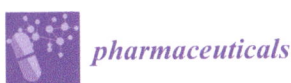

Editorial
Emerging Insights into European Markets of Biologics, Including Biosimilars

Steven Simoens * and **Isabelle Huys**

Department of Pharmaceutical and Pharmacological Sciences, KU Leuven, 3000 Leuven, Belgium; isabelle.huys@kuleuven.be
* Correspondence: steven.simoens@kuleuven.be; Tel.: +32-16-323465

Citation: Simoens, S.; Huys, I. Emerging Insights into European Markets of Biologics, Including Biosimilars. *Pharmaceuticals* 2022, 15, 615. https://doi.org/10.3390/ph15050615

Received: 11 May 2022
Accepted: 13 May 2022
Published: 17 May 2022

Publisher's Note: MDPI stays neutral with regard to jurisdictional claims in published maps and institutional affiliations.

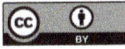

Copyright: © 2022 by the authors. Licensee MDPI, Basel, Switzerland. This article is an open access article distributed under the terms and conditions of the Creative Commons Attribution (CC BY) license (https://creativecommons.org/licenses/by/4.0/).

Biological medicinal products have revolutionised the treatment of many diseases, e.g., autoimmune diseases and cancer, by targeting key disease mediators with high specificity. As patents and other exclusivity rights on many high-selling and expensive biologics are expiring or have expired, biosimilars may enter the market. The market entry of biosimilars (the first of which was approved in the European Union in 2006) has raised questions about legal, regulatory, pricing and reimbursement procedures for these products, as well as regarding policies and incentive structures related to, for example, tendering mechanisms, gainsharing practices, physician quotas, prescribing and switching frameworks, substitutions and the education of stakeholders.

In response to this, KU Leuven (Leuven, Belgium), in collaboration with the Erasmus University Medical Center (Rotterdam, the Netherlands), established the MABEL research programme in 2016, with the aim of exploring the market environment of biologics, including biosimilars, in Europe. On the programme's fifth anniversary, we launched a Special Issue on "Biosimilars in Europe" to share some emerging insights derived from our research programme and from articles published in the Special Issue, as well as to identify unresolved questions and set out a research agenda for the future.

The Need to Reap the Rewards of Biosimilar Competition

The introduction of biosimilars may create competition, possibly resulting in lowered prices, altered market dynamics and the revision of company strategies; it might also attract new players to the biopharmaceutical market. As a result, some health care systems have embraced biosimilars as a tool to control increasing health care expenses or expand patient access to treatments. Competition between off-patent biologics and biosimilars may also induce incremental innovation and the development of next-generation biologics with, for example, a novel formulation or route of administration.

Three articles in this Special Issue provide empirical evidence concerning some of these rewards of biosimilar competition. A Spanish budget impact analysis estimated that biosimilar competition yielded a total saving of EUR 2.3 billion from 2009 to 2019, with approximately one-half of the savings originating from a reduction in list prices and the other half originating from hospital tender discounts [1]. Although total savings over this period were impressive in absolute terms, savings in relative terms amounted to less than 4% of pharmaceutical expenditures in 2019. In an analysis of the Bulgarian market for biologic disease-modifying antirheumatic medicines, Tachkov et al. showed that biosimilar market entry not only reduced prices, but also increased utilization (thus, widening patient access to treatment) and generated competition in a therapeutic class [2]. Finally, a Belgian study examined the introduction of an intravenous biosimilar in the presence of a subcutaneous reference biologic, and indicated that a cost comparison between such products needs to consider multiple factors, such as patient's body weight, discounts and intravenous vial sharing [3].

The Special Issue also confirms that not all European countries are currently reaping the full rewards of biosimilar market entry and competition. On the one hand,

Moorkens et al. suggest that the relatively high market shares of infliximab and etanercept biosimilars in Germany were attained through the implementation of biosimilar prescription quotas, variable procurement contracts between sickness funds and manufacturers, and gainsharing arrangements [4]. On the other hand, Lobo and Río-Álvarez explain how biosimilar competition in Spain is impeded by a variety of barriers, including physician and patient lack of trust in biosimilars and diverging stakeholder interest [5].

The Need to Prescribe Best-Value Biologics

There has been much debate regarding the appropriate use of off-patent reference biologics, biosimilars and next-generation biologics. Instead of promoting the use of one over the other, we believe that the focus needs to shift towards the prescription of best-value biologics. Although the latter term is not uniformly defined, countries such as Ireland and England have implemented programmes stimulating the use of best-value biologics, which may be the off-patent reference biologic, a biosimilar version or a next-generation biologic. By framing the debate in the broader context of best-value biologics, it is possible to align the interests of different stakeholders towards the common objective of maximizing population health with limited resources. However, the introduction of such a programme is not easy, as described in the article by Van Wilder concerning the 2019–2020 "Best-Value Biologics" programme in Belgium [6].

We see an important role for hospital tender procedures to achieve the selection of best-value biologics. Based on a review of tender procedures for off-patent biologics and biosimilars in Europe, Barbier et al. highlighted the importance of creating a level playing field, of timely launching tenders in accordance with public procurement laws, and of guaranteeing supply by creating room for several manufacturers to be active in the market [7]. In addition to the design of tender procedures, competition and incentives were perceived to be crucial in creating a sustainable market for best-value biologics by a panel of European experts [8]. This article makes an important contribution to the field by proposing a consensus definition and identifying some 'dos and don'ts' of a competitive, but sustainable, market for off-patent reference biologics, biosimilars and next-generation biologics. However, much more research needs to be carried out to build a comprehensive theoretical framework to understand how European competitive markets of biologics, including biosimilars, can also be sustainable.

When selecting a best-value biologic or in general terms a best-value medicine, there is a need to consider a whole therapeutic class of products. Let us take the example of rheumatoid arthritis. Although there are differences in indications and target populations, the therapeutic arsenal for rheumatoid arthritis consists of synthetic disease-modifying antirheumatic medicines (e.g., methotrexate and leflunomide), off-patent reference biologics and their biosimilars (adalimumab, infliximab and etanercept), other reference biologics (abatacept, golimumab, sarilumab, tocilizumab and certolizumab pegol) and the recent targeted synthetic Janus kinase inhibitors (tofacitinib and baricitinib). As the market entry of biosimilars and novel biologic or synthetic medicines is likely to influence the relative (cost-)effectiveness of products within a therapeutic class, treatment guidelines need to be regularly updated. However, this is not regularly performed, and, in relation to our example, there is a need for research which assesses the value of Janus kinase inhibitors versus all therapeutic alternatives for rheumatoid arthritis.

The Need to Optimise and Harmonise Regulatory Procedures

The European Medicines Agency has been a worldwide frontrunner in developing and implementing a regulatory pathway supporting the marketing authorisation of biosimilars, with the United States, Canada and Japan adopting similar pathways. The article by Ingram et al. presents a unique insight into how the regulatory agencies from these four countries responded to virtually the same set of data on eight candidate biosimilars from one company [9]. Even though authorisation decisions were the same, the authors noted some differences in how the regulatory agencies tackled the data review and benefit–risk assessment. This lack of uniformity may raise the cost of biosimilar development and may also hamper patient access.

At the time of marketing authorisation, the European Medicines Agency publishes an extensive and detailed scientific assessment report (the so-called European Public Assessment Report) concerning all aspects of a medicine. The article by Alsamil et al. evaluated the critical quality attributes in the European Public Assessment Reports of all adalimumab biosimilars, corroborating that these biosimilars have the same functions and clinical profiles, notwithstanding small variations in glycoforms and charge variants [10].

The Need to Educate Patients

Despite all the efforts and existing programmes available, informing and educating patients regarding biosimilars, there remains scepticism towards their use. Indeed, the article by Vandenplas et al. showed that biosimilar information provided by European patient organisations themselves is not always correct or sufficiently detailed [11]. Hence, this paper sends forth a call for regulatory authorities, industry associations, health care professional associations and patient organisations to jointly produce and disseminate unbiased information concerning biosimilars in a language that is accessible for patients. An additional avenue is to develop a dedicated European Commission-driven website for patients (and health care professionals) on biosimilars.

The Need for Further Research

Taking inspiration from Hippocrates, market and policy research of biologics, including biosimilars, should strive to declare the past and diagnose the present, with the intention of foretelling the future. In respect to the latter, additional research is needed, moving beyond identifying hurdles to biosimilar market entry and competition, and analysing the impact of strategies to overcome these hurdles. Furthermore, questions remain concerning the long-term sustainability of European markets of biologics, including biosimilars: how do we create a policy environment that not only promotes competition, but also safeguards economic viability and prevents shortages?

Author Contributions: Conceptualisation, S.S.; writing—review and editing: S.S. and I.H. All authors have read and agreed to the published version of the manuscript.

Funding: This research received no external funding.

Institutional Review Board Statement: Not applicable.

Informed Consent Statement: Not applicable.

Data Availability Statement: Not applicable.

Acknowledgments: The authors are grateful to Arnold Vulto and to our PhD researchers Liese Barbier, Teresa Barcina-Lacosta, Evelien Moorkens and Yannick Vandenplas for their valuable insights.

Conflicts of Interest: S.S. and I.H. are among the founders of the KU Leuven Fund on Market Analysis of Biologics and Biosimilars following Loss of Exclusivity (MABEL). S.S. was involved in a stakeholder roundtable on biologics and biosimilars sponsored by Amgen, Pfizer and MSD; he participated in advisory board meetings for Pfizer and Amgen; he contributed to studies on biologics and biosimilars for Hospira, Celltrion, Organon and Pfizer; and he had speaking engagements for Amgen, Celltrion and Sandoz. I.H. declares no competing interests.

References

1. Garcia-Goni, M.; Rio-Alvarez, I.; Carcedo, D.; Villacampa, A. Budget Impact Analysis of Biosimilar Products in Spain in the Period 2009–2019. *Pharmaceuticals* **2021**, *14*, 348. [CrossRef] [PubMed]
2. Tachkov, K.; Mitkova, Z.; Boyadzieva, V.; Petrova, G. Did the Introduction of Biosimilars Influence Their Prices and Utilization? The Case of Biologic Disease Modifying Antirheumatic Drugs (bDMARD) in Bulgaria. *Pharmaceuticals* **2021**, *14*, 64. [CrossRef] [PubMed]
3. Simoens, S.; Vulto, A.G.; Dylst, P. Simulating Costs of Intravenous Biosimilar Trastuzumab vs. Subcutaneous Reference Trastuzumab in Adjuvant HER2-Positive Breast Cancer: A Belgian Case Study. *Pharmaceuticals* **2021**, *14*, 450. [CrossRef] [PubMed]

4. Moorkens, E.; Barcina Lacosta, T.; Vulto, A.G.; Schulz, M.; Gradl, G.; Enners, S.; Selke, G.; Huys, I.; Simoens, S. Learnings from Regional Market Dynamics of Originator and Biosimilar Infliximab and Etanercept in Germany. *Pharmaceuticals* **2020**, *13*, 324. [CrossRef] [PubMed]
5. Lobo, F.; Rio-Alvarez, I. Barriers to Biosimilar Prescribing Incentives in the Context of Clinical Governance in Spain. *Pharmaceuticals* **2021**, *14*, 283. [CrossRef]
6. Van Wilder, P. The Off-Patent Biological Market in Belgium: Is the Health System Creating a Hurdle to Fair Market Competition? *Pharmaceuticals* **2021**, *14*, 352. [CrossRef]
7. Barbier, L.; Simoens, S.; Soontjens, C.; Claus, B.; Vulto, A.G.; Huys, I. Off-patent biologicals and biosimilars tendering in Europe —A proposal towards more sustainable practices. *Pharmaceuticals* **2021**, *14*, 499. [CrossRef] [PubMed]
8. Vulto, A.G.; Vanderpuye-Orgle, J.; van der Graaff, M.; Simoens, S.R.A.; Dagna, L.; Macaulay, R.; Majeed, B.; Lemay, J.; Hippenmeyer, J.; Gonzalez-McQuire, S. Sustainability of Biosimilars in Europe: A Delphi Panel Consensus with Systematic Literature Review. *Pharmaceuticals* **2020**, *13*, 400. [CrossRef] [PubMed]
9. Ingram, B.; Lumsden, R.S.; Radosavljevic, A.; Kobryn, C. Analysis of the Regulatory Science Applied to a Single Portfolio of Eight Biosimilar Product Approvals by Four Key Regulatory Authorities. *Pharmaceuticals* **2021**, *14*, 306. [CrossRef] [PubMed]
10. Alsamil, A.M.; Giezen, T.J.; Egberts, T.C.; Leufkens, H.G.; Gardarsdottir, H. Type and Extent of Information on (Potentially Critical) Quality Attributes Described in European Public Assessment Reports for Adalimumab Biosimilars. *Pharmaceuticals* **2021**, *14*, 189. [CrossRef] [PubMed]
11. Vandenplas, Y.; Simoens, S.; Van Wilder, P.; Vulto, A.G.; Huys, I. Informing Patients about Biosimilar Medicines: The Role of European Patient Associations. *Pharmaceuticals* **2021**, *14*, 117. [CrossRef] [PubMed]

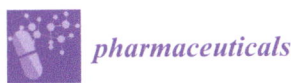

Article

Budget Impact Analysis of Biosimilar Products in Spain in the Period 2009–2019

Manuel García-Goñi [1,*], Isabel Río-Álvarez [2], David Carcedo [3] and Alba Villacampa [3]

1 Department of Applied & Structural Economics and History, Faculty of Economics and Business, Complutense University of Madrid, Campus de Somosaguas, Pozuelo de Alarcón, 28223 Madrid, Spain
2 Spanish Biosimilar Medicines Association, BioSim, 28027 Madrid, Spain; isabeldelrio@biosim.es
3 Hygeia Consulting S. L., 28046 Madrid, Spain; david.carcedo@hygeiaconsulting.com (D.C.); alba.villacampa@hygeiaconsulting.com (A.V.)
* Correspondence: mggoni@ucm.es; Tel.: +34-91-394-30-00

Abstract: Since the first biosimilar medicine, Omnitrope® (active substance somatropin) was approved in 2006, 53 biosimilars have been authorized in Spain. We estimate the budget impact of biosimilars in Spain from the perspective of the National Health System (NHS) over the period between 2009 and 2019. Drug acquisition costs considering commercial discounts at public procurement procedures (hospital tenders) and uptake data for both originator and biosimilar as actual units consumed by the NHS were the two variables considered. Two scenarios were compared: a scenario where no biosimilars are available and the biosimilar scenario where biosimilars are effectively marketed. All molecules exposed to biosimilar competition during this period were included in the analysis. The robustness of the model was tested by conducting multiple sensitivity analyses. From the payer perspective, it is estimated that the savings produced by the adoption of biosimilars would reach EUR 2306 million over 11 years corresponding to the cumulative savings from all biosimilars. Three molecules (infliximab, somatropin and epoetin) account for 60% of the savings. This study provides the first estimation of the financial impact of biosimilars in Spain, considering both the effect of discounts that manufacturers give to hospitals and the growing market share of biosimilars. We estimate that in our last year of data, 2019, the savings derived from the use of biosimilars relative total pharmaceutical spending in Spain is 3.92%. Although more research is needed, our evidence supports the case that biosimilars represent a great opportunity to the sustainability of the NHS through rationalizing pharmaceutical spending and that the full potential of biosimilar-savings has not been achieved yet, as there is a high variability in biosimilar uptake across autonomous regions.

Keywords: biologics; biosimilars; budget impact analysis; savings; pharmaceutical spending; cost containment; Spain

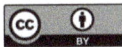

1. Introduction

Drug research and development has led to market access for many important therapeutic innovations, and undoubtedly is one of the multiple factors that influence population aging [1]. Powrie-Smith [2] points out how new therapies and vaccines have contributed to the fight against communicable diseases, resulting in a significant reduction in the incidence of viruses such as hepatitis B, as well as in infant mortality. Litchenberg [3,4] shows how those innovations have significantly improved the way health systems treat and care for the sick, increasing life expectancy and quality of life. However, those advances have come with an increase in health spending. In fact, Newhouse et al. [5] and Willeme and Dumont [6] have pointed to the advances in health technology and the therapeutic innovations developed as the most important determinants of such increases in health expenditures, and among those, pharmaceutical spending.

Trends in pharmaceutical markets have raised some concerns about the sustainability of pharmaceutical expenditure [7]. Thus, the focus should be placed on spending efficiency rather on cutting spending, to ensure the maximum return on investment in pharmaceutical products. The global pharmaceutical market will exceed USD 1.5 trillion by 2023, as it is expected to grow at a rate of between 3 and 6% per year. However, this growth will be different in different areas of the world, and in fact, in the five main markets of Europe, this growth is expected to be lower, between 1 and 4% [8]. Those expectations are based on list prices that are exclusive of discounts and rebates paid to governments. This is relevant as a divergence of 1.4 percentage points between expenditure measured at list and net prices was found in a forecast of the pharmaceutical expenditure for the EU5 countries from 2017 to 2021 [9]. Thus, considering the net prices seems critical when estimating the economic impact of any health technology, either in-patent or off-patent medicines, in pharmaceutical expenditure. In any case, a significant part of this increase in pharmaceutical spending is related to the appearance and consolidated use in clinical practice of biological medicines [10], especially for the treatment of chronic and life-threatening diseases such as cancer, multiple sclerosis or rheumatoid arthritis [11]. Many biologic products can actually slow the progress of or even prevent disease [10], but normally present a higher price than that of chemical drugs. In 2018, over 30% of all European drug spending was on biological medicines and this percentage is expected to continue to grow [12].

As in the case of generics with chemical medicines, the loss of exclusivity and the expiry of a patent on innovative biological products, hereinafter referred to as the originator, allows the entry into the market of biosimilar products. The major difference between a generic and a biosimilar is that the natural variability and more complex manufacturing of biological medicines do not allow an exact replication, as is the case with generics. Consequently, biosimilars are subjected to a more comprehensive regulatory pathway to ensure that minor differences do not affect safety or efficacy [13].

As stated by the European Medicines Agency, "a biosimilar is a biological medicine highly similar to another already approved biological medicine" and "biosimilars are approved according to the same standards of pharmaceutical quality, safety and efficacy that apply to all biological medicines" [13]. The European Medicines Agency (EMA) is responsible for evaluating the majority of applications to market biosimilars in the European Union. After the first biosimilar (the recombinant human growth hormone or somatropin) was approved in 2006, 62 biosimilar drugs corresponding to 17 active substances received marketing authorization by EMA as of 31 December 2020 [14]. In Spain, 53 biosimilar drugs for 16 active substances have been authorized for marketing to the same date [15]. However, it is worth noting that the design and implementation of pharmaceutical policies on biosimilars fall within the remit of EU Member States.

Biosimilars are lower cost alternatives of originator biologicals and are expected to bring meaningful budgetary savings to health systems. However, the spending on biosimilars is still very low, at around 1.5% of pharmaceutical expenditure in Europe in 2018 [12]. Unfortunately, there are still not many studies that estimate the savings derived from their use. Simoens et al. [16] published a review of budget impact analyses (BIA) of the use of biosimilars, although only focused mainly on two molecules, infliximab and etanercept. Furthermore, several recent studies have tried to estimate the budget impact of the introduction of recent biosimilars for either one or several molecules, at national or local levels in Italy [17–19], the UK [20,21] and Canada [22], including also in Canada a simulation exercise in which different penetration scenarios similar to the OECD average were considered [23]. In Spain, to date, the work by González Domínguez et al. [24] is the only previous study that estimated the savings due to biosimilars. They reported realized savings of EUR 478 million retrospectively from 2009 to 2016 and potential savings of EUR 1965 million in the period 2017 to 2020.

In order to understand the role of commercial discounts in price competition, it is convenient to first look at the regulation of prices for medicines in Spain (Figure 1).

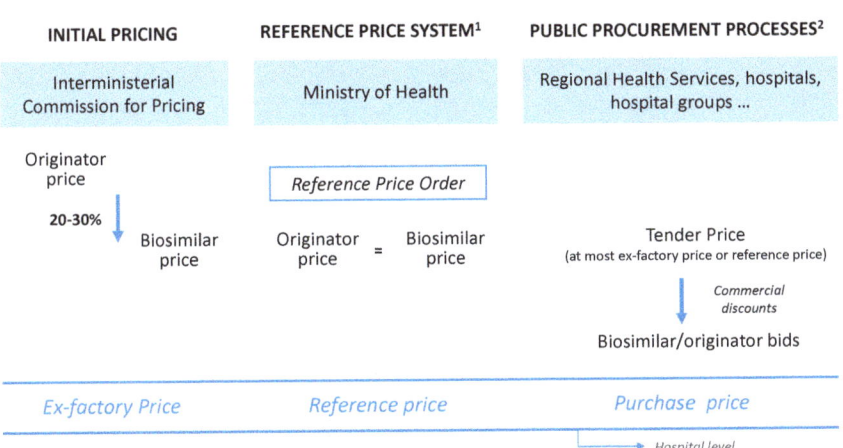

Figure 1. Price regulation of biosimilar medicines in Spain. [1] According to Royal Decree 177/2014, of 21 March, regulating the reference price system and the system of homogeneous groups of medicinal products in the National Health System. [2] According to Law 9/2017 of 8 November on public sector contracts.

After marketing authorization has been granted, the price for a biosimilar medicine is set by the Interministerial Committee on Pricing of Medicines (ICPM). In general, the ex-factory price (EFP) for the first biosimilar of a given molecule is set at around 20–30% less than the originator price [25]. The same EFP is applied to any other biosimilar of the same molecule that is authorised afterwards. Thus, the originator and biosimilar(s) have different prices for a period of time, not more than one year, since in Spain the price of off-patent medicines is regulated by the Reference Price System (RPS) [26] in the same way as in other European countries [27]. Thus, annually a Reference Price Order (RPO), published in the Official State Gazette (Spanish: Boletín Oficial del Estado, BOE), establishes the reference groups (the reference group is the basic unit of the RPS and it is constituted by at least one presentation of a biosimilar medicinal product that has the same active pharmaceutical ingredient and identical administration route) and fixes the reference price (RP) or the maximum amount of public reimbursement of the presentations of medicinal products included in the reference groups established. After the publication of the corresponding RPO, the biosimilar and originator of a particular molecule share the same RP.

EFP, or RP where applicable, is a fixed price in retail pharmacies (to which pharmacy and distributor margins and VAT are added). However, in Spain most originators and their biosimilars are dispensed at hospital pharmacies (11 of the 16 molecules with biosimilars on the Spanish market). In fact, the percentage of pharmaceutical spending on biosimilars within hospital pharmacy spending has grown continuously, from 1% in 2014 to 3% in 2018 [28]. This fact is relevant because these medicines are mainly purchased via public tenders (currently according to Law 9/2017, of 8 November, on Public Sector Contracts [29]; although previously according to Royal Legislative Decree 3/2011 [30] and before that, accordingly to Law 30/2007, of 30 October, on Public Sector Contracts [31]). Under public procurement, hospitals (or other health providers) tender a contract for the acquisition of medicines (originator and biosimilar) for a determined period and an estimated volume. Then, drug manufactures submit their bids (with a price lower or equal to the price tendered by the entity). The award of the contract depends on the economic offer, although other technical criteria are also taken into consideration. Hence, there is a variable difference between purchase price and EFP price or RP, where applicable, hereinafter referred to as "commercial discount".

This paper provides a new estimate of the budget impact generated by biosimilars in the National Health System for the years 2009 to 2019. It differs from a previous study in Spain [24] because we take into account the real acquisition scenario, that is, EFP and commercial discounts. This work is part of a wider research project analyzing the budget impact of biosimilars in the Spanish NHS, which published a report (grey literature, not indexed) in Spanish on 27th November 2020 [32].

2. Results

According to our results, the budget impact derived from the introduction of biosimilar medicines in the Spanish NHS would reach more than EUR 2306.48 million of cumulative savings in the 11-year period from 2009 to 2019 (Table 1). Somatropin (EUR 375 million), epoetin (EUR 589 million) and infliximab (EUR 450 million) biosimilars provide the greatest contribution to the aggregate savings up to 2019, which is attributable to their long presence on European pharmaceutical market (10, 10 and 5 years, respectively) and the combination of their uptake and price volumes.

Table 1. Results of the BIA (€ million savings).

Molecule [1]	Scenario without Biosimilars	Scenario with Biosimilars	Realized Savings
SOM	992.5	617.32	375.18
FIL	469.62	180.22	289.4
EPO	993.01	403.86	589.15
FOL	119.2	64.27	54.92
INF	1054.47	604.18	450.3
INS	818.41	707.87	110.54
ETA	628.39	537.91	90.48
CHO	134.67	125.34	9.32
RIT	433.39	318.76	114.62
TRA	140.89	113.26	27.63
ENO	264.86	261.25	3.62
ADA	772.46	588.69	183.77
PEG	10.77	3.2	7.57
TOTAL	6832.63	4526.15	2306.48

[1] SOM: somatropin; FIL: filgrastim; EPO: epoetin; FOL: follitropin alfa; INF: infliximab; INS: insuline glargine; ETA: etanercept; CHO: chondroitin sulfate; RIT: rituximab; TRA: trastuzumab; ENO: sodium enoxaparin; ADA: adalimumab; PEG: pegfilgrastim.

Figure 2a shows the aggregated savings over time and the annual mean savings per effectively marketed biosimilar molecule. The temporal evolution analysis showed a growing trend as more biosimilar medicines enter the market. The breakdown of the contribution by molecule (see Figure 2b) revealed that epoetin is in first position with savings of EUR 589 million, followed by infliximab (EUR 450 million) and somatropin (EUR 375 million). Taken together, these three molecules account for more than 60% of total savings in the entire period. However, the entry of biosimilars of different molecules significantly changes the market and the estimation of savings. For instance, adalimumab ranks fifth (EUR 183.77 million) in just two years in the market and a biosimilar uptake of only 18% in 2019. It is not surprising as it is the most consumed drug in the Spanish NHS in terms of hospital pharmaceutical expenditure [33]. It is also worth noting that the savings derived from the use of biosimilars are starting to account for a significant percentage of pharmaceutical spending in Spain. Figure 2c shows the percentage of annual savings caused by the use of biosimilars with respect to total pharmaceutical spending published by the Ministry of Finance in Spain [34] since 2014, calculated at ex-factory prices (EFP), without discounts. Annual savings increase from 0.67% in 2014 to 3.92% in 2019. In total, from 2014 to 2019, the savings account for 2.11% of total pharmaceutical spending.

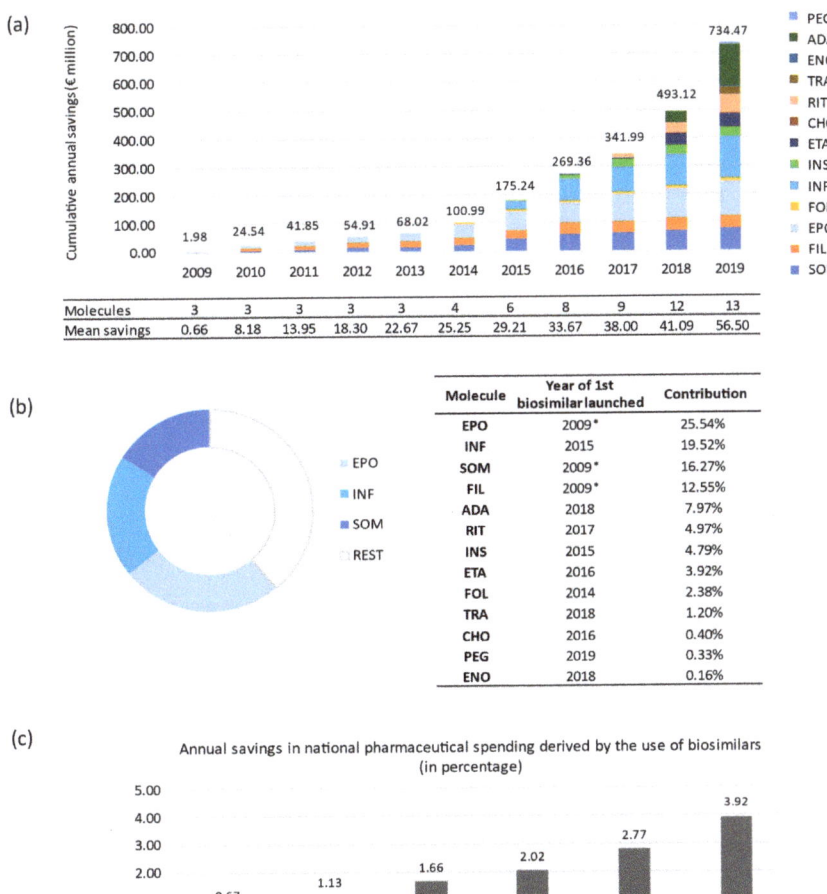

Figure 2. Distribution of aggregate savings. (**a**) Aggregate savings over time. All molecules exposed to biosimilar competition each year were included in the analysis.; (**b**) Specific contribution of each of the molecules to the total amount of savings. SOM: somatropin; FIL: filgrastim; EPO: epoetin; FOL: follitropin alfa; INF: infliximab; INS: insuline glargine; ETA: etanercept; CHO: chondroitin sulfate; RIT: rituximab; TRA: trastuzumab; ENO: sodium enoxaparin; ADA: adalimumab; PEG: pegfilgrastim. * Biosimilars marketed before 2009: somatropin, 2006; filgrastim and epoetin, 2008 (2009 is the first year with available consumption data). (**c**) Annual savings derived from the use of biosimilars, in percentages, since 2014 with respect to total pharmaceutical spending in Spain. Total pharmaceutical spending calculated by adding hospital pharmaceutical spending and spending on pharmaceuticals and medical devices per prescription, all calculated at ex-factory prices [34].

Sensitivity Analysis

The results from the analysis of alternative scenarios (see Figure 3a) show the great influence of commercial discounts at the hospital tendering on total savings. Significantly, when commercial discounts are excluded, savings realized would be reduced to EUR 1064 million from 2009 to 2019, which means about 50% reduction over the base case results. This scenario would represent the minimum savings due to biosimilar competition (application of the same PR to originator and biosimilar). The other scenario analyzed shows no significant differences from the base case estimate. The same goes for the one-way sensitivity analyses (see Figure 3b). Only the assumptions made in the absence of data (epoetin) show some relevant impact on the savings obtained in the base case, as they affect the data series of two active ingredients whose biosimilars have been on the market for a long time.

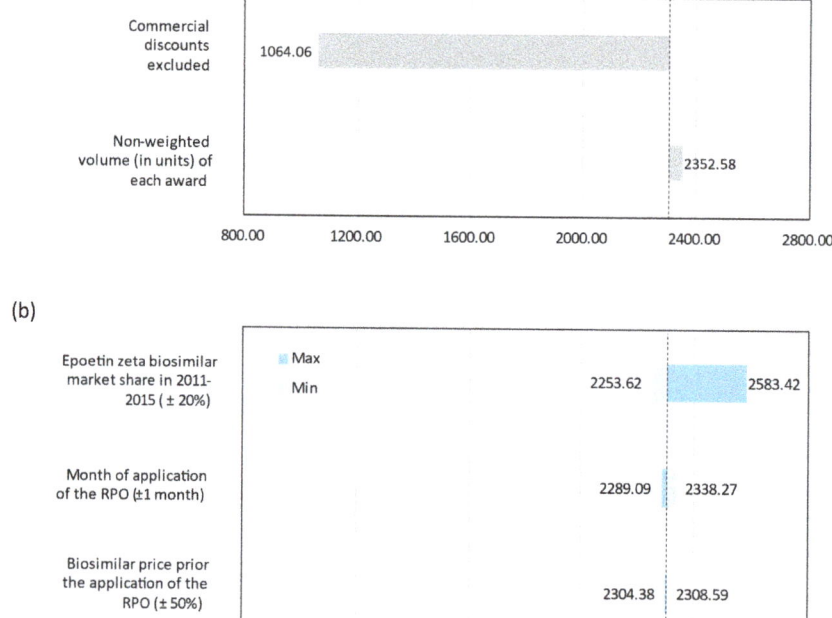

Figure 3. Results of the scenario and sensitivity analyses. (**a**) Scenario analysis. (**b**) One-way sensitivity analysis. The dotted line represents the base case value.

Finally, probabilistic sensitivity analysis provides 11-year (2009–2019) cumulative savings with an average of EUR 2310 million (95% IC: EUR 2170–EUR 2461 million) for the NHS. Overall, these results are in line with those obtained for the base case as shown in Table 2.

Figure 4 shows the 1000 Monte Carlo simulations performed in the probabilistic analysis. Each of the points represents one of the 1000 simulations carried out. Thus, a greater dispersion of the points along the axes represents a greater uncertainty of the results. As observed, a higher consumption of DDD does not always translate into higher savings, as seen with enoxaparin, chondroitin sulfate and insulin glargine. On the other hand, we see how rituximab achieves considerable savings without reaching high consumption values (in DDD).

Table 2. Results of the probabilistic sensitivity analysis (€ million).

Molecule [1]	Base Case	Probabilistic Sensitivity Analysis		
		Mean	95% CI	
SOM	375.18	377.96	348.25 -	415.67
FIL	289.40	289.27	274.55 -	303.17
EPO	589.15	590.26	546.85 -	634.32
FOL	54.92	54.92	53.71 -	56.07
INF	450.30	450.25	448.59 -	452.03
INS	110.54	110.40	106.08 -	115.03
ETA	90.48	90.60	83.26 -	99.25
CHO	9.32	9.32	8.99 -	9.68
RIT	114.62	114.63	103.36 -	126.12
TRA	27.63	27.61	26.24 -	29.04
ENO	3.62	3.61	2.27 -	4.83
ADA	183.77	184.08	161.25 -	207.42
PEG	7.57	7.57	6.79 -	8.32
TOTAL	2306.48	2310.47	2170.19 -	2460.96

[1] SOM: somatropin; FIL: filgrastim; EPO: epoetin; FOL: follitropin alfa; INF: infliximab; INS: insuline glargine; ETA: etanercept; CHO: chondroitin sulfate; RIT: rituximab; TRA: trastuzumab; ENO: sodium enoxaparin; ADA: adalimumab; PEG: pegfilgrastim.

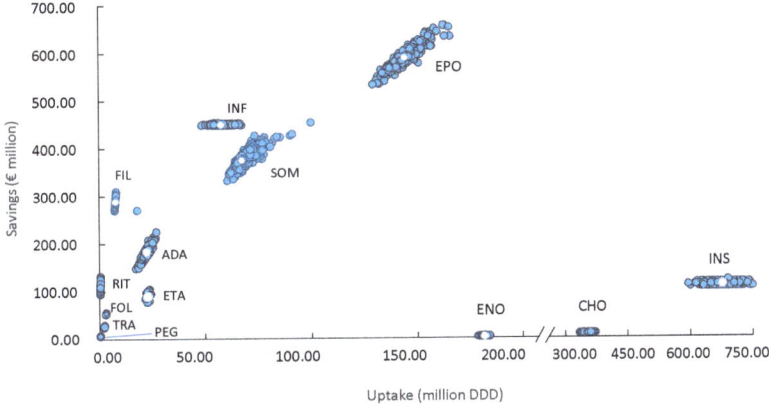

Figure 4. Scatter plot of 1000 Monte Carlo simulations. Vertical axis represents aggregated saving (€ million) for each molecule in the period 2009–2019. Horizontal axis represents the total amount of DDD (million) consumed in this period for each molecule. White dots represent the base case values. SOM: somatropin; FIL: filgrastim; EPO: epoetin; FOL: follitropin alfa; INF: infliximab; INS: insuline glargine; ETA: etanercept; CHO: chondroitin sulfate; RIT: rituximab; TRA: trastuzumab; ENO: sodium enoxaparin; ADA: adalimumab; PEG: pegfilgrastim.

3. Discussion

To our knowledge, ours is the first study that uses a BIA to estimate the retrospective savings in a European health system for the total of biosimilar molecules marketed and taking into account the real net price (EFP and commercial discounts in the hospital tenders). The only precedent for Spain is González-Domínguez et al. [24]. They estimated the savings derived from biosimilars in the NHS for the retrospective period 2009–2016 and for the prospective period 2017–2020. In order to compare our results to theirs, we have estimated the savings through the budget impact analysis according to our model for the same seven active substances (somatropin, filgrastim, epoetin, follitropin, insulin glargine, infliximab and etanercept) and in the same period (2009–2016). We estimate savings of EUR 343 million compared to EUR 478 million reported by [24]. This difference may be due to different assumptions on the price erosion, the application date of the RPO, or the estimated uptake of each molecule used and merely reflects the complexity inherent to any estimation of savings.

Few studies have calculated the real retrospective savings derived from the introduction of biosimilars in the European context. Simoens et al. [16] reviewed full publications and posters focusing on BIA of biosimilar medicines. Their work revealed the lack of peer-reviewed information on the budget impact of biosimilar products. Only three studies were considered full budget impact models according to ISPOR good practice guidelines. They all aimed to estimate the budget impact of the introduction of an infliximab biosimilar over a prospective time horizon between 1 and 3 years, also considering some type of substitution or combination.

Since then, additional BIAs of biosimilar medicines in Europe have been published. They mainly aimed to analyze the budget impact of one molecule (antiTNF class is the wider class analyzed) in a time horizon between 3 and 5 years. For instance, in Italy, Rognoni et al. [17] estimates the impact of the use of a rituximab biosimilar in the Italian National Health System in a 3- and 5-year horizon that accounts for EUR 79.2 and EUR 153.6 million, respectively. Likewise, the introduction of an adalimumab biosimilar would generate savings of EUR 260 million in 5 years [19]. In the United Kingdom, Aladul et al. [20] updated their previous study [35] including the introduction of a new antiTNF biosimilar in the areas of rheumatology and gastroenterology. According to their calculations the impact would amount, in a 3-year horizon, to GBP 285 million. Other studies expand the focus to EU5 (infliximab) [36] or a greater pool of European countries (rituximab) [37]. In a very recent study, Agirrezabal et al. [21] estimated the impact of biosimilar insulin glargine in primary care in the NHS with, specifically, savings of GBP 900,000 between October 2015 and December 2018. They also provide an estimate of the savings lost due to reduced use of biosimilars, which could have reached GBP 25.6 million, indicating that only 3.42% of the potential savings have been achieved.

Of note, most studies cited used ex-factory prices excluding discounts as cost-input. This does not reflect reality, as hospitals usually negotiate individual discounts through public tenders. By contrast, our study uses purchase prices paid by hospitals. We believe this allows for a more accurate estimation of savings due to biosimilar competition in Spain since 2009. At the same time, the large period of time we analyze, from 2009 to 2019, allows us to observe how, in general and per molecule, savings are increasing in time.

In any case, our results are broadly consistent with the observed financial impacts from other countries in that biosimilar uptake translates into significant savings and that when longer periods are considered, higher savings are realized, as expected.

It is important to note that the estimated savings are affected by the variation and level of both quantities and prices. Consequently, a higher consumption of DDD does not always translate into higher savings, as observed with enoxaparin, chondroitin sulfate and insulin glargine, due to a lower price with respect to complex biosimilar molecules such as antiTNF or monoclonal antibodies. For the same reason, rituximab achieves considerable savings without reaching high consumption values.

It is worthwhile to highlight that adalimumab (the first biosimilar launched at the end of 2018) accounts for almost 8% of the 11-year (2009–2019) cumulative savings. This figure corresponds to realized savings of EUR 187 million in scarcely one year. It is not surprising as adalimumab is responsible for the highest drug spending in Spain [33]. This suggests that higher savings in the short term may be expected. In fact, we have estimated that the percentage of annual savings caused by the use of biosimilars with respect to total pharmaceutical spending is increasing and by 2019 it was 3.92%.

An additional finding of this work is that potential savings in Spain due to biosimilars are not yet fully exploited, as the biosimilar uptake is still lower than that in other countries, at least for some active substances. For example, antiTNF biosimilar uptake in Spain was 49% in 2019 vs. Denmark (96%), Germany (61%), Italy (64%) or Norway (74%). The same pattern is observed for biosimilar monoclonal antibodies in oncology. The penetration in Spanish market barely exceeds 35% vs. Denmark (74%), Germany (49%), Italy (52%) or Norway (70%). This lower utilization proves that there is a room for improvement in the Spanish NHS [38].

In any case, it is important to note that different molecules behave differently and not all contribute equally to savings in each country, or in different countries, because of the different price and reimbursement policies, procurement procedures, and other pharmaceutical policies, which vary greatly among European countries.

In the case of Spain, a comprehensive report by the Independent Authority for Fiscal Responsibility [39] confirmed the high variability across autonomous communities in terms of uptake levels and promotion policies. This may have been a driver for the Ministry of Health's attempt to establish a national policy on biosimilars [40]. This plan, still under revision, makes recommendations to revisit those supply and demand policies put in place in Spain with the further aim of promoting the utilization of biosimilar medicines in Spain. This aim is also supported by the Advisory Committee for the Funding of the Pharmaceutical Benefit of the National Health System, a collegiate body attached to the Ministry of Health. In its analysis of this plan, the committee is of the opinion that promoting the use of biosimilars will lead to more competition and reduction of the burden of pharmaceutical spending [41]. We consider that more research is needed on the role of biosimilar competition in pharmaceutical cost containment. Given the increasing concern regarding the sustainability of healthcare systems, and the contribution biosimilars can play towards that end, in line with our findings, more ambitious or fine-tuned policies for promoting biosimilars (in general or some biosimilars specifically) may be expected.

Limitations

As in any other study, this retrospective BIA has certain limitations, mainly due to the non-availability of data, specifically among the first three biosimilar classes on the market (EPO, G-CSF, and hGH). Additional sources [42–44] were used to complete information gaps on the uptake of these biosimilars. When the price of the biosimilar prior the RPO launch was unknown, we assumed that it was a 10% higher than the price after RPO. We believe this assumption is a conservative position, as the RPO can lead to price reductions of up to 30%, as in the case of adalimumab.

Regarding the estimation of commercial discounts, as mentioned, a sample of 143 public procurement tenders (the most recent in each autonomous community) was used. Although the sample was considered to be representative, it does not include all the public procurement procedures in the country for the entire period of analysis. This is because sharing transparent information on purchase prices (tenders) is a very recent trend motivated by the EU directives on public procurement. In addition, we acknowledge that an unequal distribution of tender procedures per region might influence the estimation of actual savings in Spain. The degree of variability in the level of discounts awarded via public tenders for the same molecule within the regions is out of the scope of this research and merits itself further exploration. In addition, to overcome the lack of data on the public tenders prior to 2016, a linear regression was performed with 0% as the lower limit of discount matching the time of biosimilar launch. This would represent the evolution of price discounts derived from competition between an originator and biosimilars over the years.

The results of this BIA should be interpreted with these limitations in mind.

4. Materials and Methods

4.1. Model Design

We perform a retrospective BIA of the introduction of biosimilars from the Spanish Health System perspective covering the period from 2009 to 2019. All the molecules exposed to biosimilar competition in this period were included in the analysis (Figure 5). We adopt the third-party payer perspective and thus, we only account for direct medical costs, in particular pharmacological costs prior to and after the market introduction of biosimilars. The calculation was conducted in a Microsoft Excel-based spreadsheet model. The model was constructed in compliance with methodology guidelines for economic evaluations and analyses previously developed in Spain [45,46].

Molecule/Active substance	Year of marketing authorization	Originator®– Biosimilar®
Somatropin[1] Filgrastim[1] Epoetin[1,2]	2009	Genotropin® – Omnitrope® Neupogen® - Accofil® /Nivestim® /Zarzio® Eprex® - Binocrit® /Retacrit®
Follitropin alfa	2014	Gonal F® – Bemfola® /Ovaleap®
Infliximab Insuline glargine	2015	Remicade® – Remsima® /Inflectra® /Flixabi® /Zessly® Lantus® - Abasaglar®
Etanercept Chondrotin sulfate	2016	Enbrel® – Benepali® /Erelzi® Condrosulf®/Condrosan® - Condrotin sulfato Kern® /Abamed®
Rituximab	2017	Mabthera® – Truxima® / Rixathon®
Trastuzumab Sodium enoxaparin Adalimumab	2018	Herceptin® – Ontruzant® /Herzuma® /Kanjinti® /Trazimera® /Ogivri® Clexane® - Enoxaparina Rovi® /Hepaxane® /Inhixa® Humira® - Amgevita® /Hulio® /Hyrimoz®/Idacio® /Imraldi®
Pegfilgrastim	2019	Neulasta® – Pelgraz® / Pelmeg® /Ziextenzo®

Figure 5. Biosimilar medicines effectively marketed in Spain as of December 2019. [1] Biosimilars marketed before 2009 (2009 is the first year with available consumption data). [2] For the purpose of this study, epoetin zeta and alfa are considered as a single molecule. Bevacizumab and teriparatide biosimilars have been recently marketed in Spain (September 2019 and June 2020, respectively) but they are not included in this analysis.

To estimate the budget impact, two scenarios are compared. First, the hypothetical scenario in which biosimilar drugs are not available on the market and therefore, an originator's price would keep constant throughout the period examined. This assumption is based on a review of the price evolution of originators (anti-TNFs, trastuzumab and rituximab). We found that these originator medicines did not undergo major price changes before biosimilar entry. This could be interpreted to mean that even if other molecules generate competition in the same indication, the originator's price is rarely modified. Second, the actual scenario with biosimilars available on the market after an originator's patent expiration is examined. In this scenario, competition leads to a price reduction for originator medicines. The difference in terms of costs between the two scenarios provides the savings generated by the introduction of biosimilars.

The two main variables of the analysis are uptake (consumption data) and price for each molecule, both originator and biosimilar. To provide clarity on some specific terminology a glossary table (see Table 3) with English terms used in this manuscript and their Spanish equivalents is provided.

Table 3. Glossary of English/Spanish terms and their abbreviations.

English Term	Spanish Term	Abbreviation in Spanish
National Health System (abbreviated in text as NHS)	Sistema Nacional de Salud	SNS
Interministerial Committee on Pricing of Medicines (abbreviated in text as ICPM)	Comisión Interministerial de Precios de Medicamentos	CIPM
Ex-factory price (abbreviated in text as EFP)	Precio de venta del laboratorio	PVL
Reference price (abbreviated in text as RP)	Precio de referencia	PR
Reference Price Order (abbreviated in text as RPO)	Orden de Precios de Referencia	OPR
Reference Price System (abbreviated in text as RPS)	Sistema de Precios de Referencia	SPR
Purchase price	Precio de adquisición	-
Official State Gazette (abbreviated in text as OSG)	Boletín Oficial del Estado	BOE

4.2. Uptake Estimation

We use two sources of data on the uptake of biosimilars. For the period between 2009 and 2015, we use data provided by all manufacturers, representing the number of units effectively consumed by the NHS (BioSim, data on file) and for the period between 2016 and 2019, we use data provided by the Ministry of Health (Ministry of Health, data on file). In both scenarios (with and without biosimilars) the volumes have been converted to daily doses using the published World Health Organization (WHO) defined daily doses (DDD) [47] as previously used by Haustein et al. [48] to estimate the impact of the introduction of biosimilars in several European countries. Figure 6 shows the evolution over time of biosimilar uptake in the Spanish pharmaceutical market. In the bottom of the figure, the estimated average uptake after launch of the first biosimilar (that means, mean uptake of first year of commercialization, mean uptake of second year of commercialization, and so on) are shown.

4.3. Price Estimation

For each molecule, drug acquisition costs (EFP) for the year 2019 have been obtained from BotPlus, the Health Information database of the General Council of the Association of Official Pharmacists that provides harmonized information on medicines [49]. For the previous years, price evolution was also obtained from BotPlus, and when not available, these prices were provided by BioSim (BioSim, data on file). RPO published in the OSG from 2014 to 2019 were consulted to provide RP. RP is assumed to affect price calculations in the same month of the publication of the RPO when it is prior to the 15th day of the month, otherwise RP will apply the following month. When a biosimilar price between its commercialization and its regulation by the reference pricing system is unknown, we assume an increase of 10% over the RP, following the observation of other biosimilars for which full price data are available.

Purchase prices in hospital tenders were used to calculate discounted prices per DDD compared to the EFP for infliximab, etanercept, adalimumab, trastuzumab and rituximab (data from 143 public tenders collected by Acobur S.L. (https://www.acobur.es, accessed on 15 April 2020). This reduced price was weighted by the total volume (in units) of each award (of originator and biosimilars) to obtain the commercial discount for each molecule and year. In the case of somatropin, epoetin, filgrastim and pegfilgrastim, internal BioSim data for years 2018 and 2019 were used and a linear regression was conducted assuming a discount of 0% the year before the marketing of the first biosimilar. No discount is considered for follitropin alfa, insulin glargine, chondroitin sulfate and enoxaparin, as they are mostly dispensed by retail pharmacies, where commercial discounts do not apply. Table 4 shows the number of tenders analyzed and the level of discount for each molecule.

Table 4. Level of discount on price per molecule.

Molecule [1]	Year of First Biosimilar Launch	Public Tenders Analyzed [3]	Current Level of Discount	
			Original	Biosimilar
SOM	2009 [2]	9	++	++
FIL	2009 [2]	2	+++	+++
EPO	2009 [2]	2	+++	+++
FOL	2014	-	-	-
INF	2015	37	+	+++
INS	2015	-	-	-
ETA	2016	55	+	++
CHO	2016	-	-	-
RIT	2017	36	+	++
TRA	2018	21	+	+++
ENO	2018	-	-	-
ADA	2018	59	+	+++
PEG	2019	2	+++	+++

Level of discount on price (either EFP or RP): + (low) 0–25%; ++ (medium) 25–50%; +++ (high) >50%. [1] SOM: somatropin; FIL: filgrastim; EPO: epoetin; FOL: follitropin alfa; INF: infliximab; INS: insuline glargine; ETA: etanercept; CHO: chondroitin sulfate; RIT: rituximab; TRA: trastuzumab; ENO: sodium enoxaparin; ADA: adalimumab; PEG: pegfilgrastim; [2] Biosimilars marketed before 2009: somatropin, 2006; filgrastim and epoetin, 2008 (2009 is the first year with available consumption data). [3] The amount of public tender analyzed exceed 143 as some of them were tendered for several molecules.

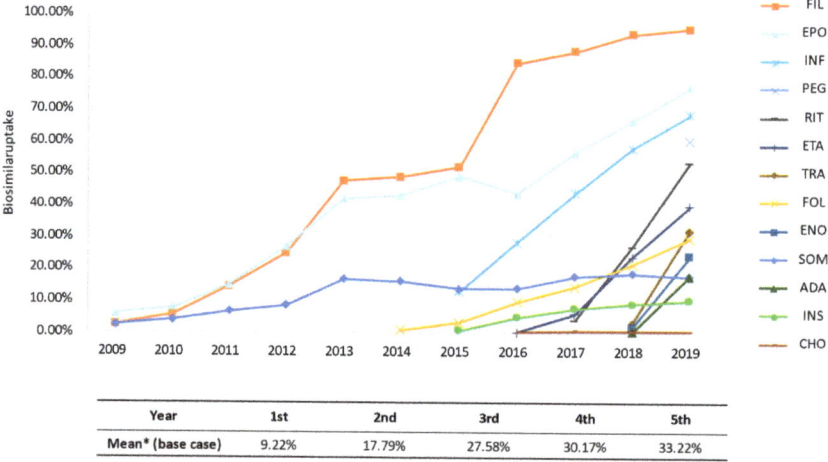

Figure 6. Biosimilar penetration in Spain over time (adapted from [29]). Biosimilar uptake (%) is calculated as volume of biosimilars over volume of biosimilars plus the originator product (DDDs). * Chondroitin sulfate and the three biosimilars marketed before 2009 (somatropin, filgrastim and epoetin) were excluded to avoid distorting the mean. SOM: somatropin; FIL: filgrastim; EPO: epoetin; FOL: follitropin alfa; INF: infliximab; INS: insuline glargine; ETA: etanercept; CHO: chondroitin sulfate; RIT: rituximab; TRA: trastuzumab; ENO: sodium enoxaparin; ADA: adalimumab; PEG: pegfilgrastim.

4.4. Molecule-Specific Assumptions

In addition to the general assumptions mentioned above, it was necessary to adopt other specific assumptions given the lack of specific information about both uptake and price variables (Table S1).

4.5. Sensitivity Analsyses

In order to evaluate the uncertainty associated with the variables used in the budget impact model and determine the robustness of the results obtained, we carried out both deterministic and probabilistic sensitivity analyses.

In the scenario analysis, some of the assumptions are modified with respect to the base case (non-additively) (Table 5). The new alternatives (non-additive) propose different ways to calculate the price variable. Scenario 1 estimates the impact on price of ignoring the discounts that manufacturers give to hospitals. Scenario 2 ignores the volume-weighting, that is to say, the purchase price only applies to the year in which the tender is awarded regardless of the duration of the contract.

Table 5. Scenario and one-way sensitivity analyses.

Scenario	Parameter	Variation with Respect to the Base Case
Scenario 1	Originator and biosimilar prices	No commercial discounts applied
Scenario 2	Commercial discounts (tenders)	No volume weighting applied
One-way	Parameter	Variation with Respect to the Base Case
One-way 1	Biosimilar price prior RPO	±50%
One-way 2	Month of application of RPO	±1 month
One-way 3	Epoetin zeta market share distribution	±20%

One-way sensitivity analysis was performed by changing, one by one, some parameters of the model: the price of some biosimilars prior the application of the RPO, the month of application of the RPO, and the market share of biosimilar epoetin in 2011–2015 (data from [42]) (Table 5).

We also performed a probabilistic sensitivity analysis using the Monte Carlo method with 1000 simulations, simultaneously modifying all parameters from base-case values following a normal distribution, in line with the recommendations of the literature [50].

5. Conclusions

The increase of health expenditures, and in particular, of pharmaceutical expenditures in Spain highlights the need for effective strategies to contain and rationalize pharmaceutical spending.

This is the first study carried out which jointly analyzes the savings for the Spanish NHS in terms of pharmaceutical expenditure derived from both the uptake of biosimilar products and the downward effect on prices resulting from competition (RPS and public tenders, with commercial discounts).

Our results show how the introduction of biosimilar drugs in the Spanish pharmaceutical market has brought competition in the market of biological products, and unquestionable, increasing and significant savings, especially at the hospital level, where the majority prescriptions for the molecules herein analyzed are issued. Thus, biosimilar medicines represent a great opportunity to promote the sustainability of the NHS through rationalization and efficiency in pharmaceutical expenditure. Our study also shows that the full potential of biosimilar savings has not been achieved yet, as there is a high variability in biosimilar uptake across autonomous regions.

This is a first approach to the impact of biosimilar medicines on the pharmaceutical market in terms of price competition, uptake and savings. However, a further research might address other issues such as level of competition, variability across molecules and within regions, relationships, if any, between market size and number of competitors or price discounts.

In any case, any pharmaceutical policy to be adopted should not only analyze its expected impact in the short-term, but also in the medium- and long-term, to promote healthy competition in the market for biological pharmaceutical products, whether originator or biosimilar. After all, the ultimate goal is the sustainability of the healthcare system with rapid access to innovative products, but also a healthy competition from biosimilars when the patent from the originators expires, resulting in better access for patients to obtain the clinical benefits derived from the treatments.

Supplementary Materials: The following are available online at https://www.mdpi.com/article/10.3390/ph14040348/s1, Table S1: Assumptions adopted for each molecule.

Author Contributions: Conceptualization, M.G.-G.; methodology, D.C. and A.V.; validation, M.G.-G.; formal analysis D.C.; investigation, D.C., M.G.-G., and I.R.-Á.; resources, I.R.-Á.; data curation, D.C.; original draft preparation, I.R.-Á., D.C., and M.G.-G.; review and editing, M.G.-G and A.V.; supervision, M.G.-G.; project administration, I.R.-Á. All authors have read and agreed to the published version of the manuscript.

Funding: The authors thank financial support for the development of this research by The Spanish Biosimilar Medicines Association, BioSim.

Institutional Review Board Statement: Not applicable.

Informed Consent Statement: Not applicable.

Data Availability Statement: Data is contained within the article.

Acknowledgments: The authors would like to thank Maria Lores (Hygeia Consulting S.L.) for her contribution to data processing. The authors also thank Marta Trapero-Bertrán (Universitat Internacional de Catalunya) her advice in the early stages of this research.

Conflicts of Interest: M.G.-G., D.C. and A.V. declare no conflicts of interest. I.R.-Á is employee of the Spanish Biosimilar Medicines Association who funded this research.

References

1. Shaw, J.; Horrace, W.; Vogel, R. The determinants of life expectancy: An analysis of the OECD health data. *South. Econ. J.* **2005**, *71*, 768–783. Available online: https://www.researchgate.net/publication/23545170_The_Determinants_of_Life_Expectancy_An_Analysis_of_the_OECD_Health_Data (accessed on 3 June 2020). [CrossRef]
2. Powrie-Smith, A. From innovation to outcomes. In *Medicines Costs in Context*; European Federation of Pharmaceutical Industries and Associations: Brussels, Belgium, 2016. Available online: https://www.efpia.eu/about-medicines/use-of-medicines/value-of-medicines/ (accessed on 3 June 2020).
3. Lichtenberg, F. Pharmaceutical innovation and longevity growth in 30 developing OECD and high-income countries, 2000–2009. *Health Policy Technol.* **2014**, *3*, 36–58. Available online: https://www.nber.org/system/files/working_papers/w18235/w18235.pdf (accessed on 3 June 2020). [CrossRef]
4. Lichtenberg, F. *The Benefits of Pharmaceutical Innovation: Health, Longevity, and Savings*; Montreal Economic Institute: Montreal, QC, Canada, 2016; ISBN 978-2-922687-66-8. Available online: http://www.vises.org.au/documents/2016_Lichtenberg_Benefits_of_Pharma_Innovation.pdf (accessed on 3 June 2020).
5. Newhouse, J.P. Medical Care Costs: How much Welfare Loss? *J. Econ. Perspect.* **1992**, *6*, 3–21. [CrossRef] [PubMed]
6. Willeme, P.; Dumont, M. Machines that go 'ping': Medical technology and health expenditures in OECD countries. *Health Econ.* **2015**, *24*, 1027–1041. [CrossRef] [PubMed]
7. OECD. *Improving Forecasting of Pharmaceutical Spending-Insights from 23 OECD and EU Countries*; OECD: Paris, France, 2019. Available online: https://ec.europa.eu/health/sites/health/files/policies/docs/pharmaceutical-expenditure-analytical-report-april-2019_en.pdf (accessed on 8 February 2021).

8. IQVIA Institute. The Global Use of Medicine in 2019 and Outlook to 2023. Forecasts and Areas to Watch. 2019. Available online: https://www.iqvia.com/insights/the-iqvia-institute/reports/the-global-use-of-medicine-in-2019-and-outlook-to-2023 (accessed on 3 June 2020).
9. Espin, J.; Schlander, M.; Godman, B.; Anderson, P.; Mestre-Ferrandiz, J.; Borget, I.; Hutchings, A.; Flostrand, S.; Parnaby, A.; Jommi, C. Projecting Pharmaceutical Expenditure in EU5 to 2021: Adjusting for the Impact of Discounts and Rebates. *Appl. Health Econ. Health Policy* **2018**, *16*, 803–817. [CrossRef] [PubMed]
10. Farfan-Portet, M.I.; Gerkens, S.; Lepage-Nefkens, I.; Vinck, I.; Hulstaert, F. Are biosimilars the next tool to guarantee cost-containment for pharmaceutical expenditures? *Eur. J. Health Econ.* **2014**, *15*, 223–228. [CrossRef] [PubMed]
11. Pugatch Consilium. Towards a Sustainable European Market for Off-Patent Biologics. Available online: https://www.pugatchconsilium.com/?p=2760 (accessed on 3 June 2020).
12. IQVIA Institute. The Impact of Biosimilar Competition in Europe. 2019. Available online: https://ec.europa.eu/docsroom/documents/38461 (accessed on 3 June 2020).
13. EMA (European Medicines Agency); European Commission. *Biosimilars in the EU. Information Guide for Healthcare Professionals*; European Medicines Agency (EMA): Amsterdam, The Netherlands, 2019. Available online: https://www.ema.europa.eu/en/documents/leaflet/biosimilars-eu-information-guide-healthcare-professionals_en.pdf (accessed on 3 June 2020).
14. Biosimilar Medicines. Available online: https://www.ema.europa.eu/en/medicines/search_api_aggregation_ema_medicine_types/field_ema_med_biosimilar (accessed on 31 December 2020).
15. Centro de Información Online de Medicamentos de la Agencia Española de Medicamentos Sanitarios (CIMA). Available online: https://cima.aemps.es/cima/publico/lista.html (accessed on 31 December 2020).
16. Simoens, S.; Jacobs, I.; Popovian, R.; Isakov, L.; Shane, L.G. Assessing the Value of Biosimilars: A Review of the Role of Budget Impact Analysis. *Pharm. Econ.* **2017**, *35*, 1047–1062. [CrossRef] [PubMed]
17. Rognoni, C.; Bertolani, A.; Jommi, C. Budget Impact Analysis of Rituximab Biosimilar in Italy from the Hospital and Payer Perspectives. *Glob. Reg. Health Technol. Assess.* **2018**, *XX*, I–II. Available online: https://journals.sagepub.com/doi/pdf/10.1177/2284240318784289 (accessed on 3 June 2020). [CrossRef]
18. Piras, M.; Naddeo, C.; Bettio, M.; Dragui, R.; Venturini, F. 1ISG-039 The cost-savings potential of biosimilar drugs: A budget impact analysis. *Eur. J. Hosp. Pharm.* **2019**, *26*, A18. Available online: https://ejhp.bmj.com/content/ejhpharm/26/Suppl_1/A18.2.full.pdf (accessed on 3 June 2020).
19. Ravasio, R.; Mazzi, S.; Esposito, M.; Fiorino, G.; Migliore, A. A Budget impact analysis of adalimumab biosimilar: The Italian context. *AboutOpen* **2019**, *5*, 16–23. Available online: https://journals.aboutscience.eu/index.php/aboutopen/article/view/280 (accessed on 3 June 2020). [CrossRef]
20. Aladul, M.I.; Fitzpatrick, R.W.; Chapman, S.R. The effect of new biosimilars in rheumatology and gastroenterology specialties on UK healthcare budgets: Results of a budget impact analysis. *Res. Soc. Adm. Pharm.* **2019**, *15*, 310–317. [CrossRef] [PubMed]
21. Agirrezabal, I.; Sánchez-Iriso, E.; Mandar, K.; Cabasés, J.M. Real-World Budget Impact of the Adoption of Insulin Glargine Biosimilars in Primary Care in England (2015–2018). *Diabetes Care* **2020**, *43*, 1767–1773. [CrossRef] [PubMed]
22. Mansell, K.; Bhimji, H.; Eurich, D.; Mansell, H. Potential cost-savings from the use of the biosimilars filgrastim, infliximab and insulin glargine in Canada: A retrospective analysis BMC. *Health Serv. Res.* **2019**, *19*, 827. [CrossRef] [PubMed]
23. Patented Medicine Prices Review Board. Biologics in Canada Part 2: Biosimilar Savings, 2018. Chartbook. National Prescription Drug Utilization Information System. 2020. Available online: https://www.canada.ca/content/dam/pmprb-cepmb/documents/reports-and-studies/chartbooks/biologics-part2-biosimilar-savings2018.pdf (accessed on 3 June 2020).
24. González Domínguez, A.; Ivanova Markova, Y.; Zozaya Gonzále, N.; Jiménez Torres, M.; Hidalgo Vega, A.; La Introducción de los Biosimilares en España. *Estimación del Ahorro Para el Sistema Nacional de Salud*; Fundación Weber: Madrid, España, 2017. Available online: http://weber.org.es/wp-content/uploads/2018/04/DT-002-Introducci%C3%B3n-de-los-Biosimilares-en-Espa%C3%B1a_vf.pdf (accessed on 3 June 2020).
25. IQVIA Institute for Human Data Science (2018). Advancing Biosimilar Sustainability in Europe. September 2018. Available online: https://www.iqvia.com/-/media/iqvia/pdfs/institutereports/advancing-biosimilar-sustainability-in-europe.pdf (accessed on 3 June 2020).
26. Real Decreto 177/2014, de 21 de Marzo, por el que se Regula el Sistema de Precios de Referencia y de Agrupaciones Homogéneas de Medicamentos en el Sistema Nacional de Salud, y Determinados Sistemas de Información en Materia de Financiación y Precios de los Medicamentos y Productos Sanitarios. Available online: https://www.boe.es/boe/dias/2014/03/25/pdfs/BOE-A-2014-3189.pdf (accessed on 3 June 2020).
27. World Health Organization. Medicines Reimbursement Policies in Europe. 2018. Available online: https://www.euro.who.int/__data/assets/pdf_file/0011/376625/pharmaceutical-reimbursement-eng.pdf (accessed on 3 June 2020).
28. IQVIA Institute. Evolución y Tendencias del Mercado Farmacéutico Español. 2019. Available online: https://staticscorreofarmaceutico.uecdn.es/cms/sites/11/2019/02/evolucionytendencias-iqvia.pdf (accessed on 3 June 2020).
29. Ley 9/2017, de 8 de Noviembre, de Contratos del Sector Público, por la que se Transponen al Ordenamiento Jurídico Español las Directivas del Parlamento Europeo y del Consejo 2014/23/UE y 2014/24/UE, de 26 de Febrero de 2014. Available online: https://www.boe.es/buscar/act.php?id=BOE-A-2017-12902 (accessed on 3 June 2020).
30. Real Decreto Legislativo 3/2011, de 14 de Noviembre, por el que se Aprueba el Texto Refundido de la Ley de Contratos del Sector Público. Available online: https://www.boe.es/buscar/act.php?id=BOE-A-2011-17887 (accessed on 3 June 2020).

31. Ley 30/2007, de 30 de Octubre, de Contratos del Sector Público. Available online: https://www.boe.es/buscar/doc.php?id=BOE-A-2007-18874 (accessed on 3 June 2020).
32. García-Goñi, M.; Carcedo, D.; Villacampa, A.; Lores, M. Análisis de Impacto Presupuestario de los Medicamentos Biosimilares en el SNS de España 2009–2022. Informe Encargado por Biosim. Madrid, 2020. Available online: https://www.biosim.es/analisis-de-impacto-presupuestario-de-los-medicamentos-biosimilares-en-el-sistema-nacional-de-salud-de-espana-2009-2022/ (accessed on 8 February 2021).
33. Ministerio de Sanidad. Prestación Farmacéutica Informe Anual del Sistema Nacional de Salud 2018. Available online: https://www.mscbs.gob.es/estadEstudios/estadisticas/sisInfSanSNS/tablasEstadisticas/InfAnualSNS2018/Cap.7_Farmacia.pdf (accessed on 3 June 2020).
34. Ministerio de Hacienda. Serie Gasto Farmacéutico y Sanitario: Periodo Junio-2014 a Enero-2021. Indicadores Sobre Gasto Farmacéutico y Sanitario. 2021. Available online: https://www.hacienda.gob.es/es-ES/CDI/Paginas/EstabilidadPresupuestaria/InformacionAAPPs/Indicadores-sobre-Gasto-Farmaceutico-y-Sanitario.aspx (accessed on 5 April 2021).
35. Aladul, M.I.; Fitzpatrick, R.W.; Chapman, S.R. Impact of Infliximab and Etanercept Biosimilars on Biological Disease-Modifying Antirheumatic Drugs Utilization and NHS Budget in the UK. BioDrugs 2017, 31, 533–544. [CrossRef] [PubMed]
36. Kanters, T.A.; Stevanovic, J.; Huys, I.; Vulto, A.G.; Simoens, S. Adoption of Biosimilar Infliximab for Rheumatoid Arthritis, Ankylosing Spondylitis, and Inflammatory Bowel Diseases in the EU5: A Budget Impact Analysis Using a Delphi Panel. Front Pharmacol. 2017, 8, 322. [CrossRef] [PubMed]
37. Gulácsi, L.; Brodszky, V.; Baji, P.; Rencz, F.; Péntek, M. The Rituximab Biosimilar CT-P10 in Rheumatology and Cancer: A Budget Impact Analysis in 28 European Countries. Adv. Ther. 2017, 34, 1128–1144. [CrossRef] [PubMed]
38. IQVIA Institute. The Impact of Biosimilar Competition in Europe. 2020. Available online: https://ec.europa.eu/health/sites/health/files/human-use/docs/biosimilar_competition_en.pdf (accessed on 3 February 2021).
39. Autoridad Independiente de Responsabilidad Fiscal (AIReF). Evaluación del Gasto Público 2019. Estudio. Gasto Hospitalario del Sistema Nacional de Salud: Farmacia e Inversión en Bienes de Equipo. 2020. Available online: https://www.airef.es/wp-content/uploads/2020/10/SANIDAD/PDF-WEB-Gasto-hospitalario-del-SNS.pdf (accessed on 3 June 2020).
40. Ministerio de Sanidad, Consumo y Bienestar Social, Plan de Acción Para Fomentar la Utilización de los Medicamentos Reguladores del Mercado en el Sistema Nacional de Salud: Medicamentos Biosimilares y Medicamentos Genéricos. 11 April 2019. Available online: https://www.mscbs.gob.es/profesionales/farmacia/pdf/PlanAccionSNSmedicamentosReguladoresMercado.pdf (accessed on 3 June 2020).
41. Comité Asesor Para la Prestación Farmacéutica. Comentarios Sobre el Documento: Plan de Acción Para Fomentar la Utilización de los Medicamentos Reguladores del Mercado en el Sistema Nacional de Salud: Medicamentos Biosimilares y Medicamentos Genéricos. Documento de Consenso (Emitido el 22 de Mayo, Finalizado el 22 de Julio de 2019). Available online: https://www.mscbs.gob.es/en/profesionales/farmacia/pdf/20190722_Documento_CAPF_consenso_genericos_biosimilares.pdf (accessed on 8 February 2021).
42. Almarza, C. Mercado de Medicamentos Biosimilares. Previsiones de Futuro e Impacto Sobre los Sistemas Nacionales de Salud. IMS Health. 2016. Available online: http://www.diariofarma.com/wp-content/uploads/2016/03/03-Concha-Almarza-IMS.pdf. (accessed on 9 April 2021).
43. Rovira, J.; Espín, J.; García, L.; de Labry, A.O. The impact of biosimilars' entry in the EU market. Andal. Sch. Public Health 2011, 30, 1–83. Available online: https://www.researchgate.net/publication/281504554_The_impact_of_biosimilars\T1\textquoteright_entry_in_the_EU_market (accessed on 3 June 2020).
44. Conselleria de Sanitat Universal I Salut Publica, Comunitat Valenciana. Memoria de Gestión de la Conselleria de Sanitat Universal i Salut Pública. Año 2015. Capítulo 10. Política Farmacéutica. Available online: http://www.san.gva.es/documents/157385/6697728/10.+Pol%C3%ADtica+Farmac%C3%A9utica.pdf (accessed on 3 June 2020).
45. Ortega Eslava, A.; Marín Gil, R.; Fraga Fuentes, M.D.; López-Briz, E.; Puigventós Latorre, F.; GENESIS-SEFH. Guía de Evaluación Económica e Impacto Presupuestario en los Informes de Evaluación de Medicamentos; Guía Práctica Asociada al Programa MADRE v 4.0; SEFH: Madrid, Spain, 2016; ISBN 978-84-617-6757-1. Available online: https://gruposdetrabajo.sefh.es/genesis/genesis/Documents/GUIA_EE_IP_GENESIS-SEFH_19_01_2017.pdf (accessed on 3 June 2020).
46. Puig-Junoy, J.; Oliva-Moreno, J.; Trapero-Bertrán, M.; Abellán-Perpiñán, J.M.; Brosa-Riestra, M.; Servei Català de la Salut (CatSalut). Guía y Recomendaciones Para la Realización y Presentación de Evaluaciones Económicas y Análisis de Impacto Presupuestario de Medicamentos en el Ámbito del CatSalut; Generalitat de Catalunya. Departament de Salut. Servei Català de la Salut: Barcelona, España, 2014. Available online: https://scientiasalut.gencat.cat/bitstream/handle/11351/1057/guia_recomanacions_avaluacions_economiques_medicaments_catsalut_2014_cas.pdf?sequence=2&isAllowed=y (accessed on 3 June 2020).
47. WHO Collaborating Centre for Drug Statistics Methodology. ATC/DDD International Language for Drug Utilization Research: The Anatomical Therapeutic Chemical (ATC) Classification System. Available online: https://www.whocc.no (accessed on 30 March 2020).
48. Haustein, R.; Christoph de Millas, A.H.; Bertram, H. Saving money in the European healthcare systems with biosimilars. GaBI J. 2012, 1, 120–126. Available online: http://gabi-journal.net/saving-money-in-the-european-healthcare-systems-with-biosimilars.html (accessed on 3 June 2020). [CrossRef]
49. Base de datos del Consejo General de Colegios Oficiales de Farmacéuticos. 2020. Available online: https://botplusweb.portalfarma.com/botplus.aspx (accessed on 30 March 2020).
50. Briggs, A.H. Handling uncertainty in cost-effectiveness models. Pharmacoeconomics 2000, 17, 479–500. [CrossRef] [PubMed]

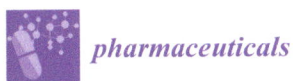

Article

Did the Introduction of Biosimilars Influence Their Prices and Utilization? The Case of Biologic Disease Modifying Antirheumatic Drugs (bDMARD) in Bulgaria

Konstantin Tachkov [1], Zornitsa Mitkova [1], Vladimira Boyadzieva [2] and Guenka Petrova [1,*]

[1] Department of Organisation and Economy of Pharmacy, Faculty of Pharmacy, Medical University of Sofia, 1000 Sofia, Bulgaria; tachkov@outlook.com (K.T.); zmitkova@pharmfac.mu-sofia.bg (Z.M.)
[2] Department of Rheumatology, Faculty of Medicine, Medical University of Sofia, 1612 Sofia, Bulgaria; vladimira.boyadzhieva@gmail.com
[*] Correspondence: gpetrova@pharmfac.mu-sofia.bg; Tel.: +359-884-222-964

Abstract: The aim of this study is to evaluate the effect of the introduction of biosimilars in Bulgaria on the prices and utilization of biologic disease modifying antirheumatic drugs (bDMARD). It is a combined qualitative and quantitative analysis of time of entry of biosimilars on the national market and the respective changes in the prices and utilization during 2015–2020. We found 58 biosimilars for 16 reference products authorized for sale on the European market by the end of 2019, but for 2 of the reference products biosimilars were not found on the national market. Only inflammatory joint disease had more than one biosimilar molecule indicated for therapy. Prices of the observed bDMARD decreased by 17% down to 48%. We noted significant price decreases upon biosimilar entrance onto the market. In total, the reimbursed expenditures for the whole therapeutic group steadily increased from 72 to 99 million BGN. Utilization changed from to 0.5868 to 2.7215 defined daily dose (DDD)/1000inh/day. Our study shows that the entrance of biosimilars in the country is relatively slow because only half of the biosimilars authorized in Europe are reimbursed nationally. Introduction of biosimilars decreases the prices and changes the utilization significantly but other factors might also contribute to this.

Keywords: biosimilars; pricing; reimbursement; utilization

Citation: Tachkov, K.; Mitkova, Z.; Boyadzieva, V.; Petrova, G. Did the Introduction of Biosimilars Influence Their Prices and Utilization? The Case of Biologic Disease Modifying Antirheumatic Drugs (bDMARD) in Bulgaria. *Pharmaceuticals* 2021, 14, 64. https://doi.org/10.3390/ph14010064

Received: 20 November 2020
Accepted: 11 January 2021
Published: 14 January 2021

Publisher's Note: MDPI stays neutral with regard to jurisdictional claims in published maps and institutional affiliations.

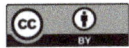

Copyright: © 2021 by the authors. Licensee MDPI, Basel, Switzerland. This article is an open access article distributed under the terms and conditions of the Creative Commons Attribution (CC BY) license (https://creativecommons.org/licenses/by/4.0/).

1. Introduction

It is largely well-established, as supported by evidence, that after the introduction of generic medicines the price of originals decreases, allowing for an increase in medicines utilization [1–4]. This is mostly valid for the synthetic medicines where the criteria for essential similarity between the originator and off-patented versions are scientifically and regulatory established [5]. Generic medicines benefit the market by offering equally high-quality treatment as originator medicines but at much lower prices [6,7]. Based on the essential similarity of medicines, countries introduce a variety of measures to stimulate generic medicines manufacturing, prescribing, dispensing, and utilization in the society [8,9]. Those measures are described as generic medicines policy [10,11]. Generic medicines policy has been promoted by the World Health Organization for many years with the main goal of encouraging governments to introduce it as part of their national drug policy [12,13]. A core element of the generic medicines policy is a list of essential drugs comprising the most widely used by the majority of people and medicines for a large number of diseases [14]. The aim of introducing generic incentives is to foster competition, decrease prices, and enlarge the utilization of essential medicines, thus, covering the needs of the majority of the population [15–17].

Biological medicines encompass a wide group of therapeutic agents that are manufactured through living organisms and include monoclonal antibodies, peptides (e.g., insulin), vaccines, blood products, RNA targeting therapies, and gene and cellular therapies [18]. A biosimilar medicine is a biological medicine that is similar to another biological medicine that has already been authorized for use [19–21]. Biosimilars have a number of important differences from generic small-molecule drugs, including manufacturing processes that are unique from their reference products (i.e., originators) [20]. There is considerable debate, still, in the scientific community about the safety and interchangeability of biological products [21]. Authors consider that the availability of biosimilars might provide an opportunity to lower health care expenditures as a result of the inherent price competition with their reference product [22]. This is due to the fact that biological products are rising as a proportion of drug expenditures globally [23]. There are estimates that over 30% of all drug spending in Europe is on biological medicines and out of them 1.5% are for biosimilars. There has been an increase by 3.4% over the last five years for all biologic medicines, and by 1.2% since 2014 for biosimilars. By the end of 2018, 16 biological molecules have had biosimilar products introduced in Europe, meaning that there is a possibility to enhance biosimilars competition with reference biological products. In countries where there is no officially introduced generic medicines policy, we can expect obstacles towards the market penetration, prescribing, and competition in the field of biological products [24,25]. This stimulated our interest towards the topic.

The aim of this study is to evaluate the effect of the introduction of biosimilars in Bulgaria on the prices and utilization of biologic disease modifying antirheumatic drugs (bDMARD) for inflammatory joint diseases therapy.

2. Results

2.1. Availability of Biosimilars in the Reimbursement Drug List

We found 58 biosimilars for 16 reference products authorised for sale on the European market by the end of 2019, but for 2 of the reference products (insulin lispro and enoxaparin) biosimilars were not found on the national market. The national market included 14 reference products for which 29 biosimilars are reimbursed (Table 1).

Fifteen biosimilars are reimbursed for the outpatient practice. Adalimumab, infliximab, etanercept, and rituximab are biologic disease modifying antirheumatic drugs (bDMARD) indicated for inflammatory joint diseases therapy for which nine biosimilars were found. The rest of the INNs for outpatient practice possess only one biosimilar reimbursed in the country, except epoetin alfa with two biosimilar (Table 1).

Trastuzumab, bevacizumab, filgrastim, pegfilgrastim, and follitropin alfa are reimbursed for inpatient practice but for different therapeutic areas and we could not compare them at a therapeutic level. Fourteen biosimilars are authorized for those INNs (Table 1).

From Table 1, it is also evident that the time period for biosimilar entry on the national reimbursed market after its marketing authorization in Europe varies from two months (infliximab first biosimilar) to nine years (bevacizumab biosimilar). It is also evident that a total six biosimilars were present in the reimbursed practice for a limited time period which were later excluded from the Positive Drug List probably due to marketing authorization holder request.

Reviewing the changes in the authorized for sale and reimbursed indications of inflammatory joint disease therapy, we found the following. Infliximab was the first reimbursed by the National Health Insurance Fund bDMARD for the indication of RA therapy, subsequently AS was added, as well as PSA as an indication. All of the indications were approved by the NCPR prior to the observed period 2015–2019. During the observed period, entrance of an infliximab biosimilar to the reimbursement practice allowed for reimbursement of all aforementioned indications immediately upon receiving approval. This was the case for other biosimilars for inflammatory joint diseases therapy as well.

Table 1. Available biosimilar in the reimbursement practice and date of entrance.

INN	Authorized Biosimilars in Europe (n)	Biosimilars Available on the National Market (n)	Authorisation Date in Europe	Date of Inclusions into the Positive Drug List (PDL)	Time Lag
			Outpatient Practice		
insulin glargine	2	1	8/09/2014	24/08/2015	11 months
adalimumab	8	1	20/03/2017	22/10/2018	1 year 5 months
		1	15/09/2018	22/03/2019	6 months
		1	25/07/2018	18/03/2019	6 months
		1	16/09/2018	20/02/2020	2 year 6 months
infliximab	4	1	9/09/2013	27/11/2013	2 months
		1	8/09/2013	27/11/2013	2 months
		1	17/05/2018	28/03/2019	10 months
etanercept	2	1	22/06/2017	19/06/2020	3 year
rituximab	5	1	16/02/2017	30/03/2018 2/11/2020 (excluded)	11 months 2 year
epoetin alfa	3	1	26/08/2007	20.03.2013 2.10.2014 (excluded)	4 year 6 months 1 year 7 months
		1	22/08/2007	26/09/2016	9 year
epoetin zeta	3	1	17/12/2007	15/06/2012	4 year 5 months
teriparatide	3	1	10/01/2017	8/11/2019 2/04/2020 (excluded)	1.9 year 6 months
somatropin	1	1	11/04/2006	3/12/2011	4 year 8 months
			Inpatient Practice		
follitropin alfa	2	1	25/03/2014	01/03/2015	1 year
filgrastim	6	1	16/09/2014	01/02/2018	3 year 5 months
		1	6/06/2010	22/08/2011 8/09/2012 (excluded)	1 year 2 months 1 year
		1	14/09/2008	21/08/2012 16/06/2014 (excluded)	4 year 2 year
		1	5/02/2009	19/09/2011	2 year 7 months
pegfilgrastim	6	1	25/04/2019	27/03/2020	11 months
		1	20/09/2018	01/03/2019	5 months
		1	21/11/2018	01/03/2019	4 months
trastuzumab	5	1	7/02/2018	12/10/2018 2/11/2020 (excluded)	8 months 2 year
		1	15/05/2018	2/02/2019	9 months
		1	11/12/2018	13/03/2019	3 months
		1	14/11/2017	21/02/2020	2 year 3 months
		1	25/07/2018	13/03/2019	6 months
bevacizumam	2	1	14/01/2018	28/09/2020	1 year 9 months

2.2. Changes in Prices and Utilization of Anti-Inflammatory Joint Diseases Medicines

During 2015–2020, a total of nine biosimilar products for four INNs were found available on the reimbursement drug list within the group of anti-inflammatory joint diseases (Table 2).

Table 2. Reference price per define daily dose (DDD) for anti-inflammatory joint diseases medicines (BGN).

INN	2015	2016	2017	2018	2019	2020	% Change (2020 to 2015)	Fisher Test
etanercept	67.08	60.49	58.69	54.55	53.75	34.39 *	48.72	
infliximab	30.61 *,*	28.68	27.018	27.02	17.92 *	17.92	41.47	
adalimumab	72.39	66.08	66.08	50.01 *	38.13 *	38.13 *,*	47.33	
cetrolizumab	63.67	57.29	57.29	53.10	53.11	50.03	21.43	
golimumab	65.56	65.24	62.05	57.50	57.50	53.34	18.63	
ustekinumab	73.70	73.24	65.53	60.65	60.65	60.65	17.71	$p < 0.0001$
tocilizumab	71.21	70.91	60.58	60.58	59.22	54.69	23.19	
rituximab	4.97	4.97	4.94	3.65 *	3.13	3.39 ↓	31.66	
secukinumab			81.04	80.88	73.08	72,58	10.44	
tofacitinib				55.51	52.94	52.94	4.63	
baricitinib					77.16	77.16	0%	

Legend: * biosimilar included; ↓ biosimilar excluded.

In 2015, infliximab had only two biosimilar alternatives available, with a third being introduced in 2019; however, this inclusion was of the originator of infliximab. Its price was influenced by the already established reference price per DDD of the corresponding biosimilars as per the active legislation requiring the reimbursing of the lowest price per DDD. The price of infliximab dropped down by nearly 41% during the period and the highest decrease was observed when the third product was included in the list. One biosimilar for etanercept entered the reimbursement practice leading to almost a 75% decrease in the reference price per DDD at the moment of entrance and total 49% price decrease during the whole period observed. Adalimumab appears to be the most competitive INN with four biosimilars introduced during the period and nearly double the decrease in the price. Originator for tocilizumab added one new dosage form leading to a small decrease in reference price per DDD. For rituximab, we found one included biosimilar and the price dropped down by 1.3 BGN per DDD. This dosage form was subsequently excluded, leading to an increase in reference price with 0.27BGN (Table 2).

Regarding the changes in prices, we observed a decrease by nearly 50% for INNs where biosimilars were introduced and with 5–21% for INNs where there was no biosimilar competitor available prior to introduction (Table 2). The decrease in the prices of the other INNs where there is no biosimilars could be explained with the regular price revision. If there is a price decrease in the reference countries it immediately affects the prices on the national market. For the period 2015–2020, all changes in prices were found to be statistically significant ($p < 0.001$). The inclusion of baricitinib resulted in a nonsignificant change in prices for the period 2019–2020 ($p = 0.1326$).

Reimbursed expenditures increased for almost all INNs in 2019 in comparison with 2015 (Table 3). Only for infliximab we noted a decrease in expenditures by 49%, which could be attributed both partly to the decreasing prices, and partly due to the entrance of new therapeutic and biosimilar competitors. Similar is the situation with adalimumab, whereby until 2018 reimbursed expenditures increased and upon the introduction of biosimilars it started to decrease. We can assume that the price decrease leads also to decrease in the reimbursed expenditures.

In total, the reimbursed expenditures for the whole therapeutic group steadily increased from 72 to 99 million BGN by the end of the observed period (nearly 36–45.9 million Euro)—Figure 1. Variations in the percent change of total reimbursed expenditures was noted between 2017 in comparison to 2016 ($p < 0.05$) when the increase is less than between 2016 and 2015 ($p > 0.05$). In 2019, we observed a decrease in total expenditures with 2.83%, which was nonsignificant. However, the change in expenditures between 2017 and 2018 were significant ($p < 0.05$), and seem to be largely influenced by the increased expenditures for secukinimab and rituximab.

Table 3. Reimbursed expenditures in monetary units (in millions of BGN).

INN	2015	2016	2017	2018	2019	% Change (2019 to 2015)	Fisher Test
Etanercept	15.87	15.78	15.27	15.47	17.19	7.69	
Infliximab	8.25	6.30	6.65	7.24	5.54	−48.77	
Adalimumab	31.86	42.24	47.70	49.99	40.08	20.51	
Cetrolizumab	3.19	3.45	4.17	4.32	4.43	27.98	
Golimumab	4.98	5.71	5.82	5.85	5.71	12.89	$p < 0.0001$
Tocilizumab	7.15	9.06	10.46	12.00	13.91	48.58	
Rituximab	0.89	0.97	1.49	11.96	10.06	91.12	
Secukinumab			1.23	7.72	11.74	89.56	
Tofacitinib				0.28	2.80	89.87	
Baricitinib					0.12	0	

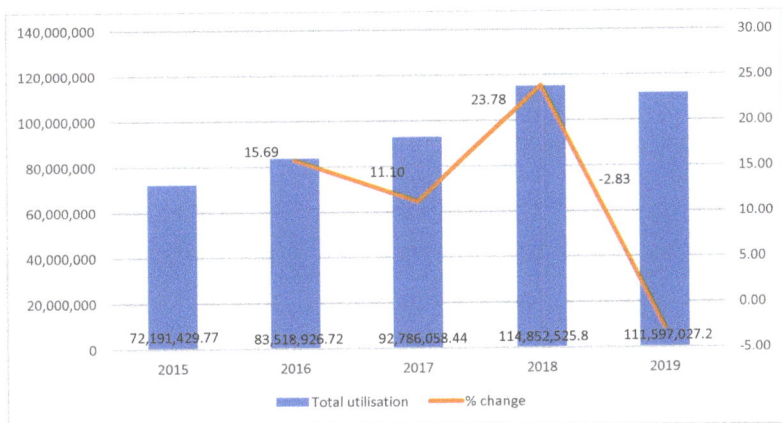

Figure 1. Total reimbursed expenditures and % change every year.

Utilization in DDD/1000inh/day is stable for most INNs, with a smooth increase except for rituximab and adalimumab (Figure 2) for which a significant increase is observed.

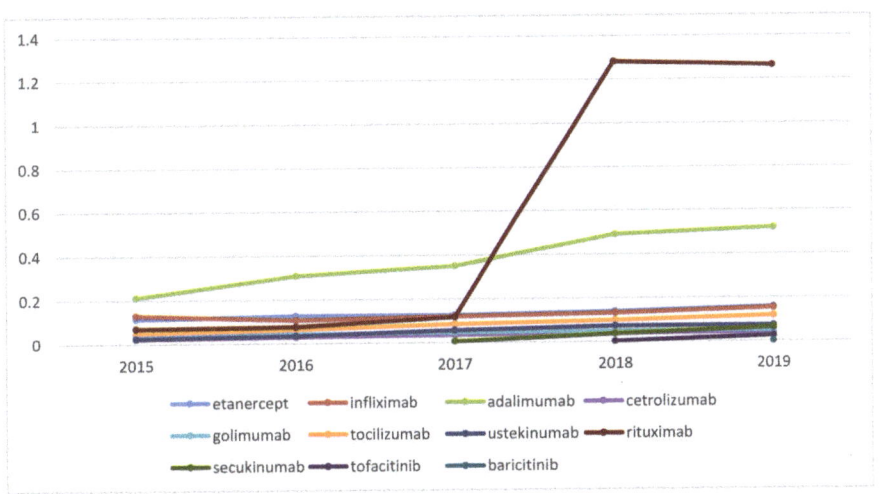

Figure 2. Utilization in DDD/1000inh/day.

As a whole, during 2015–2019 the utilization in DDD/1000inh/day increased from 0.657 to 2.395. The increase in utilization was found to be significant ($p < 0.001$). Adalimumab is definitely a leader in utilization in DDD/1000inh/day accounting for 32% to 21% of total utilization during the period (Table 4). For rituximab we noted a tremendous increase in utilization in 2018 when the first biosimilar entered the market.

Table 4. Share of utilization in DDD/1000inh/day.

	2015	% of Overall Utilization	2016	% of Overall Utilization	2017	% of Overall Utilization	2018	% of Overall Utilization	2019	% of Overall Utilization
etanercept	0.1133	17.25	0.1258	16.04	0.1263	13.41	0.1387	5.93	0.1575	6.41
infliximab	0.129	19.63	0.1059	13.50	0.1197	12.71	0.1312	5.61	0.1524	6.20
adalimmab	0.2107	32.07	0.3082	39.29	0.3506	37.22	0.489	20.91	0.5178	21.07
cetrolizumab	0.0239	3.64	0.0291	3.71	0.0353	3.75	0.0398	1.70	0.041	1.67
golimumab	0.0363	5.53	0.0423	5.39	0.0456	4.84	0.0497	2.13	0.0489	1.99
tocilizumab	0.0481	7.32	0.0616	7.85	0.0839	8.91	0.0969	4.14	0.1157	4.71
rituximab	0.0254	36.13	0.0352	4.49	0.0567	6.02	0.072	3.08	0.0726	2.95
secukinumab	0.0703	10.70	0.0764	9.74	0.1179	12.52	1.2817	54.80	1.2619	51.35
ustekinumab					0.0059	0.63	0.0374	1.60	0.0629	2.56
tofacitinib							0.0024	0.10	0.026	1.06
baricitinib									0.0007	0.03
total utilization	0.66	132.26	0.78	100.00	0.94	100.00	2.34	100.00	2.46	100.00

What is worth noting, however, is that all changes in utilization were found to be significant, even those between 2018 and 2019 ($p < 0.05$), despite the changes in total NHIF expenditures for the same time period being nonsignificant. This seems to indicate that introduction of biosimilars and the implementation of cost-containment measures is able to control for an increase in expenditures, and allow for increase in utilization of these medicines.

3. Discussion

To the best of our knowledge, this is the first national study exploring the entrance of biosimilars on the national market and their influence on the reimbursed prices and utilization of a particular therapeutic group in DDD/1000inh/day. There are two other national studies focusing on biosimilars [26,27]. The first one compared the prices of biological products for rheumatoid arthritis therapy, and found that manufacturer prices of reference biological product and biosimilars shows 36% difference for etanercept, 39% for rituximab, and 31% for infliximab, while at retail level the differences are 11%, 86%, and 143%, respectively [28]. It does not explore their reimbursement prices and utilization, but only officially published manufacturer and retail prices. Authors noted this as a limitation of the study. The second article explores the access to biotechnological drugs for rare diseases and found that they comprise a high proportion of pharmaceutical expenditures in the reimbursed biotechnological medicinal products market [29].

Similar international comparisons reviewed the requirements for reimbursement of biosimilars and compared the reimbursement status, market share, and reimbursement costs of biosimilars in Bulgaria, the Czech Republic, Croatia, Estonia, Hungary, Latvia, Lithuania, Poland, Slovakia, and Romania during 2016–2017, using a questionnaire, focusing mostly on the regulatory requirements for the pricing and reimbursement of biosimilars for each country [30]. Authors pointed out that the total expenditure on the reimbursement of biologic drugs in the CEE countries was 397,097,152 EUR in 2014 and 411,433,628 EUR in 2015, but the data for Bulgaria was scarce.

None of the national studies explore the entrance of all biosimilars. Our research found that almost half of all authorized by EMA biosimilars are available on the market but only in one therapeutic group could we establish price competition. There are still many biosimilars that are not available. In addition to this slow penetration, the time for entrance is also variable. For the earlier biosimilars it was extremely long (nine years for the epoetin alfa) but in recent years, the time of inclusion has become faster; in some cases, as quickly as two months, which indicated progress in marketing penetration. This might be also due to the fact that in the area of bDMARD for inflammatory joint diseases therapy not only is biosimilar competition increasing, but also therapeutic competition, and the range of improved indications has expanded to cover other forms of arthritis. The first bDMARD (infliximab) for joint diseases therapy were positioned for rheumatoid arthritis in 2000, subsequently the indications increased to allow for other types of inflammatory joint diseases (RA, PSA, AS). In 2003, the indication AS was added, and in 2004 the indication of psoriatic arthritis (PSA) was approved. Despite the approval received by EMA for the treatment of RA in 2000 for etanercept and 2003 for adalimumab, the NHIF added both bDMARDS with a significant delay at the end of 2009, but for the three inflammatory joint diseases (RA, PSA, AS). In 2010, the NHIF included in the list two new molecules: anti-IL-6-tocilizumab and anti-CD20-rituximab with indication RA (rituximab received approval also for Wegener's disease in 2015). One year later, certolizumab pegol was included in the therapeutic arsenal, approved by the NHIF, for the indication RA, and in 2015 for the other two inflammatory joint diseases. In 2012, golimumab received approval for the three diagnoses and ustekinumab a year later, but only for the indication of psoriatic arthritis. The last two bDMARDs received approval in 2017 for secukinumab and in 2019 for ixekizumab. A new group of medicines-target synthetic DMARDS has entered widely in the practice of rheumatologists in 2018. Tofacitinib was the first approved by the NHIF in March 2018, followed by baricitinib in 2019. To date, no biosimilar products of these have been presented but we found that their entrance changes the utilization in the group as a whole.

It is also important to note that biosimilars entrance is delayed also by the market exclusivity practices of the pharmaceutical companies [31].

A limitation of our study is that we focused only on the therapeutic group for outpatient practice, because the reimbursed prices of medicines for hospitals are an object of tenders and all of them are also subject of confidential rebate negotiation so the real market price could not be established.

Regarding the prices, we confirmed the hypothesis that the biosimilars decrease the prices of biological product even at the moment of their entrance in the reimbursement system. The prices are highly competitive and in comparison with the INNs, where there is no biosimilars, prices are falling down at twice the rate [27]. The pricing policy in Bulgaria is oriented towards lower costs and lower prices. External reference pricing is applied for price approval and lowest ex-manufacturing price is used out of 10 reference countries. After the reimbursement approval, the lowest price per DDD is used as a reference price for reimbursement within the INN. The fact that the years with the most included biosimilars (2018–2019) had a nonsignificant change in total expenditures indicates that these cost-containment measures are effective.

We also confirm that the entrance of biosimilars influences the utilization in a positive direction, except for infliximab, with significant changes being observed for all INNs. The decrease in utilization of infliximab could be attributed to the constantly lowering prices and entrance of new bDMARDS within the group. This is probably influenced by adalimumab who is the leader in the group. Adalimumab is one of the most commonly prescribed blockers of TNFa due to its well-established long-term safety profile [28], tolerability, and effectiveness compared to other bDMARDS [32]. It is one of the first three bDMARDS approved for treatment by the NHIF with 18 indications to date. Recent studies reveal that adalimumab is one of the most prescribed biologics in the United States after an analysis of the treatment of 40,373 RA patients [33].

A study of the utilization of biosimilars was conducted in Korea, where authors found an increasing market share for infliximab biosimilars at over 30%, while rituximab and trastuzumab had a share of 12.89% and 13.93%, respectively [34]. They also found savings over six years after the biosimilar entry to the market. A similar study explores the utilization of infliximab and filgrastim on the US market and it was one of the first matching the importance of biosimilar products [35]. The cost savings are considered as benefits from the introduction of biosimilars [36]. Other authors also prove that biosimilars not only decrease the prices but also increase the utilization but still there are concerns for their interchangeability [37,38].

The other study discussed the market drivers for biosimilars [39]. The authors confirm that there is a correlation between the biosimilar penetration and price decrease. They consider that incentive policies to enhance uptake remain an important driver of biosimilar penetration. The only incentive that is available at the moment in Bulgaria is that the price of biosimilar should be no more than 80% of the price of originator, but it was introduced in the legislation just in 2018 so it does not affect the whole period studied [40]. Therefore, we could not consider that this change in regulation is influencing the price decrease during the whole period.

4. Materials and Methods

The study utilized a combined quantitative and qualitative analysis of time of entry of biosimilars on the national market and the respective changes in the prices and utilization of biologic disease modifying antirheumatic drugs (bDMARD).

4.1. Qualitative Analysis

The qualitative analysis included comparisons of market entry of biosimilars—their time of approval and entry onto the Bulgarian market. Information regarding all authorized biosimilars and approval of their new indications till the end of 2019 was taken from the EMA webpage [41]. Subsequently, the Internet page of the National Council of Prices and Reimbursement (NCPR) [42] was searched for reimbursed biosimilars up until the end of 2020.

The availability was presented as the number of biosimilars per international non-proprietary name (INN), authorized by EMA and available on the European market, which was then compared to the date of product entry into the reimbursement list on the national market.

4.2. Quantitative Analysis

After the qualitative analysis, we selected a single therapeutic group-biologic disease modifying antirheumatic drugs (bDMARs) for further analysis. The choice was based upon the fact that this therapeutic group had the largest number of reimbursed biological and biosimilar products for the longest duration of time. Under inflammatory joint diseases we encompass rheumatoid arthritis (RA), psoriatic arthritis (PSA), and ankylosing spondylitis (AS) because those are the most often reimbursed diagnoses.

Two data sources were accessed for the quantitative analysis—the National Health Insurance Fund (NHIF) and the NCPR. From the NHIF we extracted data on the reimbursed expenditures for the period 2015–2019 of bDMARD for inflammatory joint disease medicines. The changes in expenditures for every year are presented in national currency (BGN) at the exchange rate of 1 BGN = 0.95 Euro. The exchange rate of BGN to Euro in Bulgaria has been fixed since 1997.

The NCPR database was accessed retrospectively to follow changes in medicine reference prices per defined daily dose (DDD) and per INN throughout the period 2015–2020. The reference price per DDD is the lowest reimbursed price per DDD.

Utilization of the medicines for inflammatory joint diseases was analyzed in monetary units and in DDD/1000inh/day by using the WHO formula ((Sales data/DDD/number of inhabitants/365) $\times$ 1000) [43].

4.3. Statistical Analysis

Friedman's variant of ANOVA was applied for all years for which data was available to follow the changes in prices and utilization. Where a new medicine was introduced, and data was available only for two years, a Wilcoxon nonparametric analysis was applied to analyze the changes in therapy for all biologics. p-values of less than 0.05 were considered statistically significant. The software package MedCalc version 19.6 was used.

5. Conclusions

Our study shows that the entrance of biosimilars in the country is relatively slow because only half of the authorized biosimilars in Europe are reimbursed. Introduction of biosimilars decreases the prices and changes the utilization significantly but other factors might also contribute to this.

Author Contributions: Conceptualization, G.P. and K.T.; methodology, Z.M., K.T.; formal analysis, K.T., Z.M., V.B., G.P., data curation G.P., Z.M.; statistical analysis, K.T.; writing, K.T., Z.M., V.B., G.P.; supervision, G.P. All authors have read and agreed to the published version of the manuscript.

Funding: This research received no external funding.

Institutional Review Board Statement: Not applicable.

Informed Consent Statement: Not applicable.

Data Availability Statement: Data sharing not applicable.

Conflicts of Interest: The authors declare no conflict of interest.

References

1. Kaplan, W.A.; Ritz, L.S.; Vitello, M.; Wirtz, V.J. Policies to promote use of generic medicines in low and middle income countries: A review of published literature, 2000–2010. *Health Policy* **2012**, *106*, 211–224. [CrossRef]
2. Dylst, P.; Simoens, S. Does the Market Share of Generic Medicines Influence the Price Level? *PharmacoEconomics* **2011**, *29*, 875–882. [CrossRef]
3. King, D.; Kanavos, P. Encouraging the use of generic medicines: Implications for transition economies. *Croat. Med. J.* **2002**, *43*, 462–469. [PubMed]
4. Gama, H.; Torre, C.; Guerreiro, J.P.; Azevedo, A.; Costa, S.; Lunet, N. Use of generic and essential medicines for prevention and treatment of cardiovascular diseases in Portugal. *BMC Health Serv. Res.* **2017**, *17*, 449. [CrossRef]
5. European Commission. Directive 2001/83/EC of the European Parliament and of the Council of 6 November 2001 on the Community code relating to medicinal products for human use. *OJ L* **2001**, *311*, 67–128. Available online: http://data.europa.eu/eli/dir/2001/83/oj (accessed on 12 January 2021).
6. Dylst, P.; Vulto, A.G.; Godman, B.; Simoens, S. Generic Medicines: Solutions for a Sustainable Drug Market? *Appl. Health Econ. Health Policy* **2013**, *11*, 437–443. [CrossRef]
7. Spinks, J.; Chen, G.; Donovan, L. Does generic entry lower the prices paid for pharmaceuticals in Australia? A comparison before and after the introduction of the mandatory price-reduction policy. *Aust. Health Rev.* **2013**, *37*, 675–681. [CrossRef]
8. Elek, P.; Harsányi, A.; Zelei, T.; Csetneki, K.; Kaló, Z. Policy objective of generic medicines from the investment perspective: The case of clopidogrel. *Health Policy* **2017**, *121*, 558–565. [CrossRef]
9. Dylst, P.; Vulto, A.; Simoens, S. Societal value of generic medicines beyond cost-saving through reduced prices. *Expert Rev. Pharm. Outcomes Res.* **2015**, *15*, 701–711. [CrossRef]
10. Salmane-Kulikovska, I.; Poplavska, E.; Ceha, M.; Mezinska, S. Use of generic medicines in Latvia: Awareness, opinions and experiences of the population. *J. Pharm. Policy Pract.* **2019**, *12*, 1. [CrossRef]
11. Steele, J.W. Generic Competition in Canada. *Pharmacoeconomics* **1994**, *6*, 480–482. [CrossRef]
12. WHO. *Guideline for National Drug Policies*; World Health Organization: Geneva, Switzerland, 1988.
13. Rietveld, A.H.; Haaijer-Ruskamp, F.M. Policy options for cost-containment of pharmaceuticals. *Int. J. Risk Saf. Med.* **2002**, *15*, 29–54.
14. WHO. *The Selection of Essential Drugs*; World Health Organization: Geneva, Switzerland, 1977.
15. Kemp, A.; Roughead, E.E.; Kim, D.-S.; Ong, B. Pricing policies for generic medicines in Australia, New Zealand, the Republic of Korea and Singapore: Patent expiry and influence on atorvastatin price. *WHO South-East Asia J. Public Health* **2018**, *7*, 99–106. [CrossRef]
16. Miguel, P.Z. Legal and policy foundations for global generic competition: Promoting affordable drug pricing in developing societies. *Glob. Public Health* **2015**, *10*, 1–16. [CrossRef]

17. Mossialos, E.; Mrazek, M.; Walley, T. *Regulating Pharmaceuticals in Europe: Striving for Efficiency, Equity and Quality*; Open University Press: Berkshire, UK, 2004.
18. European Medicines Agency. Biosimilar Medicines. Retrieved 17 June 2015. Available online: http://www.ema.europa.eu/ema/index.jsp?curl=pages/special_topics/document_listing/document_listing_000318.jsp (accessed on 1 November 2020).
19. Berkowitz, S.A.; Engen, J.R.; Mazzeo, J.R.; Jones, B.G. Analytical tools for characterizing biopharmaceuticals and the implications for biosimilars. *Nat. Rev. Drug Discov.* **2012**, *11*, 527–540. [CrossRef]
20. Harvey, R.D. Science of Biosimilars. *J. Oncol. Pract.* **2017**, *13*, 17s–23s. [CrossRef]
21. Li, E.; Ramanan, S.; Green, L. Pharmacist Substitution of Biological Products: Issues and Considerations. *J. Manag. Care Spéc. Pharm.* **2015**, *21*, 532–539. [CrossRef]
22. Nabhan, C.; Parsad, S.; Mato, A.R.; Feinberg, B.A. Biosimilars in Oncology in the United States. *JAMA Oncol.* **2018**, *4*, 241. [CrossRef]
23. Troen, P.; Newton, M.; Patel, J.; Scott, K. *The Impact of Biosimilar Competition in Europe*; White paper; IQVIA: Durham, NC, USA, 2019.
24. Moorkens, E.; Vulto, A.G.; Huys, I.; Dylst, P.; Godman, B.; Keuerleber, S.; Claus, B.; Dimitrova, M.; Petrova, G.; Sović-Brkičić, L.; et al. Policies for biosimilar uptake in Europe: An overview. *PLoS ONE* **2017**, *12*, e0190147. [CrossRef]
25. Cazap, E.; Jacobs, I.; McBride, A.; Popovian, R.; Sikora, K. Global Acceptance of Biosimilars: Importance of Regulatory Consistency, Education, and Trust. *Oncologist* **2018**, *23*, 1188–1198. [CrossRef]
26. Manova, M.; Savova, A.; Vasileva, M.; Terezova, S.; Kamusheva, M.; Grekova, D.; Petkova, V.; Petrova, G. Comparative Price Analysis of Biological Products for Treatment of Rheumatoid Arthritis. *Front. Pharmacol.* **2018**, *9*, 1070. [CrossRef]
27. Kamusheva, M.; Manova, M.; Savova, A.T.; Petrova, G.I.; Mitov, K.; Harsányi, A.; Kaló, Z.; Márky, K.; Kawalec, P.; Angelovska, B.; et al. Comparative Analysis of Legislative Requirements About Patients' Access to Biotechnological Drugs for Rare Diseases in Central and Eastern European Countries. *Front. Pharmacol.* **2018**, *9*, 795. [CrossRef]
28. Stiff, K.M.; Cline, A.; Feldman, S. Tracking the price of existing biologics when drugs enter the market. *Expert Rev. Pharm. Outcomes Res.* **2019**, *19*, 375–377. [CrossRef]
29. Burmester, G.-R.; Gordon, K.B.; Rosenbaum, J.T.; Arikan, D.; Lau, W.L.; Li, P.; Faccin, F.; Panaccione, R. Long-Term Safety of Adalimumab in 29,967 Adult Patients from Global Clinical Trials Across Multiple Indications: An Updated Analysis. *Adv. Ther.* **2019**, *37*, 364–380. [CrossRef]
30. Kawalec, P.; Stawowczyk, E.; Tesar, T.; Skoupa, J.; Turcu-Stiolica, A.; Dimitrova, M.; Petrova, G.I.; Rugaja, Z.; Männik, A.; Harsanyi, A.; et al. Pricing and Reimbursement of Biosimilars in Central and Eastern European Countries. *Front. Pharmacol.* **2017**, *8*, 288. [CrossRef]
31. Rome, B.N.; Lee, C.C.; Kesselheim, A.S. Market Exclusivity Length for Drugs with New Generic or Biosimilar Competition, 2012–2018. *Clin. Pharmacol. Ther.* **2020**. [CrossRef]
32. Sator, P. Safety and tolerability of adalimumab for the treatment of psoriasis: A review summarizing 15 years of real-life experience. *Ther. Adv. Chronic Dis.* **2018**, *9*, 147–158. [CrossRef]
33. Atzinger, C.B.; Guo, J.J. Biologic Disease-Modifying Antirheumatic Drugs in a National, Privately Insured Population: Utilization, Expenditures, and Price Trends. *Am. Health Drug Benefits* **2017**, *10*, 27–36.
34. Lee, H.-J.; Han, E.; Kim, H. Comparison of Utilization Trends between Biosimilars and Generics: Lessons from the Nationwide Claims Data in South Korea. *Appl. Health Econ. Health Policy* **2020**, *18*, 557–566. [CrossRef]
35. Dutcher, S.K.; Fazio-Eynullayeva, E.; Eworuke, E.; Carruth, A.; Dee, E.C.; Blum, M.D.; Nguyen, M.D.; Toh, S.; Panozzo, C.A.; Lyons, J.G. Understanding utilization patterns of biologics and biosimilars in the United States to support postmarketing studies of safety and effectiveness. *Pharmacoepidemiol. Drug Saf.* **2020**, *29*, 786–795. [CrossRef]
36. Dutta, B.; Huys, I.; Vulto, A.G.; Simoens, S. Identifying Key Benefits in European Off-Patent Biologics and Biosimilar Markets: It is Not Only about Price! *BioDrugs* **2020**, *34*, 159–170. [CrossRef]
37. Kim, Y.; Kwon, H.-Y.; Godman, B.; Moorkens, E.; Simoens, S.; Bae, S. Uptake of Biosimilar Infliximab in the UK, France, Japan, and Korea: Budget Savings or Market Expansion Across Countries? *Front. Pharmacol.* **2020**, *11*, 970. [CrossRef]
38. O'Callaghan, J.; Barry, S.P.; Bermingham, M.; Morris, J.M.; Griffin, B.T. Regulation of biosimilar medicines and current perspectives on interchangeability and policy. *Eur. J. Clin. Pharmacol.* **2018**, *75*, 1–11. [CrossRef]
39. Rémuzat, C.; Dorey, J.; Cristeau, O.; Ionescu, D.; Radière, G.; Toumi, M. Key drivers for market penetration of biosimilars in Europe. *J. Mark. Access Health Policy* **2017**, *5*, 1272308. [CrossRef]
40. Ministry Council. *Regulation on the Conditions, Rules and Order of Regulating and Registering of the Prices of Medicinal Product*; State Gazette No 40/2013; Last amended: State Gazette 19/2020; Council of Ministers: Sofia, Bulgaria, 2020.
41. EMA. Science, Medicines, Health. Biosimilar Medicines: Marketing Authorization. Available online: https://www.ema.europa.eu/en/human-regulatory/marketing-authorisation/biosimilar-medicines-marketing-authorisation (accessed on 12 January 2021).
42. National Council of Prices and Reimbursement. Electronic Registries. Available online: http://portal.ncpr.bg/registers/pages/register/list-medicament.xhtml (accessed on 12 January 2021).
43. WHO. Essential Medicines and Health Products. DDD Indicators. Available online: https://www.who.int/medicines/regulation/medicines-safety/toolkit_indicators/en/index1.html (accessed on 12 January 2021).

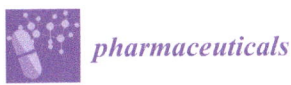

Article

Simulating Costs of Intravenous Biosimilar Trastuzumab vs. Subcutaneous Reference Trastuzumab in Adjuvant HER2-Positive Breast Cancer: A Belgian Case Study

Steven Simoens [1,*], Arnold G. Vulto [1,2] and Pieter Dylst [3]

1 Department of Pharmaceutical and Pharmacological Sciences, KU Leuven, 3000 Leuven, Belgium; a.vulto@gmail.com
2 Hospital Pharmacy, Erasmus University Medical Center, 3000 CA Rotterdam, The Netherlands
3 EG nv/sa, 1020 Brussels, Belgium; pieter.dylst@eg.be
* Correspondence: steven.simoens@kuleuven.be; Tel.: +32-16-323465

Abstract: This study aimed to compare drug costs and healthcare costs of a 1 year adjuvant course with intravenous biosimilar trastuzumab vs. subcutaneous reference trastuzumab in HER2-positive breast cancer from the Belgian hospital perspective. Our simulation is based on the methodology used by Tjalma and colleagues, and considered costs of drugs, healthcare professional time and consumables. We calculated intravenous drug costs for different body weights, and computed drug costs and healthcare costs to treat 100 patients with either trastuzumab formulation, assuming a binomial body weight distribution in this sample. Scenarios were run to account for drug discounts and intravenous vial sharing. Drug costs amounted to €1,431,282 with intravenous biosimilar trastuzumab and €1,522,809 with subcutaneous reference trastuzumab for a sample of 100 patients in the base case analysis. When healthcare professional time and consumables were also considered, healthcare costs with intravenous biosimilar trastuzumab were similar to those with subcutaneous reference trastuzumab. Differences in healthcare costs between intravenous biosimilar trastuzumab and subcutaneous reference trastuzumab depended on the level of discounts on these formulations and on intravenous vial sharing. Our case study demonstrates that comparing costs of intravenous vs. subcutaneous formulations is complex and multifactorial, and entails more than a simple cost comparison of products.

Keywords: trastuzumab; biosimilar; intravenous; subcutaneous; HER2-positive breast cancer; drug costs; healthcare costs; cost simulation

Citation: Simoens, S.; Vulto, A.G.; Dylst, P. Simulating Costs of Intravenous Biosimilar Trastuzumab vs. Subcutaneous Reference Trastuzumab in Adjuvant HER2-Positive Breast Cancer: A Belgian Case Study. *Pharmaceuticals* **2021**, *14*, 450. https://doi.org/10.3390/ph14050450

Academic Editor: Jean Jacques Vanden Eynde

Received: 16 April 2021
Accepted: 7 May 2021
Published: 11 May 2021

Publisher's Note: MDPI stays neutral with regard to jurisdictional claims in published maps and institutional affiliations.

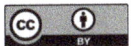

Copyright: © 2021 by the authors. Licensee MDPI, Basel, Switzerland. This article is an open access article distributed under the terms and conditions of the Creative Commons Attribution (CC BY) license (https://creativecommons.org/licenses/by/4.0/).

1. Introduction

Trastuzumab has played, and continues to play, a pivotal role in the standard first-line treatment of HER2-positive breast cancer for approximately two decades. Initial approval was based on the significant overall survival advantage demonstrated in key clinical trials in both the metastatic [1–3] and adjuvant [4,5] breast cancer settings. Until relatively recently, trastuzumab was administered using intravenous (IV) regimens either as monotherapy or, more usually, in combination with chemotherapy or biologic therapy. A subcutaneous (SC) formulation of trastuzumab was subsequently developed and was approved for use in Europe. The IV and SC formulations of trastuzumab show comparable pharmacokinetics [6–8], and have been reported to have equivalent (non-inferior) efficacy and tolerability in the HannaH, PrefHer and MetaspHer clinical studies [9–11]. In 2020, the global ex-factory turnover of reference trastuzumab accounted for more than US$4 billion [12].

A drug cost comparison at 2017 ex-factory prices in Belgium has been performed for the IV and SC formulations of reference trastuzumab for patients in different weight categories [13]. The calculation for a total of 18 cycles of adjuvant trastuzumab showed higher drug costs with the SC formulation for patients weighing >75 kg and with the IV formulation for those weighing <75 kg. The main reason for this was the single fixed available dose for the SC formulation (600 mg).

A biosimilar is a biological medicine that is highly similar to another already approved biological medicine (the "reference medicine") and does not show clinically meaningful differences from the reference medicine with respect to pharmaceutical quality, efficacy, and safety [14]. Several IV trastuzumab biosimilars have reached advanced stages of clinical development globally [15], some of which are available in Europe.

The aim of this case study was to compare drug costs and healthcare costs of IV biosimilar trastuzumab vs. SC reference trastuzumab (Herceptin®, Roche) as adjuvant treatment for one year in women with HER2-positive breast cancer from the hospital perspective in Belgium as an example to show the multifactorial character of an at-first-sight simple comparison. Our study is based on the methodology used by Tjalma and colleagues [13,16].

2. Results

Drug costs for a 1 year course of adjuvant treatment with IV biosimilar trastuzumab (at 2020 Belgian list prices) ranged from €17,858 for a patient weighing 87.5 kg to €10,244 for a patient weighing 50 kg (see Figure 1). In the case of a 1 year course with SC reference trastuzumab, drug costs amounted to €15,228, irrespective of patient body weight. Thus, treatment with IV biosimilar trastuzumab was less expensive in terms of drug costs than with SC reference trastuzumab for patients weighing up to 75 kg (see Figure 1).

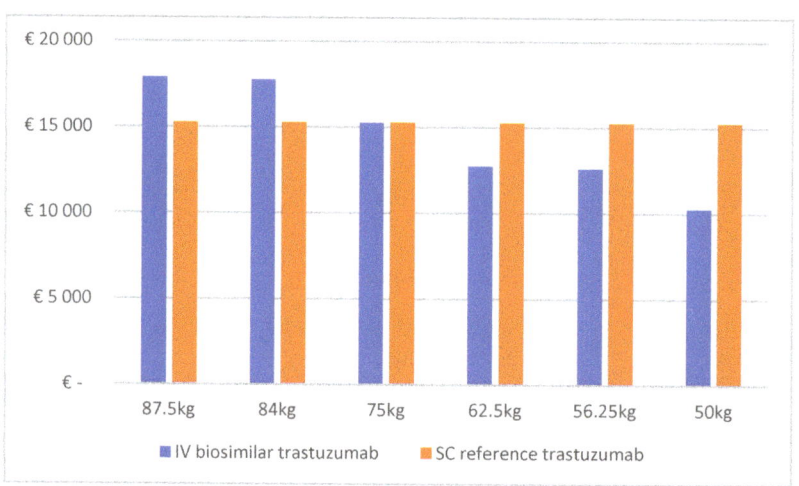

Figure 1. Drug costs for 1 year course of adjuvant treatment with IV biosimilar trastuzumab or with SC reference trastuzumab.

We next determined the difference in healthcare costs (i.e., drug costs, healthcare professional time costs and consumables costs) between the IV and SC formulations. This calculation took into account that the IV trastuzumab administration was previously estimated to cost €907.20 per course more than SC administration in terms of healthcare professional time costs and consumables costs [16]. Figure 2 shows that healthcare costs for a 1 year course of adjuvant treatment with IV biosimilar trastuzumab were lower than costs with SC reference trastuzumab for a patient weighing 50 kg, for a patient weighing 56.25 kg and for a patient weighing 62.5 kg. Healthcare costs with IV biosimilar trastuzumab exceeded those with SC reference trastuzumab for a patient weighing 75 kg, for a patient weighing 84 kg and for a patient weighing 87.5 kg; the reason being that IV trastuzumab is dosed on a mg/kg basis and the SC formulation has a fixed dose for all body weights.

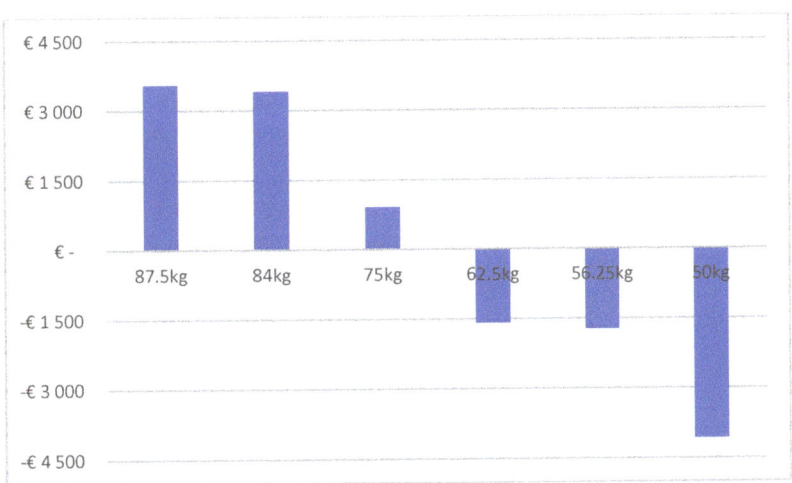

Figure 2. Difference in healthcare costs of 1 year course of adjuvant treatment with IV biosimilar trastuzumab as compared with SC reference trastuzumab.

When calculated for a sample of 100 patients, the difference in drug costs between the IV and SC formulations amounted to €91,527 (see Table 1). When also considering healthcare professional time and consumables, healthcare costs for a 1 year course of adjuvant treatment with IV biosimilar trastuzumab were similar to those with SC reference trastuzumab (i.e., savings of €807 with IV biosimilar trastuzumab). Furthermore, Table 1 shows that differences in healthcare costs between IV biosimilar trastuzumab and SC reference trastuzumab depended on the level of discounts on these formulations. In a scenario assuming a discount of 50% on IV biosimilar trastuzumab and 20% on SC reference trastuzumab, savings in healthcare costs of €411,886 were generated by treating 100 patients with IV biosimilar trastuzumab as compared to SC reference trastuzumab. These savings increased to €430,192 when IV vial sharing is considered.

Table 1. Drug costs and healthcare costs of treating 100 patients with IV biosimilar trastuzumab vs. SC reference trastuzumab.

	Base Case	Scenario with 20% Discount on IV Biosimilar and on SC Reference Trastuzumab	Scenario with 35% Discount on IV Biosimilar and 20% Discount on SC Reference Trastuzumab	Scenario with 35% Discount on IV Biosimilar and on SC Reference Trastuzumab	Scenario with 50% Discount on IV Biosimilar and 20% Discount on SC Reference Trastuzumab
Drug costs					
IV	€1,431,282	€1,145,026	€930,333	€930,333	€715,641
SC	€1,522,809	€1,218,247	€1,218,247	€989,826	€1,218,247
IV-SC	−€91,527	−€73,222	−€287,914	−€59,493	−€502,606
Healthcare costs					
IV-SC	−€807	€17,498	−€197,194	€31,227	−€411,886

3. Discussion

This study has simulated drug costs and healthcare costs for a 1 year course of adjuvant treatment with either IV biosimilar trastuzumab or SC reference trastuzumab in HER2-positive breast cancer patients in Belgium. Our results indicated that the cost difference between IV and SC formulations depends on patient body weight, drug discounts and IV vial sharing.

In our base case analysis, drug costs were less for IV biosimilar trastuzumab for a patients weighing less than 75 kg. The median weight of women with breast cancer is invariably <75 kg and has ranged from 64 to 72 kg in European studies comparing IV and SC reference trastuzumab administration [17–20]. Therefore, it can be expected that drug costs of IV biosimilar trastuzumab would be lower than for SC reference trastuzumab for the majority of patients.

When considering healthcare costs, our base case analysis took into account that IV administration is associated with more costs related to healthcare professional time and consumables than SC administration, in addition to differences in drug costs. However, savings in healthcare professional time and consumables with SC administration might not be as high when trastuzumab is given in combination with chemotherapy. When trastuzumab is administered in combination with chemotherapy, this is usually for the first 6–8 cycles of 18 cycles during adjuvant therapy. During these 6–8 cycles, there are potential cost savings with respect to healthcare professional time and consumables with IV trastuzumab administration by piggy backing on the costs that must be applied for IV chemotherapy administration during concurrent or sequential administration. The combination of trastuzumab with chemotherapy is usual practice (94%) during adjuvant therapy across German hospitals [21], whereas trastuzumab monotherapy is the norm in the Southeast Netherlands (100%) [22] and most common in Southeast Wales (83%) [23].

Multiple studies have reported that SC reference trastuzumab administration is associated with less indirect costs related to productivity loss than IV administration [16,19,20]. Our analysis did not consider productivity loss and, hence, underestimated savings of SC vs. IV trastuzumab administration. However, such indirect costs associated with trastuzumab administration (irrespective of administration route) are relatively low (1–4%) when compared to total costs [24].

When we applied healthcare cost estimates to a sample of 100 patients, lower drug costs with IV biosimilar trastuzumab as compared to SC reference trastuzumab offset higher costs of healthcare professional time and consumables in our base case analysis. Also, we ran scenario analyses accounting for drug discounts and for the re-use of IV vial leftovers. We believe that these scenarios more accurately reflect market and clinical practices in Belgium, even though the related input parameters are associated with more uncertainty and resulting cost difference estimates are illustrative rather than exact. In terms of generalizability to other healthcare systems, healthcare cost differences between these trastuzumab formulations of course depend on the difference between the drug procurement cost and reimbursement rate, on local healthcare professional and consumable costs, and on the hospital or retail setting in which IV and SC formulations are typically provided.

Our results are in line with those of an Italian study [25], which found that treatment with IV biosimilar trastuzumab was less expensive than with SC reference trastuzumab in patients weighing less than a specific threshold. Also, this study corroborated our finding that, when vial leftovers are used for other patients, savings with IV biosimilar trastuzumab grew.

We hope that our case study contributes to a more differentiated view on the difference between IV and SC formulations beyond the bare price of the products alone. Indeed, we acknowledge that other factors may also play important roles like the business models of hospitals and the earning system of physicians. A hospital that is short in IV administration capacity, and gains limited earnings from IV administrations, may like to avoid investments to expand such (expensive) capacity. On the other hand, if physician reimbursement for IV administration is higher than for SC administration, then it will be attractive for physicians to favor the former. In a number of countries, parenteral drugs are increasingly being administered outside the hospital, closer to where patients are living. Such initiatives are more dependent on the availability of SC formulations.

There are a number of limitations in our study. The estimate of cost savings related to healthcare professional time and consumables with SC trastuzumab administration related to 2017 [16], while drug prices related to 2020. Although the former are likely to have increased since then, this is unlikely to change our result that healthcare cost differences between IV and SC trastuzumab formulations depend on patient body weight. Also, any analysis is dependent on the potential for changing prices and discounts that might be offered in particular situations for both IV biosimilar trastuzumab and SC reference trastuzumab, as underlined by our sensitivity analysis.

Few studies have explored cost differences between IV biosimilar trastuzumab and SC reference trastuzumab [26]. More research is required that replicates our cost estimates in healthcare systems that are organized and financed differently than in Belgium and that takes into account market dynamics and shifts in prescribing practices between different trastuzumab formulations.

4. Materials and Methods

Calculations of drug costs for IV biosimilar trastuzumab vs. SC reference trastuzumab were conducted in the same manner and following the same methods as reported for the comparison of IV vs. SC reference trastuzumab in the study by Tjalma and colleagues [13]. Drug costs were compared for a 1 year trastuzumab course in the adjuvant HER2-positive breast cancer setting in Belgium. For IV biosimilar trastuzumab, there is an initial loading dose of 8 mg/kg infused over 90 min, followed by maintenance doses of 6 mg/kg infused over 30 min every 3 weeks for a total of 18 cycles. For SC reference trastuzumab, the equivalent schedule of 600 mg SC is administered by slow injection over 2–5 min every 3 weeks for 18 cycles. For each treatment (IV biosimilar vs. SC reference), the number of vials required per patient was determined for different patient body weights (87.5, 84, 75, 62.5, 56.25 and 50 kg) and was rounded to the next highest half vial (as is usual practice). The number of vials was then multiplied by the ex-factory list price in 2020 to calculate drug costs. List prices were reduced by 15% given that Belgian hospitals can only invoice 85% of a drug's list price to the National Institute for Health and Disability Insurance once a biosimilar is available [27]. All prices were exclusive of tax. The 85% list price of IV biosimilar trastuzumab (Herzuma®) was €276.87 per 150 mg vial and that for SC reference trastuzumab (Herceptin®) was €846.01 per 600 mg vial [28].

Next, we compared healthcare costs for IV biosimilar trastuzumab vs. SC reference trastuzumab at the previously defined different patient body weights (see above) by taking into consideration potential savings through SC use that have been previously estimated by Tjalma and colleagues [16]. They estimated savings at 2017 prices of SC vs. IV administration of €907.20 per course related to healthcare professional (i.e., nurse, pharmacist and assistant) and consumables (e.g., syringes, needles, alcohol, swabs, etc.) costs. Oncologist time was not included as a healthcare professional cost as this consultation visit was assumed to be the same for both the IV and SC reference formulations.

Drug costs and healthcare costs to treat 100 patients with either trastuzumab formulation were then calculated assuming the following numbers of patients in each body weight category: 87.5 kg ($n = 7$); 84.0 kg ($n = 16$); 75.0 kg ($n = 25$); 62.5 kg ($n = 25$); 56.25 kg ($n = 20$); and 50.0 kg ($n = 7$). This distribution of patients by body weight category was based on the binomial distribution normally found among patients with early-stage HER2-positive breast cancer [17–20].

In addition to the base case analysis, we conducted a sensitivity analysis that accounts for discounts offered by the manufacturer to the hospital. As discounts are confidential, we ran multiple scenarios, but the scenario assuming a discount of 50% on the IV biosimilar formulation and 20% on the SC reference formulation was deemed most realistic after consultation with an industry expert.

The base case analysis used an IV vial (or half a vial for IV trastuzumab in Belgium) as the unit of measurement. Hence, costs associated with the total number of vials administered over 18 cycles were calculated, even if some of the last vial's contents had to be discarded. However, in clinical practice, any drug not used may not necessarily be wasted but rather used for other patients scheduled for treatment in parallel on the same day [20]. This practice is common in many countries [24] and also appears to be the practice in

Belgian hospitals. If hospitals use the potentially wasted drug in other patients, it will generate savings from the hospital perspective. Therefore, we ran a second scenario in which cost estimates accounted for discounts and reflected actual use of the IV biosimilar formulation (i.e., not rounded to the next half vial).

All calculations were performed in Microsoft Excel 2016.

Author Contributions: Conceptualization and methodology, P.D.; formal analysis: P.D. and S.S.; writing—review and editing: S.S., A.G.V. and P.D. All authors have read and agreed to the published version of the manuscript.

Funding: This research received no external funding.

Institutional Review Board Statement: Not applicable.

Informed Consent Statement: Not applicable.

Data Availability Statement: Access to data supporting reported results can be requested from the corresponding author.

Acknowledgments: Medical writing support was provided by Peter Todd of Tajut Ltd. (Kaiapoi, New Zealand) and was funded by Mundipharma Comm. VA (Mechelen, Belgium).

Conflicts of Interest: S.S. and A.G.V. are among the founders of the KU Leuven Fund on Market Analysis of Biologics and Biosimilars following Loss of Exclusivity (MABEL). S.S. was involved in a stakeholder roundtable on biologics and biosimilars sponsored by Amgen, Pfizer and MSD; he has participated in advisory board meetings for Pfizer and Amgen; he has contributed to studies on biologics and biosimilars for Hospira, Celltrion and Pfizer; and he had speaking engagements for Amgen, Celltrion and Sandoz. P.D. was an employee of Mundipharma at the time of conceptualizing and conducting the analysis.

References

1. Gianni, L.; Dafni, U.; Gelber, R.D.; Azambuja, E.; Muehlbauer, S.; Goldhirsch, A.; Untch, M.; Smith, I.; Baselga, J.; Jackisch, C.; et al. Treatment with trastuzumab for 1 year after adjuvant chemotherapy in patients with HER2-positive early breast cancer: A 4-year follow-up of a randomised controlled trial. *Lancet Oncol.* **2011**, *12*, 236–244. [CrossRef]
2. Marty, M.; Cognetti, F.; Maraninchi, D.; Snyder, R.; Mauriac, L.; Tubiana-Hulin, M.; Chan, S.; Grimes, D.; Anton, A.; Lluch, A.; et al. Randomized phase II trial of the efficacy and safety of trastuzumab combined with docetaxel in patients with human epidermal growth factor receptor 2-positive metastatic breast cancer administered as first-line treatment: The M77001 study group. *J. Clin. Oncol.* **2005**, *23*, 4265–4274. [CrossRef] [PubMed]
3. Slamon, D.J.; Leyland-Jones, B.; Shak, S.; Fuchs, H.; Paton, V.; Bajamonde, A.; Fleming, T.; Eiermann, W.; Wolter, J.; Pegram, M.; et al. Use of chemotherapy plus a monoclonal antibody against HER2 for metastatic breast cancer that overexpresses HER2. *N. Engl. J. Med.* **2001**, *344*, 783–792. [CrossRef] [PubMed]
4. Piccart-Gebhart, M.J.; Procter, M.; Leyland-Jones, B.; Goldhirsch, A.; Untch, M.; Smith, I.; Gianni, L.; Baselga, J.; Bell, R.; Jackisch, C.; et al. Trastuzumab after adjuvant chemotherapy in HER2-positive breast cancer. *N. Engl. J. Med.* **2005**, *353*, 1659–1672. [CrossRef] [PubMed]
5. Romond, E.H.; Perez, E.A.; Bryant, J.; Suman, V.J.; Geyer, C.E., Jr.; Davidson, N.E.; Tan-Chiu, E.; Martino, S.; Paik, S.; Kaufman, P.A.; et al. Trastuzumab plus adjuvant chemotherapy for operable HER2-positive breast cancer. *N. Engl. J. Med.* **2005**, *353*, 1673–1684. [CrossRef]
6. Ismael, G.; Hegg, R.; Muehlbauer, S.; Heinzmann, D.; Lum, B.; Kim, S.B.; Pienkowski, T.; Lichinitser, M.; Semiglazov, V.; Melichar, B.; et al. Subcutaneous versus intravenous administration of (neo)adjuvant trastuzumab in patients with HER2-positive, clinical stage I-III breast cancer (HannaH study): A phase 3, open-label, multicentre, randomised trial. *Lancet Oncol.* **2012**, *13*, 869–878. [CrossRef]
7. Jackisch, C.; Hegg, R.; Stroyakovskiy, D.; Ahn, J.S.; Melichar, B.; Chen, S.C.; Kim, S.B.; Lichinitser, M.; Staroslawska, E.; Kunz, G.; et al. HannaH phase III randomised study: Association of total pathological complete response with event-free survival in HER2-positive early breast cancer treated with neoadjuvant-adjuvant trastuzumab after 2 years of treatment-free follow-up. *Eur. J. Cancer* **2016**, *62*, 62–75. [CrossRef]
8. Quartino, A.L.; Hillenbach, C.; Li, J.; Li, H.; Wada, R.D.; Visich, J.; Li, C.; Heinzmann, D.; Jin, J.Y.; Lum, B.L. Population pharmacokinetic and exposure-response analysis for trastuzumab administered using a subcutaneous "manual syringe" injection or intravenously in women with HER2-positive early breast cancer. *Cancer Chemother. Pharmacol.* **2016**, *77*, 77–88. [CrossRef]
9. Jackisch, C.; Stroyakovskiy, D.; Pivot, X.; Ahn, J.S.; Melichar, B.; Chen, S.C.; Meyenberg, C.; Al-Sakaff, N.; Heinzmann, D.; Hegg, R. Subcutaneous vs Intravenous Trastuzumab for Patients With ERBB2-Positive Early Breast Cancer: Final Analysis of the HannaH Phase 3 Randomized Clinical Trial. *JAMA Oncol.* **2019**, *5*, e190339. [CrossRef]

10. Pivot, X.; Spano, J.P.; Espie, M.; Cottu, P.; Jouannaud, C.; Pottier, V.; Moreau, L.; Extra, J.M.; Lortholary, A.; Rivera, P.; et al. Patients' preference of trastuzumab administration (subcutaneous versus intravenous) in HER2-positive metastatic breast cancer: Results of the randomised MetaspHer study. *Eur. J. Cancer* **2017**, *82*, 230–236. [CrossRef]
11. Pivot, X.; Verma, S.; Fallowfield, L.; Muller, V.; Lichinitser, M.; Jenkins, V.; Sanchez Munoz, A.; Machackova, Z.; Osborne, S.; Gligorov, J.; et al. Efficacy and safety of subcutaneous trastuzumab and intravenous trastuzumab as part of adjuvant therapy for HER2-positive early breast cancer: Final analysis of the randomised, two-cohort PrefHer study. *Eur. J. Cancer* **2017**, *86*, 82–90. [CrossRef] [PubMed]
12. Roche. Roche Reports Solid Results in 2020. Available online: https://www.roche.com/dam/jcr:6014f1d7-ea74-4f59-bbbc-25e0 71a6866f/en/210204_IR_FY2020_EN.pdf (accessed on 15 March 2021).
13. Tjalma, W.; Huizing, M.T.; Papadimitriou, K. The smooth and bumpy road of trastuzumab administration: From intravenous (IV) in a hospital to subcutaneous (SC) at home. *Facts Views Vis. Obgyn* **2017**, *9*, 51–55. [PubMed]
14. Kadam, V.; Bagde, S.; Karpe, M.; Kadam, V. A Comprehensive Overview on Biosimilars. *Curr. Protein Pept. Sci.* **2016**, *17*, 756–761. [CrossRef]
15. Barbier, L.; Declerck, P.; Simoens, S.; Neven, P.; Vulto, A.G.; Huys, I. The arrival of biosimilar monoclonal antibodies in oncology: Clinical studies for trastuzumab biosimilars. *Br. J. Cancer* **2019**, *121*, 199–210. [CrossRef] [PubMed]
16. Tjalma, W.A.A.; Van den Mooter, T.; Mertens, V.; Bastiaens, V.; Huizing, M.T.; Papadimitriou, K. Subcutaneous trastuzumab (Herceptin) versus intravenous trastuzumab for the treatment of patients with HER2-positive breast cancer: A time, motion and cost assessment study in a lean operating day care oncology unit. *Eur. J. Obstet Gynecol. Reprod. Biol.* **2018**, *221*, 46–51. [CrossRef]
17. Farolfi, A.; Silimbani, P.; Gallegati, D.; Petracci, E.; Schirone, A.; Altini, M.; Masini, C. Resource utilization and cost saving analysis of subcutaneous versus intravenous trastuzumab in early breast cancer patients. *Oncotarget* **2017**, *8*, 81343–81349. [CrossRef]
18. Lazaro Cebas, A.; Cortijo Cascajares, S.; Pablos Bravo, S.; Del Puy Goyache Goni, M.; Gonzalez Monterrubio, G.; Perez Cardenas, M.D.; Ferrari Piquero, J.M. Subcutaneous versus intravenous administration of trastuzumab: Preference of HER2+ breast cancer patients and financial impact of its use. *J. BUON* **2017**, *22*, 334–339.
19. Lopez-Vivanco, G.; Salvador, J.; Diez, R.; Lopez, D.; De Salas-Cansado, M.; Navarro, B.; De la Haba-Rodriguez, J. Cost minimization analysis of treatment with intravenous or subcutaneous trastuzumab in patients with HER2-positive breast cancer in Spain. *Clin. Transl. Oncol.* **2017**, *19*, 1454–1461. [CrossRef]
20. Olofsson, S.; Norrlid, H.; Karlsson, E.; Wilking, U.; Ragnarson Tennvall, G. Societal cost of subcutaneous and intravenous trastuzumab for HER2-positive breast cancer—An observational study prospectively recording resource utilization in a Swedish healthcare setting. *Breast* **2016**, *29*, 140–146. [CrossRef]
21. Dall, P.; Koch, T.; Gohler, T.; Selbach, J.; Ammon, A.; Eggert, J.; Gazawi, N.; Rezek, D.; Wischnik, A.; Hielscher, C.; et al. Trastuzumab without chemotherapy in the adjuvant treatment of breast cancer: Subgroup results from a large observational study. *BMC Cancer* **2018**, *18*, 51. [CrossRef]
22. Seferina, S.C.; Lobbezoo, D.J.; de Boer, M.; Dercksen, M.W.; van den Berkmortel, F.; van Kampen, R.J.; van de Wouw, A.J.; de Vries, B.; Joore, M.A.; Peer, P.G.; et al. Real-Life Use and Effectiveness of Adjuvant Trastuzumab in Early Breast Cancer Patients: A Study of the Southeast Netherlands Breast Cancer Consortium. *Oncologist* **2015**, *20*, 856–863. [CrossRef]
23. Webster, R.M.; Abraham, J.; Palaniappan, N.; Caley, A.; Jasani, B.; Barrett-Lee, P. Exploring the use and impact of adjuvant trastuzumab for HER2-positive breast cancer patients in a large UK cancer network. Do the results of international clinical trials translate into a similar benefit for patients in South East Wales? *Br. J. Cancer* **2012**, *106*, 32–38. [CrossRef] [PubMed]
24. Inotai, A.; Agh, T.; Karpenko, A.W.; Zemplenyi, A.; Kalo, Z. Behind the subcutaneous trastuzumab hype: Evaluation of benefits and their transferability to Central Eastern European countries. *Expert Rev. Pharmacoecon. Outcomes Res.* **2019**, *19*, 105–113. [CrossRef]
25. Agirrezabal, I.; Gaikwad, I.; Cirillo, L.; Lothgren, M. Predicted treatment costs and savings per patient of Kanjinti (trastuzumab biosimilar) vs. subcutaneous (SC) and intravenous (IV) Herceptin and other trastuzumab biosimilars in Italy. *Value Health* **2018**, *21*, S31–S32. [CrossRef]
26. Simoens, S. How do biosimilars sustain value, affordability, and access to oncology care? *Expert Rev. Pharmacoecon. Outcomes Res.* **2020**, 1–3. [CrossRef] [PubMed]
27. National Institute for Health and Disability Insurance. Reduction to 85% for the Purpose of Invoicing of Specific Medicines in Hospital. Available online: https://www.riziv.fgov.be/nl/professionals/andere-professionals/farmaceutische-industrie/Paginas/terugbetaling-geneesmiddelen-01042019.aspx (accessed on 17 February 2021).
28. Belgian Centre for Pharmacotherapeutic Information. Your Independent Medicines Guide. Available online: https://www.bcfi.be/nl/start (accessed on 16 February 2021).

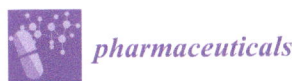

Article

Learnings from Regional Market Dynamics of Originator and Biosimilar Infliximab and Etanercept in Germany

Evelien Moorkens [1,†], Teresa Barcina Lacosta [1,†], Arnold G. Vulto [1,2,*], Martin Schulz [3,4,5], Gabriele Gradl [5], Salka Enners [5], Gisbert Selke [6], Isabelle Huys [1,‡] and Steven Simoens [1,‡]

1. Department of Pharmaceutical and Pharmacological Sciences, KU Leuven, 3000 Leuven, Belgium; evelien.moorkens@kuleuven.be (E.M.); teresa.barcina@kuleuven.be (T.B.L.); isabelle.huys@kuleuven.be (I.H.); steven.simoens@kuleuven.be (S.S.)
2. Hospital Pharmacy, Erasmus University Medical Center, 3015 Rotterdam, The Netherlands; a.vulto@erasmusmc.nl
3. Institute of Pharmacy, Freie Universität Berlin, 14195 Berlin, Germany; m.schulz@fu-berlin.de
4. Department of Medicine, ABDA—Federal Union of German Associations of Pharmacists, 10557 Berlin, Germany; m.schulz@abda.de
5. Deutsches Arzneiprüfungsinstitut e. V. (DAPI), 10557 Berlin, Germany; m.schulz@dapi.de (M.S.); G.Gradl@dapi.de (G.G.); S.Enners@dapi.de (S.E.)
6. AOK Research Institute (WIdO), 10178 Berlin, Germany; gisbert.selke@wido.bv.aok.de
* Correspondence: a.vulto@gmail.com; Tel.: +31-653-455-720
† Joint first author. These authors contributed equally to this work.
‡ Joint last author.

Received: 7 August 2020; Accepted: 17 October 2020; Published: 21 October 2020

Abstract: Drug budget and prescription control measures are implemented regionally in Germany, meaning that the uptake of pharmaceuticals, including biosimilars, can vary by region. We examine regional market dynamics of tumor necrosis factor alpha (TNFα) inhibitor originators and biosimilars in Germany and studied the influence of biosimilar policies on these dynamics. This study is based on: (1) a literature review in which German biosimilar policies are identified, (2) the analysis of dispensing data (2010–2018) for the class of TNFα inhibitors, and (3) ten semi-structured interviews investigating prescribers' and insurers' views on factors potentially influencing biosimilar uptake. The analysis of biosimilar market shares of infliximab and etanercept revealed wide variations across the 17 German Regional Associations of Statutory Health Insurance Accredited Physicians (PA regions). Quantitative analyses indicated that biosimilar market shares for infliximab and etanercept were significantly lower in former East Germany when compared to former West Germany regions. Through qualitative interview analyses, this study showed that the use of infliximab and etanercept biosimilars across Germany is primarily influenced by (1) the regional-level implementation of biosimilar quotas and the presence of monitoring/sanctioning mechanisms to ensure adherence to these quotas, (2) the different insurer-manufacturer discount contracts, and (3) gainsharing arrangements established at the insurer-prescriber level.

Keywords: infliximab; etanercept; TNFα inhibitors; biologics; biosimilars; Germany; policies; incentives; uptake; market dynamics

1. Introduction

The incorporation of biologic therapies into clinical practice has positively transformed health outcomes for many patients diagnosed with severe and highly debilitating chronic conditions [1–3].

As a result, these therapies have represented a growing market in recent decades (accumulated global sales of USD 312 billion in 2018) [4]. Being approved for an increasing number of disease areas, high-cost biologic therapies constitute an important budget impact to be managed by healthcare systems across Europe [5]. However, with the expiration of patents and other exclusivity rights for biologics, non-innovator and therapeutically equivalent versions, i.e., biosimilars, enter the market with the potential to create competition within the therapeutic classes [6]. This leads to altered market dynamics and potentially to decreasing treatment costs and increasing patient access to biologic therapies [7].

Germany, with 83 million inhabitants [8], is the most populous country of the European Union and is an important market for biologics and biosimilars [9,10]. Here, sales of biologics amounted to EUR 11 billion in 2017 [11]. An important class of biologics that has been subject to competition by biosimilars is that of TNFα inhibitors (sales of EUR 2.2 billion in 2017 for Germany) [4]. Five active substances with a TNFα neutralizing activity (infliximab, etanercept, adalimumab, golimumab and certolizumab pegol) are available for the treatment of immune-mediated inflammatory diseases [12]. The originator products—Remicade® (infliximab), Enbrel® (etanercept) and Humira® (adalimumab)—have been present in the German pharmaceuticals market for more than 15 years now. In 2013, infliximab biosimilars under the names Inflectra® and Remsima® received marketing authorization by the European Medicines Agency (EMA) and accessed different European markets. Consequently, in 2015, Inflectra® and Remsima® were launched in Germany. They were followed by the market entry of infliximab biosimilars Flixabi® (2016) and Zessly® (2018). In the case of etanercept, biosimilar products Benepali® and Erelzi® were brought to the German market in 2016 and 2017, respectively [11]. The offer of TNFα inhibitors has been expanded with the incorporation of adalimumab biosimilars Imraldi®, Hyrimoz®, Amgevita®, Hulio® in the last quarter of 2018 and the posterior market launch of Idacio® (2019) and awaits further developments, once exclusivity rights for Cimzia® (certolizumab pegol) and Simponi® (golimumab) have expired in 2021 and 2024, respectively [13,14].

The German law for more safety in the supply of pharmaceuticals (German: Gesetz für mehr Sicherheit in der Arzneimittelversorgung, GSAV June 2019) has been recently amended to optimize the use of biosimilar products as a cost-containment tool [15]. The introduced changes would provide a more favorable environment for the close monitoring of biosimilar regional market dynamics at the federal level. This is of relevance based on the decentralized organization of the German healthcare system, where the German regions are responsible for managing prescription and drug budget control activities. Regional differences in biosimilar policies and practices have been associated with the heterogeneous uptake of biosimilars between product classes and across regions [15–18]. In Germany, differences in biosimilar market shares were described for TNFα inhibitors at the end of 2018: in Westphalia-Lippe and Lower Saxony, biosimilar uptake was two times higher than in Baden-Württemberg. However, reasons behind the variable uptake of biosimilars across the 17 German Regional Associations of Statutory Health Insurance Accredited Physicians (PA regions; German: Kassenärztliche Vereinigungen (KV)) have not been examined in detail [19].

In this study, we analyze the regional market dynamics of TNFα inhibitors following the entry of biosimilars for infliximab and etanercept, and investigate the influence of diverse factors, especially biosimilar policies and practices, on biosimilar uptake. This study builds on previous research analyzing regional market dynamics of infliximab and etanercept originators and biosimilars in Sweden (see Box 1) [17,18].

Box 1. Summary of what is already known about this topic and the added value of the study.

What is already known about this topic
- Regional variations in the use of TNFα inhibitor biosimilars in Sweden have been attributed to the extent of actual (discounted/rebated) price differences between biosimilars and the originator product, the engagement of key opinion leaders, the issuance of local guidelines and to gainsharing arrangements [17,18].
- In Germany, biosimilar uptake is also known to vary at the regional level. This was investigated by Blankart et al. for erythropoiesis-stimulating substances, filgrastim and somatropin. Variations in biosimilar uptake were partly attributed to the presence of explicit regional cost-control measures, such as quota regulations [54].
What this study adds
- Although previous studies have characterized regional variations in the uptake of TNFα inhibitor biosimilars in Germany, the reasons behind this variable uptake have not been examined in detail [19].
- This study highlights the influence of prescription and budget control activities (organized at the regional and insurer level) on the variable uptake of infliximab and etanercept biosimilars.

2. Results

2.1. Overview of TNFα Inhibitor Dynamics in the German Healthcare System

2.1.1. The German Market for TNFα Inhibitors

In Germany, the federal and regional governments delegate certain healthcare responsibilities to self-regulated organizations of payers and providers that can operate within the Statutory Health Insurance (SHI; German: Gesetzliche Krankenversicherung (GKV)) scheme or the substitutive Private Health Insurance (PHI; German: Private Krankenversicherung (PKV)) scheme. Within SHI, the main payers are multiple membership-based not-for-profit insurance companies (sickness funds; German: Krankenkassen), which may function nationwide or at the regional level [20]. According to SHI data, originator products Humira®, Enbrel® and Simponi® and a biosimilar version of Enbrel® (Benepali®) still ranked in 2018 among the top 30 contributors to pharmaceutical expenditure [19]. Due to the scheme for care delivery in Germany, most of this expenditure is managed by the ambulatory sector, through which the majority of prescriptions for TNFα inhibitors are issued. In Germany, there is a clear distinction in the provision of outpatient and hospital care. Outpatient care is delivered by individual doctor practices and specialized medical centers, where services are provided that are usually a hospital competence across Europe [21,22]. In this sense, most prescriptions for intravenous infliximab (70% issued by gastroenterologists) and subcutaneous etanercept (87% issued by rheumatologists) go through the German ambulatory sector [11]. Within this sector, sickness funds negotiate overall prescription budgets with the Federal Association of Statutory Health Insurance Physicians (German: Kassenärztliche Bundesvereinigung (KBV)). They also contract prescription budgets for the regions through negotiations with the 17 German PA regions. Although Germany is divided into 16 federal states (German: Bundesländer), the areas Northrhine and Westphalia-Lippe within the state of Northrhine-Westphalia are represented by two independent PA regions [19].

2.1.2. Regulations of the German Market for TNFα Inhibitors

TNFα inhibitor therapies entered the German market under a free-pricing and full reimbursement scheme (up to a patient co-payment of at most EUR 10 per pack dispensed). However, lower list prices are expected for biosimilars when compared to the originator. While price setting for pharmaceuticals in the hospital market is unregulated and established through direct hospital-manufacturer negotiations, some instruments for regulation are applicable to the retail market [19]. For example, reference price groups were established for infliximab and etanercept in accordance with §35 German Social Code Book V (German: Sozialgesetzbuch V (SGB V)) [23]; the reference price acts as a reimbursement limit, with any overshooting cost borne by the patient. The inclusion of all infliximab-containing products into a reference price group resulted in a 22% reduction in Remicade®'s selling price at the end of

2018 [19]. Until recently, the German Legislation (§129 SBG V) only allowed automatic substitution for bioidenticals (i.e., biosimilars made by the same production site and process, as is the case for Inflectra® and Remsima®) [19]. Modifications of the law for more safety in the supply of pharmaceuticals (GSAV) have extended these regulations to non-bioidentical biosimilars, provided that the Federal Joint Committee (German: Gemeinsamer Bundesausschuss (G-BA)) recognizes interchangeability [15]. Based on the restrictions for automatic substitution of biologics, the type of procurement contract (§130a SGB V) usually applied to generics has been deemed inadequate for biosimilars. Despite the various alternative procurement mechanisms possible (e.g., tendering), insurance companies mostly rely on the organization of "open-house rebate contracts" (German: Open-House-Rabattverträge) in which all suppliers of originator biologics and biosimilars can participate. Participants in "open-house rebate contracts" qualify to sign a supply contract if they adhere to certain pre-defined contractual conditions, including mandatory discounts on list prices. These conditions are freely set by the insurer and cannot depend on individual negotiations with certain suppliers [19].

The market for TNFα inhibitors is indirectly regulated through the establishment of prescribing targets. Every year, the National Association of Statutory Health Insurance Funds (German: Gesetzliche Krankenversicherung-Spitzenverband (GKV-SV) and KBV agree on target areas for prescribing control (biosimilars included). For these areas, they use the previous year's prescription rates to set recommendations. The output of this negotiation is reflected in a non-binding contract (German: Bundesrahmenvorgaben für die Arzneimittelvereinbarungen) that serves as a guideline for regional agreements. Insurer companies and regional physician associations look at the national advisory agreement and define implementation details for contracts which are binding at the regional level (German: Arzneimittelvereinbarungen). Minor deviations are allowed, as long as the overall cost-containment effect is achieved. This means that regional physician associations are not forced to rely on biosimilar prescription quotas. Instead, they can give more importance to alternative cost-containment mechanisms that still meet the general objective [19].

2.2. Analysis of Dispensing Data for TNFα Inhibitors

2.2.1. TNFα Inhibitor Products: Evolution in Sales Volume

Overall, in Germany, the sales volume of TNFα inhibitor products has increased over time (from 17.68M defined daily doses (DDDs) in 2010 to 42.06M DDDs in 2018). From 2010 to 2018, sales volume for infliximab and adalimumab increased over two-fold, and 1.8-fold for etanercept (see Figure 1). The rise in the sales volume of TNFα inhibitors has been attributed to several factors (e.g., the lower threshold at which treatment with biologics is initiated, changes in the dosing regimen) [24,25]. In the case of infliximab and etanercept, the data in this study showed that year-over-year increases (%) in use occurred shortly after biosimilar entry (13.4% increase for infliximab and 13.7% increase for etanercept).

The compound annual growth rate (CAGR) of sales volume (DDDs) indicated different growth trends for infliximab and etanercept (see Figure 1). While growth intensified for etanercept in the last few years, it decreased in the case of infliximab. This suggests a saturation of the market for infliximab, which has been subject to the competitive pressure of TNFα inhibitor therapies with a different administration profile and approval for an extended range of indications [7].

Figure 2 shows the composition of the market for TNFα inhibitors in terms of individual products from 2010 until 2018. In 2010, the greatest volume share corresponded to adalimumab (40%), while the shares for infliximab and etanercept were 21% and 34%, respectively. The volume share for the innovative products Cimzia® and Simponi® amounted to 5%. During a nine-year time period, the volume share for adalimumab remained stable, while the shares for infliximab and etanercept decreased in favor of the originator therapies Cimzia® and Simponi®. The data represented in Figure 2 indicate that the market entry of infliximab biosimilars (2015) has not induced a shift in prescribing trends from other TNFα inhibitor originator products (Enbrel®, Humira®, Cimzia®, Simponi®) towards infliximab-containing products. This observation also applies to the entry of etanercept biosimilars in 2016.

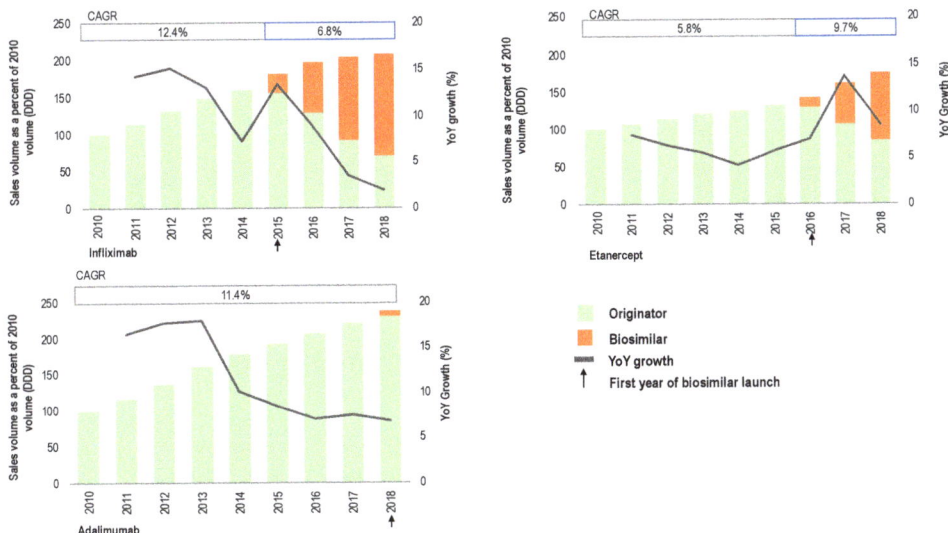

Figure 1. Sales volume evolution (2010–2018) expressed as a percentage of 2010 volume and measured as defined daily doses (DDDs) for originator and biosimilar products containing infliximab, etanercept and adalimumab (primary axis). Year-over-year (YoY) growth (%) is represented on the secondary axis. Compound annual growth rate (CAGR) is calculated before and after biosimilar launch. The graphical representation of the data is based on a figure published by IQVIA [26].

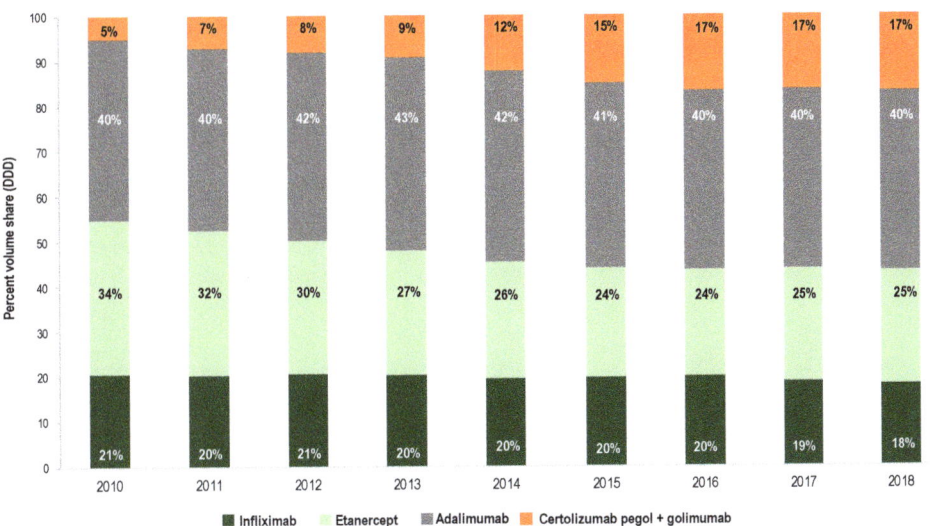

Figure 2. Composition of the market for TNFα inhibitors in terms of individual products from 2010 to 2018. The sales volume (DDDs) for infliximab (originator + biosimilars), etanercept (originator + biosimilars), adalimumab (originator + biosimilars), certolizumab pegol and golimumab is expressed as a share of the total volume of TNFα inhibitors.

2.2.2. Infliximab and Etanercept Biosimilars and Originators: Evolution in Market Shares for the German Regions

At the end of 2018, the combination of biosimilar products for infliximab and etanercept represented, in terms of sales volume (DDDs), 25% of the German market for TNFα inhibitors (see Figure 3).

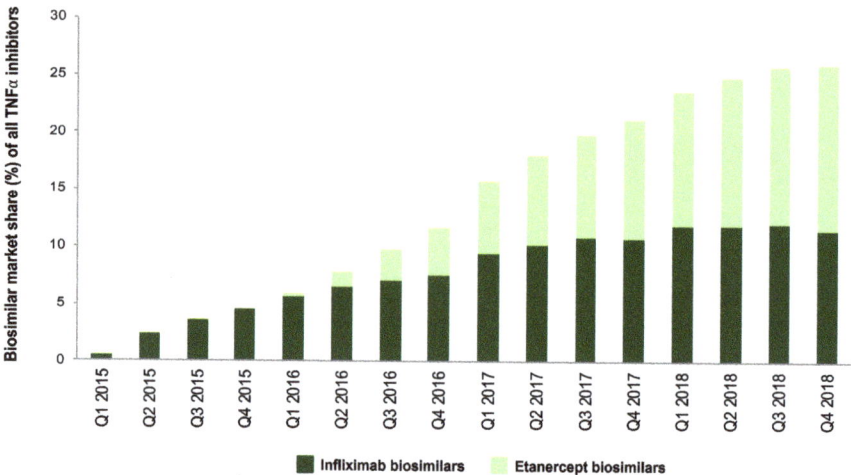

Figure 3. Composition of the market for TNF α inhibitors in terms of biosimilar products (2015–2018). Biosimilar market shares (%) for infliximab and etanercept are calculated in relation to the total volume of TNFα inhibitors.

The level of biosimilar penetration for infliximab and etanercept was comparable (56% and 61%, respectively) in Germany at the end of the third year after biosimilar market entry (see Figure 4). However, regional data on the uptake of infliximab and etanercept biosimilars (Q4 2018) pointed to a wide variation in biosimilar market shares between the 17 German PA regions (see Table 1). In the case of infliximab, the lowest biosimilar market share was observed for Brandenburg (33%), while the largest value was observed for Lower Saxony (87%). In a similar way, there was large variance of market shares for etanercept, with Brandenburg being the region with the lowest biosimilar uptake (33%) and Westphalia-Lippe being the highest (77%). The time evolution analysis of market shares showed that in general, regions with an early adoption of biosimilars (e.g., Northrhine, Westphalia-Lippe) also reached high biosimilar uptake levels (Q4 2018). Exceptions to this trend were identified (e.g., Brandenburg). While Brandenburg behaved as an early adopter of infliximab biosimilars, uptake levels at the end of 2018 were low.

Table 1. Market shares (%) of biosimilar infliximab and etanercept in Germany's 17 PA regions. Colors gradually change from red to green with increasing biosimilar market shares.

	Q1 2015	Q2 2015	Q3 2015	Q4 2015	Q1 2016	Q2 2016	Q3 2016	Q4 2016	Q1 2017	Q2 2017	Q3 2017	Q4 2017	Q1 2018	Q2 2018	Q3 2018	Q4 2018
INFLIXIMAB																
Lower Saxony	2%	11%	17%	24%	26%	34%	40%	48%	74%	76%	83%	84%	88%	88%	87%	87%
Westphalia-Lippe	3%	20%	25%	33%	40%	49%	57%	64%	68%	73%	77%	79%	83%	84%	86%	86%
Bavaria	2%	12%	18%	25%	30%	37%	38%	42%	55%	66%	70%	72%	75%	77%	78%	78%
Bremen	0%	3%	14%	21%	24%	10%	22%	38%	37%	48%	53%	58%	61%	71%	74%	77%
Schleswig Holstein	2%	9%	12%	13%	20%	21%	25%	27%	33%	40%	38%	47%	55%	63%	73%	76%
Rhineland Palatinate	1%	11%	17%	25%	25%	37%	41%	47%	55%	59%	60%	69%	69%	70%	62%	70%
Northrhine	1%	13%	27%	32%	40%	46%	50%	53%	57%	57%	61%	62%	63%	67%	69%	70%
Saarland	3%	24%	22%	24%	31%	33%	44%	49%	61%	57%	61%	63%	65%	67%	67%	69%
Hesse	6%	19%	28%	38%	44%	42%	43%	45%	47%	52%	51%	55%	55%	56%	58%	60%
Mecklenburg Western Pomerania	0%	0%	7%	8%	11%	12%	12%	25%	22%	28%	46%	43%	42%	43%	48%	58%
Thuringia	1%	3%	8%	15%	22%	26%	24%	23%	27%	36%	39%	50%	54%	56%	59%	53%
Hamburg	0%	1%	6%	11%	17%	14%	16%	21%	22%	25%	31%	34%	39%	43%	49%	52%
Baden-Württemberg	1%	3%	8%	12%	14%	14%	16%	21%	27%	30%	34%	41%	42%	48%	47%	49%
Berlin	0%	2%	5%	10%	15%	26%	29%	31%	36%	36%	38%	40%	43%	45%	44%	49%
Saxony-Anhalt	8%	29%	35%	31%	27%	27%	27%	25%	31%	42%	43%	46%	51%	53%	53%	48%
Saxony	0%	3%	4%	9%	10%	14%	14%	16%	18%	20%	22%	29%	33%	36%	40%	45%
Brandenburg	7%	21%	25%	25%	27%	30%	29%	31%	30%	29%	28%	29%	30%	33%	34%	33%
ETANERCEPT																
Westphalia-Lippe	0%	0%	0%	0%	0%	22%	38%	47%	55%	59%	62%	66%	71%	75%	76%	77%
Lower Saxony	0%	0%	0%	0%	0%	3%	9%	25%	48%	55%	61%	65%	69%	70%	73%	74%
Bavaria	0%	0%	0%	0%	0%	4%	10%	17%	34%	46%	50%	55%	61%	63%	65%	68%
Northrhine	0%	0%	0%	0%	0%	8%	14%	20%	28%	33%	39%	47%	54%	59%	63%	67%
Hamburg	0%	0%	0%	0%	0%	1%	5%	11%	17%	21%	22%	27%	40%	49%	57%	62%
Schleswig Holstein	0%	0%	0%	0%	0%	4%	7%	11%	17%	22%	28%	31%	44%	53%	57%	60%
Rhineland Palatinate	0%	0%	0%	0%	0%	5%	11%	19%	30%	35%	40%	46%	51%	53%	56%	59%
Bremen	0%	0%	0%	0%	0%	3%	8%	18%	28%	29%	37%	39%	47%	47%	54%	55%
Hesse	0%	0%	0%	0%	0%	4%	13%	15%	19%	22%	24%	28%	32%	35%	41%	50%
Saxony-Anhalt	0%	0%	0%	0%	0%	2%	5%	7%	11%	16%	21%	28%	39%	44%	43%	46%
Baden-Württemberg	0%	0%	0%	0%	0%	4%	11%	16%	23%	26%	30%	32%	37%	38%	42%	46%
Saarland	0%	0%	0%	0%	0%	4%	8%	10%	18%	19%	19%	25%	26%	34%	34%	42%
Saxony	0%	0%	0%	0%	0%	1%	3%	6%	9%	13%	17%	24%	31%	37%	39%	40%
Berlin	0%	0%	0%	0%	0%	2%	6%	11%	16%	19%	22%	26%	28%	32%	35%	37%
Mecklenburg Western Pomerania	0%	0%	0%	0%	0%	2%	4%	8%	13%	16%	18%	21%	26%	30%	36%	37%
Thuringia	0%	0%	0%	0%	0%	1%	2%	4%	5%	9%	11%	17%	23%	25%	33%	35%
Brandenburg	0%	0%	0%	0%	0%	3%	6%	10%	12%	14%	16%	19%	24%	25%	31%	33%

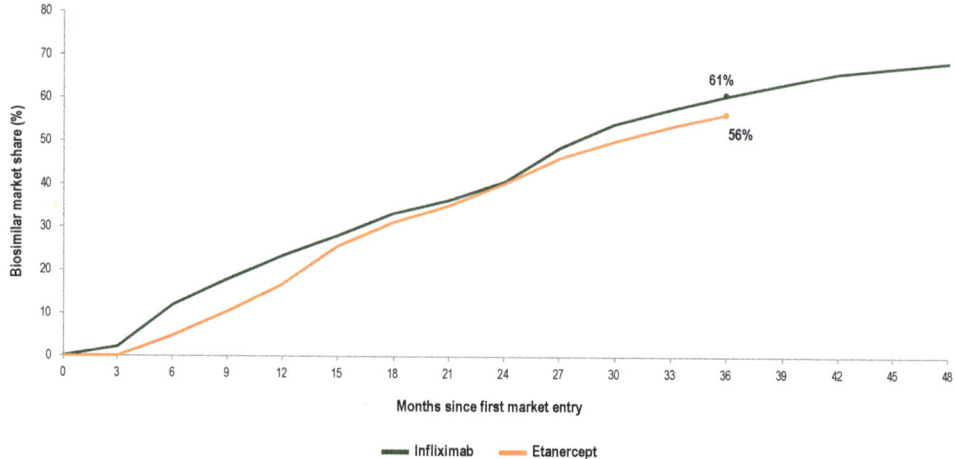

Figure 4. Biosimilar penetration for infliximab and etanercept in Germany over time. Biosimilar market shares (%) are calculated as volume of biosimilars over volume of biosimilars plus the originator product (DDDs).

Biosimilar uptake patterns for infliximab and etanercept were similar across Germany in Q4 2018 (see Figure 5). Indeed, regional biosimilar market shares for infliximab and etanercept were positively correlated (adjusted $R^2 = 0.64$). This allowed us to identify common low- and high-biosimilar uptake regions. Saxony, Saxony-Anhalt, Brandenburg, Berlin and Baden-Württemberg showed low uptake for both infliximab and etanercept biosimilars. On the contrary, Lower Saxony, Westphalia-Lippe, Bavaria and Northrhine showed high uptake for both infliximab and etanercept biosimilars (see Figure 5c).

Figure 5 shows a predominant location of low-uptake regions within the regions formerly forming East Germany (Brandenburg, Mecklenburg Western Pomerania, Saxony, Saxony-Anhalt and Thuringia). The statistical analysis conducted (see Section 4) indicated that biosimilar market shares were significantly lower in former East Germany when compared to former West Germany. The dichotomous variable East/West location has been considered a potential co-founder in this study. In order to identify underlying predictor variables behind variable biosimilar uptake, multiple bivariate regression models were conducted to study the statistical association between a number of determinants of socio-economic welfare and regional biosimilar market shares. This is further detailed in Section 4. None of the chosen socio-economic predictor variables were found to be significantly correlated to regional biosimilar market shares.

2.3. The Role of Biosimilar Policies and Practices on Biosimilar Uptake: Interview Results

Physician associations regard biosimilars as a tool for economic prescribing and recommend that physicians initiate eligible patients on biosimilars and switch from the reference product to the biosimilar when possible. The view of physician associations has been generally consistent across Germany, with some discrepancies on the importance given to maintaining the prescriber's choice over an argument of prescribing more economically. Relatively high price differences between the biosimilar and the originator product after discounting were regarded by interviewees as a driver for increased biosimilar use (see Table 2). Sickness fund representatives from the Saxony/Thuringia area signaled that physicians may prefer to prescribe discounted originators over biosimilars when price differences are small. This may explain the comparatively low biosimilar infliximab and etanercept market shares in this area and, in general, in regions formerly forming East Germany. When asked for reasons behind the lower biosimilar uptake in former East Germany regions, interviewees pointed to the past reliance of eastern Germany physicians on the strategies applied by originator companies to increase customer fidelity. This may have created stronger historical bonds between physicians and originator manufacturers that are still present today. It was also signaled that low biosimilar market shares do not necessarily reflect inefficiency regarding economic prescribing, but reliance on alternative cost-containment mechanisms.

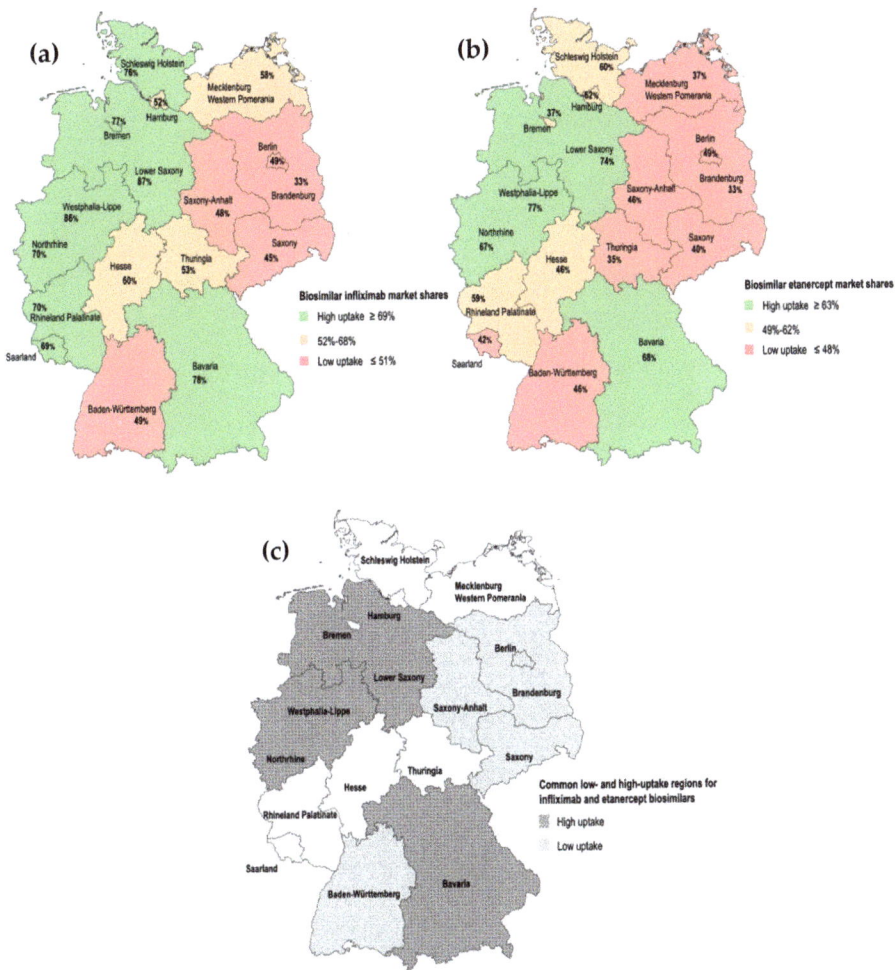

Figure 5. (**a**) Market shares (%) of biosimilar infliximab in Q4 2018. (**b**) Market shares (%) of biosimilar etanercept in Q4 2018. (**c**) Low- and high-uptake PA regions which are common for infliximab and etanercept biosimilars in Q4 2018. The dotted pattern refers to regions with high biosimilar uptake for both infliximab and etanercept. The crossed pattern refers to regions with low biosimilar uptake for both infliximab and etanercept. The map templates were extracted from mapchart.net.

Table 2. Summary of factors identified to drive biosimilar use and facilitate biosimilar acceptance in Germany. These factors have been identified through the qualitative analysis of interview data.

Drivers of Biosimilar Use	Factors Facilitating Biosimilar Acceptance
Biosimilar prescription quotas: -Efficient monitoring -Presence of a sanctioning mechanism	Efficient communication between stakeholders -Robust reporting capability of regional physician associations
Greater cost-savings potential associated to biosimilars	
Gainsharing contracts	
Position statements/guidelines on the safety of switching	

In contrast, physician and sickness fund representatives from Westphalia-Lippe supported the prescription of biosimilars over originators, regardless of the real price difference realized after discount agreements. Here, the strategic long-term perspective relied on viewing biosimilars as a tool to reduce the increasing economic pressure that threatens the sustainability of the German Healthcare System.

Incentives for Increased Biosimilar Use

As stated by interviewees, certain policies/practices may affect the market penetration of biosimilars. These can differ between regions and be associated with regional variations in biosimilar market shares. Table 2 summarizes the identified drivers and facilitators for increased biosimilar use in Germany.

The establishment of biosimilar quotas was consistently identified as an important control instrument to drive biosimilar use. Interviewees indicated that the success of quotas depends on the effectiveness of the mechanisms put in place to monitor adherence to these quotas, as well as on the presence of mechanisms to sanction non-adherence. Interviewees agreed on the importance of setting out effective communication strategies to inform physicians about their accomplished prescribing rates and to facilitate biosimilar acceptance. The effectiveness of these strategies would depend to a certain extent on the robustness of the reporting capability of the regional physician associations. Interviewees also indicated that the preferential use of biosimilars over originator products has been driven by the organization of gainsharing contracts between groups of physicians and insurers. An example is the BioLike initiative, launched by the insurer company Barmer GEK for gastroenterologists and rheumatologists in different PA regions (e.g., Hamburg, Saarland, Saxony, Schleswig-Holstein, Thuringia, Westphalia-Lippe). This initiative has led to an increased use of TNFα inhibitor biosimilars and has allowed sharing the realized savings through biosimilar prescriptions between groups of prescribers and the insurer companies [27]. One of the interviewed experts signaled the positive experience of physicians with this initiative in Westphalia-Lippe.

Several German organizations, including the Drug Commission of the German Medical Association (German: Arzneimittelkommission der deutschen Ärzteschaft (AkdÄ)), the Federal Association of German Hospital Pharmacists (German: ADKA - Bundesverband Deutscher Krankenhausapotheker) and the Paul Ehrlich Institute (German: Paul Ehrlich Institut (PEI)), have published favorable statements on the safety of switching between a reference product and its corresponding biosimilars, as well as between biosimilars [28–30]. Interviewees mentioned that the publication of these statements may especially drive biosimilar acceptance in regions where biosimilar uptake has historically been low (e.g., Baden-Württemberg). The views of stakeholders with respect to the benefits of allowing the pharmacy-level automatic substitution of biologics (GSAV) are more divided. While physician representatives have mostly expressed doubts about the added benefit of implementing this policy, insurers have regarded it as an instrument for increased biosimilar use.

Interviewees participating in this study were also asked to identify factors primarily associated to regional variations in biosimilar uptake. Both the differing regional-level implementation of biosimilar quotas and the varying characteristics of procurement contracts appeared as important contributors. Through a comparative analysis of regional agreements for biosimilar prescription quotas, the current study showed variability in the way the national recommendations have been implemented regionally (see Table 3). Most regions have established binding biosimilar quotas. However, other regions have defined prescribing targets to be interpreted as recommendations. While biosimilar quotas for Westphalia-Lippe and Northrhine have historically been more ambitious than the national reference, Baden-Württemberg has only established non-binding recommendations for specialists known to be more familiar with TNFα inhibitor biosimilars (gastroenterologists and rheumatologists).

Table 3. Comparative analysis of regional quota agreements for TNFα inhibitors, based on information available on the websites of the 17 German PA regions [31–47]. Quotas were set either generally for biosimilars or more specifically for the therapeutic group or for each of the active substances within the therapeutic group. Quotas may apply to all prescribers or to specific medical specialties.

Regions	Quota Agreements: Characteristics					
	Early Quota Adoption: (Before 2016)	Set Unspecifically for Biosimilars	Set for the Category of TNFα Inhibitors	Set for the Active Substance	Applied Generally to All Prescribers	Applied Differently per Specialty
Baden-Württemberg				√		√
Bavaria	√		√			√
Berlin				√	√	
Brandenburg			√			√
Bremen				√	√	
Hamburg			√			√
Hesse				√	√	
Mecklenburg Western Pomerania: (missing data)						
Lower Saxony	√			√	√	
Northrhine			√			√
Rhineland Palatinate			√			√
Saarland				√	√	
Saxony			√			√
Saxony-Anhalt		√				√
Schleswig Holstein				√	√	
Thuringia			√			√
Westphalia-Lippe	√			√		√

A certain flexibility has been allowed as well in the design and implementation of "open-house rebate contracts" established at the insurer-manufacturer level. Interviewees indicated that this may lead to intra- and inter-regional variability in biosimilar uptake. Interviewees in Westphalia-Lippe, Saxony and Thuringia reported the possibility of sickness funds to follow more or less aggressive strategies, depending on the magnitude of the pre-specified discount set as an entry requirement. Contract participants may be asked to offer the maximum level of discount possible and entry requirements may be set in a way that the differences in prices between the contract participants are minimized. These strategies may discourage the participation of originator manufacturers, leading to no discounts being negotiated for the originator. This limits the cost-savings potential that insurers could have attained through lower net prices for originator products. Therefore, insurers may adopt a less aggressive strategy where they ask for the maximum discount that the originator company is willing to provide. This strategy, although it may meet the insurer's cost-containment objectives, results in lower than expected reductions of prices after biosimilar market entry.

3. Discussion

Across Europe, the level of market penetration for biosimilars has been described to be country- and product-class-specific [7,48]. In Germany, we have found similar levels of market penetration for infliximab and etanercept biosimilars at the end of 2018. However, we had expected higher biosimilar market penetration for etanercept due to the experience already gained by the market presence of infliximab biosimilars. The lower than expected market penetration of etanercept biosimilars could be partly explained by the different competition strategies followed by originator companies, which were reported to be more aggressive in the case of etanercept. Interviewees also indicated that the different administration routes for infliximab (intravenous) and etanercept (subcutaneous) may have played a role. The switch from Enbrel® to etanercept biosimilars implies changes in the administration device used by patients when self-administering the drug, while this is not the case for the switch from Remicade® to infliximab biosimilars.

Previous biosimilar uptake studies in Sweden [17,18] and the current study for Germany have shown that biosimilar market penetration is also region-specific and that there are wide regional variations in biosimilar market shares for TNFα inhibitors [19]. Our study of biosimilar market shares across the German regions showed common high and low uptake regions for infliximab and etanercept biosimilars. The data on market shares for adalimumab biosimilars (up to 2020) [49] indicate that regions where the uptake of infliximab and etanercept biosimilars has been high, also behaved as early adopters for adalimumab biosimilars. Therefore, we presume that biosimilar incentive policies applied regionally have had a consistent effect on the incorporation of biosimilars for the whole class of TNFα inhibitors. This observation might not be applicable to other biologic therapies (e.g., filgrastim, follitropin α) for which biosimilar uptake patterns differ from the patterns described along this study [49]. Several studies have investigated biosimilar policies implemented across Europe to qualitatively assess their impact on biosimilar uptake [50,51]. Instead, the current study examined regional variations in biosimilar uptake in order to derive practices/incentives influencing biosimilar use. Studies published by Moorkens et al. [17,18] followed this approach and were among the first to identify factors driving biosimilar use through quantitative analysis [52–54]. According to Moorkens et al., the absolute/relative difference in discounted price between originator and biosimilars influence decision-making regarding biosimilar use in Sweden [17]. We have not quantitatively evaluated price effects on biosimilar uptake, as information on discounted/rebated prices was not available. However, as described in the following section, we have been able to identify a set of incentive measures driving the use of infliximab and etanercept biosimilars in Germany.

3.1. Incentives for Increased Biosimilar Use

This study described different approaches taken by the German regions to implement a system of biosimilar prescription quotas. More active (e.g., Westphalia-Lippe) and less active (e.g., Baden-Württemberg) approaches were identified. Baden-Württemberg constituted an example of a region where the implementation of biosimilar quotas was lenient and biosimilar uptake levels were low. The role of lenient approaches on lack of adherence to biosimilar quotas has been commonly reported [27,48]. The current study, however, indicates the importance of setting instruments to support adherence with biosimilar quotas. Interviewees identified that these instruments are an effective monitoring and sanctioning system and an effective communication strategy to bridge the objectives of insurers, physician associations and individual prescribers. The capacity of regional physician associations to actively communicate with physicians and to regularly report on achieved uptake levels has been suggested as a factor driving biosimilar use in Westphalia-Lippe [55].

In Germany, the discounts realized through the establishment of "open-house rebate contracts" are confidential. The real price difference between biosimilars and the respective originator product is usually not known by prescribers. However, sickness funds are aware of the magnitude of the discounted price difference between the originator and the biosimilar alternatives. Interviewees indicated that this may define the commitment of insurers to incentivize biosimilar use over the use of discounted originator products. Based on this, the investment in educational and other resources needed to encourage biosimilar use may vary for the different sickness funds and for the different regions. Gainsharing initiatives established across Germany are an example of the active involvement of sickness funds with the promotion of biosimilars. Some of these initiatives have opted to inform participating physicians on net prices realized through discounting. It has been suggested that this approach might increase the interest of physicians on the principles of cost-effective prescribing [27]. The publication of favorable statements on the safety of switching between reference products and biosimilars is also an example of the active involvement of scientific expert committees. We hypothesize that these committees operate as opinion leaders in Germany, having an influence on prescriber's decision-making regarding biosimilars.

Finally, the proposal to implement a policy for the automatic substitution of biologics at the pharmacy level (GSAV) has elicited conflicting views among stakeholders in healthcare [19]. We hypothesize that this measure may have a considerable impact on biosimilar uptake, potentially equalizing differences in biosimilar market shares across Germany. Further research would be needed to evaluate whether the implementation of this measure substantially changes the situation described in this study.

3.2. Study Limitations

The analysis of market dynamics for the class of TNFα inhibitors was based on the availability of data from ambulatory prescriptions covered by the SHI funds. The lack of information on prescriptions issued by the PHI system or at the hospital level was not expected to affect the comprehensiveness of the analysis, as most sales volume for TNFα inhibitors has been generated within the ambulatory care sector and the SHI scheme is covering 87% of Germany's population [8,56].

We conducted a regression analysis to assess the statistical relationship between several variables chosen as predictors and the outcome variable (biosimilar market shares). We could only include descriptors of socio-economic welfare and performance indicators for the different regional healthcare systems as explanatory variables. Due to the lack of publicly available data, we could not study the association between procurement contract conditions/real differences in discounted prices between originators and biosimilars and regional biosimilar market shares. According to the view of the experts interviewed for this study, we hypothesize that these factors may better explain regional-level variability in biosimilar market shares. The availability of a limited number of observations (N = 16; we combined the data from Northrhine and Westphalia-Lippe) also conditioned the analysis: only the association between two predictor variables and market shares could be modelled simultaneously.

The qualitative analysis of interview data supplemented findings from the quantitative analysis and identified regional predictors of biosimilar uptake that could not have been easily quantified or proxied. However, it must be noted that these interviews were carried out only in nine of the 17 German PA regions. The lack of representation of every region is expected to have only a moderate impact on the generalizability of the study findings, as the interviewed regions represent > 50% of the sales volume for TNFα inhibitors in Germany.

3.3. Future Research

The current study provides an overview of market dynamics for the class of TNFα inhibitors in Germany and especially evaluates the evolution in sales volume for all TNF α inhibitors after the market entry of infliximab and etanercept biosimilars. To accurately evaluate the impact of biosimilar entry within the class of TNFα inhibitors, we would have needed to study the evolution in costs per molecule and per patient before and after the market launch of TNFα inhibitor biosimilars. This analysis could not be conducted due to the lack of publicly available data, but it constitutes an interesting starting point for future studies.

As part of this study, we have stressed the influence of biosimilar policies/practices for prescription and budget control on biosimilar uptake. However, the implementation success for these policies has varied across the German regions. It might be useful for future analyses to evaluate the cumulative effect of implementing multiple incentive policies/practices and to see how this effect relates to observed biosimilar market shares for the regions.

4. Materials and Methods

The methodology chosen for this study is based on previous studies that investigated factors influencing biosimilar uptake in Sweden [17,18]. We first conducted a literature review to describe the main characteristics of the German market for TNFα inhibitors. For reasons of international comparability, we refer to German-specific terminology identified through the literature search by using the English equivalent term. A glossary table (see Table 4) with English terms used in this manuscript and their German equivalent is provided below. Then, we examined dispensing data on sales volume and biosimilar market shares for this drug class. In order to investigate potential factors behind the variable regional uptake of infliximab and etanercept biosimilars, we relied on quantitative and qualitative analyses conducted in parallel, as detailed in the following subsections.

Table 4. Glossary of English/German terms and abbreviations.

English Term	German Term	German Abbreviation
Drug Commission of the German Medical Association	Arzneimittelkommission der deutschen Ärzteschaft	AkdÄ
Federal Association of Statutory Health Insurance Physicians	Kassenärztliche Bundesvereinigung	KBV
ADKA - Federal Association of German Hospital Pharmacists	ADKA - Arbeitsgemeinschaft Deutscher Krankenhaus Apotheker e.V.	-
Federal Joint Committee	Gemeinsamer Bundesausschuss	G-BA
Federal Ministry of Justice and Consumer Protection	Bundesministerium der Justiz und für Verbraucherschutz	BMJV
ABDA - Federal Union of German Associations of Pharmacists	ABDA - Bundesvereinigung Deutscher Apothekerverbände e.V.	-
German Institute for Drug Use Evaluation	Deutsches Arzneiprüfungsinstitut e.V.	DAPI
German law for more safety in the supply of pharmaceuticals	Gesetz für mehr Sicherheit in der Arzneimittelversorgung	GSAV
German federal states	Bundesländer	-
German Regional Associations of Statutory Health Insurance Accredited Physicians (also referred to in text as PA regions): **To be noted**: -This paper makes a distinction between the 16 German federal states and the 17 PA regions. Although Germany is divided into 16 federal states, the areas Northrhine and Westphalia-Lippe within the state Northrhine-Westphalia are represented by two independent PA regions. -Dispensing data have been provided/analysed per PA region and the univariate regression study has been conducted with data at the state level. This was due to limitations in data availability for the univariate regression analyses. -When referring to regions formerly forming East Germany, we include Brandenburg, Mecklenburg Western Pomerania, Saxony, Saxony-Anhalt and Thuringia, but not Berlin. This is because we do not have sub regional data to analyze uptake differences between areas formerly forming East and West Berlin.	Kassenärztliche Vereinigungen	KV
National Association of Statutory Health Insurance Funds	Gesetzliche Krankenversicherung-Spitzenverband	GKV-SV
National advisory agreement on spending targets: (also referred to in text as national-level agreements on prescription targets)	Bundesrahmenvorgaben für die Arzneimittelvereinbarungen	-
"Open-house rebate" contracts	Open-House-Rabattverträge	-
Private Health Insurance (abbreviated in text as PHI)	Private Krankenversicherung	PKV
Regional agreements on prescribing spending targets, supply and economy targets (also referred to in text as regional-level contracts to establish prescribing quotas)	Arzneimittelvereinbarungen	-
Sickness Funds (also referred to in text as insurer organizations or insurers)	Krankenkassen	-
Social Code Book V (Statutory Health Insurance)	Sozialgesetzbuch V (Gesetzliche Krankenversicherung)	SGB V
Statutory Health Insurance (abbreviated in text as SHI)	Gesetzliche Krankenversicherung	GKV

4.1. Literature Review

The main characteristics of the German healthcare system in dealing with biologics, including biosimilars, were extracted from a literature review. PubMed, Embase and Scopus were searched up to December 2019 to yield information on combined searches including the terms: policies, practices, measures, biosimilars and Germany. Studies in English and German were accepted. The website of the Federal Ministry of Justice and Consumer Protection (German: Bundesministerium der Justiz und für Verbraucherschutz (BMJV)) was accessed to retrieve relevant articles from the German Social Code Book (SGB) V [57]. Additionally, the websites of the KBV [58], the different KVs [31–47], and the GKV-SV were consulted [59].

4.2. Analysis of Dispensing Data for TNFα Inhibitors

Regional data on sales volume and uptake of TNFα inhibitor originators and biosimilars were provided by the database of the German Institute for Drug Use Evaluation (German: Deutsches Arzneiprüfungsinstitut e.V. (DAPI)). This database contains anonymous claims data of drugs prescribed and subsequently dispensed by community pharmacies at the expense of the SHI Funds. Nearly 87% of Germany's population is insured by the SHI system [8,56]. The DAPI database covers all claims data from a representative sample of more than 80% of the community pharmacies throughout all regions. Dispensing data were linked to the database of the ABDA – Federal Union of German Associations of Pharmacists (German: ABDA—Bundesvereinigung Deutscher Apothekerverbände e.V.) containing information about the (brand) name, composition, active ingredient, strength, package size, dosage form, and route of administration of German medicinal products [60]. Defined daily doses (DDDs) [61] were calculated from dispensing data and extrapolated by regional factors to 100% of all community pharmacies, and thus 100% of the SHI insured population.

For this analysis, drug use data were examined from the first quarter (Q1) of 2010 to the last quarter (Q4) of 2018. The study of the evolution of sales volume (DDDs) for all marketed TNFα inhibitors allowed us to visualize the effect of the market entry of infliximab and etanercept biosimilars. In addition, shifts in drug utilization trends across the class of TNFα inhibitors were described following biosimilar incorporation, as well as after the market entry of the innovator therapies Cimzia® and Simponi®. Biosimilar market shares were calculated from volume data (DDDs) and represented the volume of biosimilars over the volume of biosimilars plus the respective originator product. The evolution of biosimilar market shares for infliximab and etanercept was studied at the national level and across the 17 PA regions from the quarter in which the biosimilar entered the market (Q1 2015 for infliximab; Q1 2016 for etanercept) to the last quarter of 2018. The regional analysis of market shares allowed the identification of high- and low-biosimilar uptake regions. Uptake was considered to be high in regions where biosimilar market shares were ≥69% for infliximab and ≥63% for etanercept, and low in regions where market shares were ≤51% for infliximab and ≤48% for etanercept. (These thresholds correspond to the lower and upper third of the maximum difference in market shares observed for Q4 2018).

The predominant location of low-uptake regions within the former East Germany, i.e., Brandenburg, Mecklenburg Western Pomerania, Saxony, Saxony-Anhalt and Thuringia, led us to evaluate the statistical relationship between regional biosimilar market shares (dependent variable; N = 16) and the East/West location of the regions at a level of significance of 0.05. This univariate regression analysis was conducted with SPSS (IBM SPSS Statistics 26). Two regression models, one accounting for infliximab data and another for etanercept were built and used as a baseline for a more exhaustive statistical analysis. As the East/West location of the regions was considered to be a co-founding variable, the objective of conducting a more exhaustive analysis was to identify underlying predictor variables (socio-economic factors) behind variable biosimilar uptake. We built various bivariate regression models to examine the statistical relationship between biosimilar market shares and a set of predictors describing: (1) the variable level of socio-economic welfare across the 16 German federal states (e.g., gross domestic product (GDP) per capita, human development index) and (2) the performance of the different regional healthcare systems (e.g., number of healthcare workers employed per 1000 inhabitants, total healthcare expenditure and healthcare expenditure calculated as a share of GDP) [62]. Furthermore, we studied the correlation between regional biosimilar market shares for infliximab and etanercept to evaluate whether biosimilar uptake patterns were similar within the class of TNFα inhibitors.

4.3. Interviews

A total of ten semi-structured interviews (12 participants) were organized from October 2018 to February 2020 with a view to gain insight into factors potentially influencing biosimilar uptake. The conduction of interviews allowed us to complement the findings from the quantitative analysis and to investigate determinants of biosimilar uptake that could not have be evaluated quantitatively.

A selective sampling methodology was followed to achieve representation from physician associations and health insurance companies operating at the national and regional level. The interviewed representatives from these two stakeholder groups have been involved in decision-making regarding drug budget and prescription control activities and have expertise in the field of biosimilars. Participation from representatives in Baden-Württemberg, Bremen, Hamburg, Mecklenburg Western Pomerania, Lower Saxony, Saxony, Schleswig-Holstein, Thuringia and Westphalia-Lippe was achieved.

For data collection, an interview guide was drafted, validated and approved (August 2018) by the UZ/KU Leuven ethics committee (reference number: MP006423). The interview guide followed the structure of a guide previously developed by the department to study regional management of biosimilars in Sweden [17,18]. The topics were adapted for Germany through a literature search conducted as part of a master's thesis [63]. Interview questions were organized into questions on dispensing data for TNFα inhibitors and questions on national and regional-level biosimilar policies. All interviewees received an email with an attached informed consent form and were asked for permission to record the interviews. All interviews were conducted in English via telephone calls. The recorded interviews were transcribed ad verbatim and processed using the software QSS NVivo 12. For content analysis, we built a thematic framework based on previous knowledge and findings emerging from the interviews. The results of the qualitative study were shared with the contacted interviewees for a validation exercise.

5. Conclusions

Variation in market penetration of TNFα inhibitor biosimilars between German regions depends on a complex interplay of multiple factors.

Experts interviewed for this study have highlighted the influence of prescription and budget control activities (organized at the regional and insurer level) on the variable uptake of infliximab and etanercept biosimilars across Germany. The use of biosimilars has been found to depend on: the regional-level implementation of biosimilar quotas, the presence of an effective monitoring and sanctioning system to regulate adherence to biosimilar quotas, the effectiveness of the communication between regional physician associations and individual prescribers, the different conditions for discount contracts established at the insurer-manufacturer level and the organization of initiatives for gainsharing. The allowance of pharmacy-level automatic substitution for biologics is expected to play a decisive role in the evolution of biosimilar consumption patterns across Germany.

Availability of Data and Materials: The datasets generated during and/or analyzed during the current study are available from the corresponding author on reasonable request.

Ethics Approval: The interview guide and methodology for this study was approved by the Research Ethics Committee UZ/KU Leuven on 28 August 2018 (MP006423).

Consent to Participate: Informed consent was obtained from all individual participants included in the study.

Author Contributions: I.H., S.S., A.G.V. and E.M. were involved in the conceptualization of this study. G.G. and M.S. took part in data provision and analysis. E.M. and T.B.L. were involved in data collection and analysis.

E.M. and T.B.L. drafted the initial version of the manuscript. I.H., S.S., A.G.V., M.S., G.G., S.E. and G.S. critically reviewed the manuscript. All authors have read and agreed to the published version of the manuscript.

Funding: This study was supported by KU Leuven and by the Fund on Market Analysis of Biologics and Biosimilars following Loss of Exclusivity (MABEL).

Acknowledgments: The authors would like to thank Irene Langner for her insights into the German healthcare system and into the quota system for biosimilars in Germany. The authors also thank the participating interviewees for their contribution to this study and for their feedback on the manuscript. In addition, the authors acknowledge the Leuven Biostatistics and Statistical Bioinformatics Centre for statistical advice during the project and Yannick Mouha for his help with data collection in the context of his master's thesis.

Conflicts of Interest: S.S., I.H. and A.G.V. have founded the KU Leuven Fund on Market Analysis of Biologics and Biosimilars following Loss of Exclusivity (MABEL). S.S. was involved in a stakeholder roundtable on biologics and biosimilars sponsored by Amgen, Pfizer and MSD; he has participated in advisory board meetings for Pfizer and Amgen; he has contributed to studies on biologics and biosimilars for Hospira (together with A.G.V. and I.H.), Celltrion, Mundipharma and Pfizer, and he has had speaking engagements for Amgen and Sandoz. A.G.V. is involved in consulting, advisory work and speaking engagements for a number of companies, a.o. AbbVie, Accord, Amgen, Biogen, EGA, Pfizer/Hospira, Mundipharma, Roche, Sandoz. E.M., T.B.L., G.G., S.E., M.S. and G.S. declare no conflict of interest.

References

1. Baumgart, D.C.; Misery, L.; Naeyaert, S.; Taylor, P.C. Biological Therapies in Immune-Mediated Inflammatory Diseases: Can Biosimilars Reduce Access Inequities? *Front. Pharmacol.* **2019**, *10*. [CrossRef] [PubMed]
2. Edwards, C.J.; Fautrel, B.; Schulze-Koops, H.; Huizinga, T.W.J.; Kruger, K. Dosing down with biologic therapies: A systematic review and clinicians' perspective. *Rheumatology* **2018**, *57*, 589. [CrossRef] [PubMed]
3. Smolen, J.S.; Braun, J.; Dougados, M.; Emery, P.; FitzGerald, O.; Helliwell, P.; Kavanaugh, A.; Kvien, T.K.; Landewé, R.; Luger, T.; et al. Treating spondyloarthritis, including ankylosing spondylitis and psoriatic arthritis, to target: Recommendations of an international task force. *Ann. Rheum. Dis.* **2014**, *73*, 6–16. [CrossRef] [PubMed]
4. IQVIA. *Fokus Biosimilars, Ausgabe 5*; IQVIA Commercial GmbH & Co. OHG: Frankfurt am Main, Germany, 2019.
5. Organisation for Economic Co-Operation and Development (OECD). *Improving Forecasting of Pharmaceutical Spending—Insights from 23 OECD and EU Countries*; OECD: Paris, France, 2019.
6. European Medicines Agency (EMA). *Guideline on Similar Biological Medicinal Products*; European Medicines Agency: London, UK, 2014.
7. IQVIA. *The Impact of Biosimilar Competition in Europe*; IQVIA Commercial GmbH & Co. OHG: Frankfurt am Main, Germany, 2018.
8. Statistisches Bundesamt (Destatis). Genesis-Online, dl-de/by-2-0. Available online: https://www-genesis.destatis.de/genesis/online (accessed on 30 May 2019).
9. IQVIA. *Fokus Biosimilars, Ausgabe 1*; IQVIA Commercial GmbH & Co. OHG: Frankfurt am Main, Germany, 2018.
10. Grand View Research. *Biosimilars Market Size, Share & Trends Analysis by Product, Application & Region—Global Segment Forecasts 2018-2025*; Grand View Research, Inc.: San Francisco, CA, USA, 2018.
11. IQVIA. *Fokus Biosimilars, Ausgabe 2*; IQVIA Commercial GmbH & Co. OHG: Frankfurt am Main, Germany, 2018.
12. European Medicines Agency (EMA). Medicines. Anti-TNF Alpha. Available online: https://www.ema.europa.eu/en/search/search/field_ema_web_categories%253Aname_field/Human/search_api_aggregation_ema_medicine_types/field_ema_med_biosimilar?search_api_views_fulltext=ANTI%20TNF%20ALPHA%20 (accessed on 6 October 2019).
13. IQVIA. *Fokus Biosimilars, Ausgabe 4*; IQVIA Commercial GmbH & Co. OHG: Frankfurt am Main, Germany, 2019.
14. GaBI Journal Editor; GaBI Online Editor. Patent expiry dates for biologicals: 2018 update. *Generics Biosimilars Initiat. J.* **2019**, *8*, 24–31. [CrossRef]
15. Bundesministerium für Gesundheit. *Gesetzentwurf der Bundesregierung. Entwurf Eines Gesetzes Für Mehr Sicherheit in der Arzneimittelversorgung (GSAV)*; Bundesministerium für Gesundheit: Bonn, Germany, 2019.

16. Dranitsaris, G.; Jacobs, I.; Kirchhoff, C.; Popovian, R.; Shane, L.G. Drug tendering: Drug supply and shortage implications for the uptake of biosimilars. *Clin. Outcomes Res.* **2017**, *9*, 573–584. [CrossRef] [PubMed]
17. Moorkens, E.; Simoens, S.; Troein, P.; Declerck, P.; Vulto, A.G.; Huys, I. Different Policy Measures and Practices between Swedish Counties Influence Market Dynamics: Part 1-Biosimilar and Originator Infliximab in the Hospital Setting. *BioDrugs* **2019**, *33*, 285–297. [CrossRef] [PubMed]
18. Moorkens, E.; Simoens, S.; Troein, P.; Declerck, P.; Vulto, A.G.; Huys, I. Different Policy Measures and Practices between Swedish Counties Influence Market Dynamics: Part 2-Biosimilar and Originator Etanercept in the Outpatient Setting. *BioDrugs* **2019**, *33*, 299–306. [CrossRef] [PubMed]
19. Schwabe, U.; Paffrath, D.; Ludwig, W.D.; Klauber, J. *Arzneiverordnungs-Report 2019*; Springer: Berlin/Heidelberg, Germany, 2019.
20. Busse, R.; Blümel, M. Germany: Health System Review. *Health Systems in Transition*; WHO Regional Office for Europe: Copenhagen, Denmark, 2014; Volume 16.
21. KPMG. *Improving Healthcare Delivery in Hospitals by Optimized Utilization of Medicines. A Study into 8 European Countries*; KPMG Advisory N.V.: Amstelveen, The Netherlands, 2019.
22. Simon-Kucher & Partners. *Biosimilars im Krankenhaus—Potenziale Besser Nutzen*; Simon-Kucher & Partners: Berlin, Germany, 2017.
23. Gemeinsamer Bundesausschuss. *Zusammenfassende Dokumentation über die Änderung der Arzneimittel-Richtlinie (AM-RL): Anlage IX—Festbetragsgruppenbildung*; Gemeinsamer Bundesausschuss: Berlin, Germany, 2017.
24. Brandes, A.; Groth, A.; Gottschalk, F.; Wilke, T.; Ratsch, B.A.; Orzechowski, H.D.; Fuchs, A.; Deiters, B.; Bokemeyer, B. Real-world biologic treatment and associated cost in patients with inflammatory bowel disease. *Z. Für Gastroenterologie* **2019**, *57*, 843–851. [CrossRef] [PubMed]
25. Emery, P.; Solem, C.; Majer, I.; Cappelleri, J.C.; Tarallo, M. A European chart review study on early rheumatoid arthritis treatment patterns, clinical outcomes, and healthcare utilization. *Rheumatol. Int.* **2015**, *35*, 1837–1849. [CrossRef] [PubMed]
26. IQVIA. *Advancing Biosimilar Sustainability in Europe. A Multi-Stakeholder Assessment*; IQVIA Commercial GmbH & Co. OHG: Frankfurt am Main, Germany, 2018.
27. Arbeitsgemeinschaft Probiosimilars. Handbuch Biosimilars. Available online: https://probiosimilars.de/img_upload/2019/10/Handbuch-Biosimilars_Oktober-2019.pdf (accessed on 17 October 2019).
28. Arzneimittelkommission der Deutschen Ärzteschaft; Wissenschaftlicher Fachausschuss der Bundesärztekammer. Leitfaden "Biosimilars", 1. Auflage. Available online: https://www.akdae.de/Arzneimitteltherapie/LF/Biosimilars/ (accessed on 17 October 2019).
29. Bundesverband Deutscher Krankenhausapotheker e.V. Pressemeldung zu Biosimilars. Available online: https://www.adka.de/en/news/details/pressemeldung-zu-biosimilars-2017-09-01/ (accessed on 17 October 2019).
30. Paul-Ehrlich-Institut; Federal Institute for Vaccines and Biomedicines. Position of Paul-Ehrlich-Institut Regarding the Use of Biosimilars. Available online: https://www.pei.de/EN/medicinal-products/antibodies/mab/monoclonal-antibodies-node.html?cms_tabcounter=1 (accessed on 17 October 2019).
31. KV Bavaria. Arzneimittelvereinbarung nach § 84 Abs. 1 SGB V für das Jahr 2018. Available online: https://www.kvb.de/fileadmin/kvb/dokumente/Praxis/Rechtsquellen/Arzneimittelvereinbarungen/KVB-RQ-AMV-2018-Arzneimittelvereinbarung.pdf (accessed on 13 October 2019).
32. KV Berlin. Arzneimittelvereinbarung nach § 84 Abs. 1 SGB V für das Jahr 2018 für Berlin. Available online: https://www.kvberlin.de/20praxis/60vertrag/10vertraege/arznei_und_heilmittel/arzneimittel_vb_2018.pdf (accessed on 13 October 2019).
33. KV Westphalia-Lippe. Arzneimittelvereinbarung nach § 84 Abs. 1 SGB V für das Jahr 2018 für Westfalen-Lippe. Available online: https://www.kvwl.de/arzt/recht/kvwl/amv_hmv/amv_wl_2018.pdf (accessed on 13 October 2019).
34. KV Brandenburg. Vereinbarung des Ausgabenvolumens für Arznei- und Verbandmittel nach § 84 Abs. 1 in Verbindung mit Abs. 6 SGB V (Arzneimittelvereinbarung) für das Jahr 2018. Available online: https://www.kvbb.de/praxis/verordnungen/arzneimittel/ (accessed on 13 October 2019).
35. KV Baden-Württemberg. Arzneimittelvereinbarung nach § 84 Abs. 1 SGB V für den Bereich der KV Baden-Württemberg für das Jahr 2018. Available online: https://www.kvbawue.de/praxis/vertraege-recht/vertraege-von-a-z/arzneimittel/ (accessed on 13 October 2019).

36. KV Bremen. Vereinbarung zur Sicherstellung der Arzneimittelversorgung im Jahr 2018. Available online: https://www.kvhb.de (accessed on 13 October 2019).
37. KV Hamburg. Wirkstoffvereinbarung nach § 106b Abs. 1 SGB V i. d. F. des 2. Nachtrages. Available online: https://www.kvhh.net/kvhh/pages/index/p/177/0/g_id/428 (accessed on 13 October 2019).
38. KV Mecklenburg Western Pomerania. Kassenärztlichen Vereinigung Mecklenburg-Vorpommern. Available online: https://www.kvmv.de/startseite/ (accessed on 13 October 2019).
39. KV Lower Saxony. Arzneimittelvereinbarung 2016, Anlage 1. Available online: https://www.kvn.de/Patienten/Arztsuche.html (accessed on 13 October 2019).
40. KV Saxony. Arzneimittelvereinbarung gemäß § 84 SGB V. für das Jahr 2018. Available online: https://www.kvs-Saxony.de/mitglieder/vertraege/arzneimittelvereinbarung-fuer-das-jahr-2018-gem-84-sgb-v/ (accessed on 13 October 2019).
41. KV Saxony-Anhalt. Arzneimittelvereinbarung 2019 zur Sicherstellung der Vertragsärztlichen Versorgung mit Arzneimitteln Gemäß § 84 Abs. 1 SGB V für das Jahr 2019. Available online: https://www.kvsa.de/fileadmin/user_upload/PDF/Praxis/Arznei_Heilmittelvolumen_Richtgroessen/20190409_Arzneimittelvereinbarung_2019.pdf (accessed on 13 October 2019).
42. KV Schleswig-Holstein. Zielvereinbarung zur Steuerung der Arzneimittelversorgung 2018. Available online: https://www.kvsh.de/fileadmin/user_upload/dokumente/Praxis/Vertraege/Arzneimittelvertraege/Zielvereinbarungen/2018_01_01_Zielvereinbarung_AM_OCR.pdf (accessed on 13 October 2019).
43. KV Thuringia. Arzneimittelvereinbarung für das Jahr 2018 nach § 84 Abs. 1 SGB V. Available online: https://www.kv-thuringia.de (accessed on 13 October 2019).
44. KV Northrhine. Vereinbarung. Available online: https://www.kvno.de/downloads/verordnungen/arzneimittelvereinbarung2019.pdf (accessed on 13 October 2019).
45. KV Rhineland Palatinate. Arzneimittelvereinbarung. Anlage 1. Available online: https://www.kv-rlp.de/mitglieder/vertraege/arznei-und-heilmittel/ (accessed on 13 October 2019).
46. KV Saarland. Arznei-, Verband- und Heilmittelvereinbarung für das Jahr 2018. Available online: https://www.kvsaarland.de (accessed on 13 October 2019).
47. KV Hesse. Arzneimittel-Vereinbarung nach § 84 SGB V für das Jahr 2018. Available online: https://www.kvHesse.de/fileadmin/user_upload/kvHesse/Mitglieder/Recht_Vertrag/VERTRAG_Arzneimittel-Vereinbarung-2018_17082018.pdf (accessed on 13 October 2019).
48. Bocquet, F.; Loubière, A.; Fusier, I.; Cordonnier, A.-L.; Paubel, P. Competition Between Biosimilars and Patented Biologics: Learning from European and Japanese Experience. *Pharm. Econ.* **2016**, *34*, 1173–1186. [CrossRef] [PubMed]
49. Arbeitsgemeinschaft Probiosimilars. Biosimilars in Zahlen. Marktdaten 2019. Available online: https://probiosimilars.de/publikationen/?id=33&date= (accessed on 13 October 2019).
50. Moorkens, E.; Vulto, A.G.; Huys, I.; Dylst, P.; Godman, B.; Keuerleber, S.; Claus, B.; Dimitrova, M.; Petrova, G.; Sovic-Brkicic, L.; et al. Policies for biosimilar uptake in Europe: An overview. *PLoS ONE* **2017**, *12*, e0190147. [CrossRef] [PubMed]
51. Rémuzat, C.; Kapuśniak, A.; Caban, A.; Ionescu, D.; Radière, G.; Mendoza, C.; Toumi, M. Supply-side and demand-side policies for biosimilars: An overview in 10 European member states. *J. Mark. Access Health Policy* **2017**, *5*. [CrossRef]
52. Rémuzat, C.; Dorey, J.; Cristeau, O.; Ionescu, D.; Radière, G.; Toumi, M. Key drivers for market penetration of biosimilars in Europe. *J. Mark. Access Health Policy* **2017**, *5*, 1272308. [CrossRef] [PubMed]
53. Olry de Labry, A.G.E.; Linder, L.; García, L.; Espín, J.; Rovira, J. Biosimilars in the European market. *Generics Biosimilars Initiat. J.* **2013**, *2*, 30–35. [CrossRef]
54. Blankart, K.E.; Arndt, F. Physician-Level Cost Control Measures and Regional Variation of Biosimilar Utilization in Germany. *Int. J. Environ. Res. Public Health* **2020**, *17*, 4113. [CrossRef] [PubMed]
55. Flume, M. Regional management of biosimilars in Germany. *Generics Biosimilars Initiat. J.* **2016**, *5*, 125–127. [CrossRef]
56. Federal Ministry of Health. KM6-statistics. Available online: http://www.gbe-bund.de. (accessed on 30 May 2019).
57. Federal Ministry of Justice and Consumer Protection. Available online: https://www.bmjv.de/EN/Home/home_node.html (accessed on 9 November 2019).

58. Kassenärztliche Bundesvereinigung (KBV). Available online: https://www.kbv.de/html/about_us.php (accessed on 13 October 2019).
59. GKV Spitzenverband. Available online: https://www.gkv-spitzenverband.de (accessed on 15 December 2019).
60. ABDATA Pharma Daten Service; ABDA Datenbank and ABDA Artikelstamm. *Bi-Monthly Update*; Avoxa-Mediengruppe Deutscher Apotheker GmbH: Eschborn, Germany, 2017.
61. WHO Collaborating Centre for Drug Statistics Methodology. ATC/DDD International Language for Drug Utilization Research: The Anatomical Therapeutic Chemical (ATC) Classification System. Available online: https://www.whocc.no/ (accessed on 30 May 2019).
62. Statistische Ämter der Bundes und der Länder; Gemeinsames Statistikportal. Gesundheitswirtschaft. Länderergebnisse Bruttowertschöpfung und Erwerbstätige der Gesundheitswirtschaft 2018. Available online: http://www.statistikportal.de/de/ggrdl/ergebnisse/wertschoepfungs-erwerbstaetigen-ansatz (accessed on 30 May 2019).
63. Mouha, Y. Biosimilars: How can We Explain Regional Variations in Their Use?—Market Dynamics of Originator Biological and Biosimilar Infliximab and Etanercept in Germany. Master's Thesis, KU Leuven, Leuven, Belgium, 2019.

Publisher's Note: MDPI stays neutral with regard to jurisdictional claims in published maps and institutional affiliations.

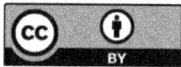

© 2020 by the authors. Licensee MDPI, Basel, Switzerland. This article is an open access article distributed under the terms and conditions of the Creative Commons Attribution (CC BY) license (http://creativecommons.org/licenses/by/4.0/).

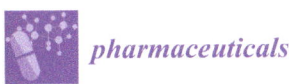

Review

Barriers to Biosimilar Prescribing Incentives in the Context of Clinical Governance in Spain

Félix Lobo [1,*] and Isabel Río-Álvarez [2]

[1] Department of Economics, University Carlos III de Madrid and Funcas, 28903 Getafe, Madrid, Spain
[2] Spanish Biosimilar Medicines Association, BioSim, 28027 Madrid, Spain; isabeldelrio@biosim.es
* Correspondence: flobo@eco.uc3m.es

Citation: Lobo, F.; Río-Álvarez, I. Barriers to Biosimilar Prescribing Incentives in the Context of Clinical Governance in Spain. *Pharmaceuticals* **2021**, *14*, 283. https://doi.org/10.3390/ph14030283

Academic Editors: Arnold G. Vulto, Steven Simoens and Isabelle Huys

Received: 22 January 2021
Accepted: 19 March 2021
Published: 22 March 2021

Publisher's Note: MDPI stays neutral with regard to jurisdictional claims in published maps and institutional affiliations.

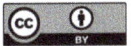

Copyright: © 2021 by the authors. Licensee MDPI, Basel, Switzerland. This article is an open access article distributed under the terms and conditions of the Creative Commons Attribution (CC BY) license (https://creativecommons.org/licenses/by/4.0/).

Abstract: Incentives contribute to the proper functioning of the broader contracts that regulate the relationships between health systems and professionals. Likewise, incentives are an important element of clinical governance understood as health services' management at the micro-level, aimed at achieving better health outcomes for patients. In Spain, monetary and non-monetary incentives are sometimes used in the health services, but not as frequently as in other countries. There are already several examples in European countries of initiatives searching the promotion of biosimilars through different sorts of incentives, but not in Spain. Hence, this paper is aimed at identifying the barriers that incentives to prescribe biosimilars might encounter in Spain, with particular interest in incentives in the framework of clinical governance. Both questions are intertwined. Barriers are presented from two perspectives. Firstly, based on the nature of the barrier: (i) the payment system for health professionals, (ii) budget rigidity and excessive bureaucracy, (iii) little autonomy in the management of human resources (iv) lack of clinical integration, (v) absence of a legal framework for clinical governance, and (vi) other governance-related barriers. The second perspective is based on the stakeholders involved: (i) gaps in knowledge among physicians, (ii) misinformation and distrust among patients, (iii) trade unions opposition to productivity-related payments, (iv) lack of a clear position by professional associations, and (v) misalignment of the goals pursued by some healthcare professionals and the goals of the public system. Finally, the authors advance several recommendations to overcome these barriers at the national level.

Keywords: incentives; clinical governance; biosimilars; Spain; barriers

1. Introduction

This paper is aimed at identifying the barriers that incentives to prescribe biosimilars might encounter in Spain. Incentives were chosen as one of the main policy actions to stimulate biosimilar use in Spain because they have an important potential leverage, they are relatively underdeveloped in Spain, and they may be controversial in promoting prescription patterns.

We particularly focus on incentives in the framework of clinical governance as they are intertwined concepts. Clinical governance would be impossible to implement without incentives, and incentives, if not impossible, would be difficult to establish in different frameworks.

Biosimilar medicines significantly help to improve patient access to biological therapies that have revolutionised the prognosis of multiple serious diseases, while contributing to price competition in the market and the sustainability of healthcare systems. If one of the main current problems in health policy is to make access to new medicines compatible with sustainability, biosimilars are part of the solution by freeing up very considerable resources [1] (p. 7).

Biosimilar medicines have a long history in the Spanish pharmaceutical market. Since the approval of the first biosimilar medicine in 2006, within the European regulatory framework [2–6], there are currently 54 authorised medicines (42 effectively marketed) for 17 active ingredients [7]. Biosimilar uptake varies greatly between Autonomous Communities, hospitals, and clinical services. There is also high variability in uptake between molecules regardless of their time on the market [8]. Even so, a budget impact analysis published by the end of 2020 quantifies the savings generated by biosimilars in the National Health System (NHS) at over €2300 million over the 2009–2019 period: "This shows how the entry of biosimilars into the Spanish pharmaceutical market has led to unquestionable and significant savings, especially in hospital pharmacy" [9] (p. 11). The same study estimates that unless major changes occur in market behaviour, the expected savings for 2020–2022 would exceed €2800 million.

However, the uptake of biosimilars in Spain is below the European neighbouring countries' average. This is observed in the antiTNF group, epoetin and human growth hormone, three of the six active ingredients for which there are data available, which means that there is room for improvement in their use [8]. Thus, the aforementioned budgetary impact analysis estimates that if biosimilar uptake reached 80% in 2022, the €2800 million would be increased by an additional €430 million. The French government set a similar objective in its National Health Strategy for 2018–2022 [10].

The promotion of biosimilars is part of most Pharmaceutical policy strategies. The Independent Authority for Fiscal Responsibility (Autoridad Independiente de Responsabilidad Fiscal, AIReF), which is responsible for ensuring the sustainability of public finances, considers the promotion of biosimilars the most relevant tool for controlling hospital pharmaceutical expenditure [8]. This institution suggests the establishment of biosimilar prescribing incentives to maximise this savings opportunity.

The "Action Plan to promote the use of market regulating medicines in the National Health System: biosimilar medicines and generic medicines" of the Ministry of Health states that "In the Autonomous Communities [...] actions will be carried out to link financial or other incentives" [11] (p. 38). This two-level (national and regional) approach is because the Spanish NHS is a decentralised system since health competences are transferred to the 17 Autonomous Communities. Coordination, strategy for pharmaceutical policy and medicine pricing and financing decisions, among others, lie essentially with the Ministry of Health, and with Autonomous Communities when it comes to budgeting, purchasing and provision [12].

Further, the Commission for Social and Economic Reconstruction of the *Congreso de los Diputados* (the lower Parliament chamber) dealing with the reform of the NHS to tackle with the Covid-19 pandemic included in its report the need to "significantly increase the proportion of biosimilars" [13] (p. 25).

In short, the promotion of biosimilars in general, and the establishment of prescribing incentives in particular, seem to be unavoidable tasks according to decision-makers and policy makers in the short-term.

Therefore, this paper is aimed at identifying the barriers that a model of incentives to prescribe biosimilars might encounter in the context of clinical governance in Spain. Both concepts are intertwined as incentives are the instrument and clinical governance the organisational form.

This is a pioneering approach, as the research literature on this topic is very scarce.

This work is based on a broader study of the incentives that, in the context of clinical governance, can lead to greater use of biosimilar medicines in healthcare [14]. This study reviews and presents the most outstanding experiences of this sort developed in high income countries and examines the possible barriers to their implementation in Spain.

2. Incentives and Clinical Governance

Incentivising health professionals, especially prescribing physicians, is a crucial issue for the organisation and reform of the NHS and for policies to promote biosimilars. Payment systems, including pay for performance, and competition, including benchmarking and yardstick competition, are typical financial incentives [15,16]. However, the incentives that move people are not only financial, nor, of course, only monetary. In the health sector there are other very powerful motivations such as: dedication to service, altruism, professional satisfaction, and reputation; scientific curiosity, the feeling of belonging to a group, etc. [17].

Before moving on, it should be noted that in this study we refer to a very narrow definition of incentive. Specifically, financial incentives that are not necessarily monetary or exclusive to the prescriber. This is critical since many studies about European biosimilar landscape refer to "incentive policies" that are not necessarily financial incentives. For instance, educational campaigns, quotas, or tendering practices are considered incentive tools to increase the uptake of biosimilars and financial incentive would be just another mechanism for that purpose [18–21]. An important study carried out by the European Commission considers that one of the challenges for the Spanish NHS in the future is "to align the incentives of the different service providers with the system's quality and efficiency goals. For example, staff incentives could be improved." [22] (p. 253).

The use of incentives to influence physicians' prescribing patterns and encourage their alignment with organisational goals is a policy that has been embodied in various experiences over time and across countries. In Spain, towards the end of the 1990s, financial incentives related to prescription were already applied in several Autonomous Communities. By 2018, there were at least seven autonomous communities applying them. The AIReF, in its 2018 review of public expenditure on medication dispensed through prescription, recommends establishing prescription incentives [23]. The same recommendation is made in its recent evaluation of the pharmaceutical spending in the public hospital setting in Spain, but now directly linked to biosimilar prescription: "in view of the success of international experiences, it is proposed to implement a gain-sharing incentive system for hospitals, care services and health professionals" [8] (p. 89). A gain-sharing incentive system (also called gainshare agreement) is based on sharing savings associated with more efficient use of medicines at the same time as any efficiencies made will be invested back into patient care to improve their health outcomes [24].

However, when it comes to promoting biosimilars, there are doubts about the most appropriate type of incentives. Some voices are in favour of financial incentives and argue in their support, for example, their contribution to the progress of biosimilars in Germany. "Prescribers need confidence in outcomes, and they and/or the health system need to benefit financially from using biosimilars" [25]. Other opinions consider that it is better to motivate physicians through schemes that avoid direct financial incentives [26].

Incentives are easier to implement in well-organised broader contexts such as health services following the lines of what is known as "clinical governance". We acknowledge that there is no consensus definition for clinical governance. Our vision of the concept is as follows: This is an organisational form of health services at the micro-level, aimed at achieving better outcomes in terms of patient health, characterised by the following elements:

- Involvement of health professionals not only in treatments but in the whole management.
- Decentralisation of decisions and autonomy of services.
- Restructuring of services in a multidisciplinary manner aimed at the management of high-quality clinical processes.
- Measurement and evaluation of performance and remuneration that may include monetary and non-monetary incentives.

Some biosimilar prescribing incentives have been put in place in Europe. Although it is not the scope of this research, we summarise in Table 1 the more relevant initiatives to our view, the British experiences being those closer to our approach of clinical governance.

Table 1. European initiatives on biosimilar prescribing incentives.

Country	Level	Incentive Program	Description
France [27]	National-Ministry of Health Hospital and retail pharmacies	Instruction no DSS/1C/DGOS/PF2/2018/42 du 19 février 2018 relative à l'incitation à la prescription hospitalière de médicaments biologiques similaires […].	Hospitals can earn 20% or even 30% of the difference between the public price of the originator and its biosimilars.
Germany [28,29]	Regional-Saxonia Regional physician association and sick fund	"Biolike" initiative. Agreement between KV Westfalen-Lippe and sick fund Barmer.	Physicians who reach a certain biosimilar uptake are eligible to bill additional services for their patients.
Italy [30]	Regional-Campania Regional Health Service	DGR n.66 del 14.07.2016. Misure di incentivazione dei farmaci a brevetto scaduto e dei biosimilari. Monitoraggio delle prescrizioni attraverso la piattaforma Sani.ARP	Centres can earn 50% of the difference between the public price of the originator and its biosimilars to invest in high-cost innovator medicines; while a 5% will be invested back in the centre which generated the savings.
United Kingdom [31–34]	Local-Hospital Trusts and Clinical Commissioning Groups	Gainshare agreement between the Trust and the Clinical Commissioning Groups (50:50)	Hospitals can earn 50% of the difference between the public price of the originator and its biosimilars that are reinvested in patient care.

The gainshare agreements reached with regional or local leadership in the United Kingdom [32–34], mostly between 2015 and 2017, under a well-established framework [35] are examples of what we mean by biosimilar prescribing incentives in the context of clinical governance. However, in 2018, NHS England began to link the concept of best-value drug to drug procurement as part of a wider strategy to increase savings [36,37]. While this measure might be effective, it does not fall under our definition.

In Spain, a good example of combining incentives and clinical governance is the "Área del Corazón" (Heart area) of the University Hospital of La Coruña, coordinated by Dr Alfonso Castro Beiras in the 1990s [38]. The project was based on the willingness to cooperate from the cardiology and cardiac surgery services. This clinical management model was based on four elements: (i) Process standardisation; (ii) Strengthening of information systems; (iii) Use of diagnosis-related groups as patient classification systems and (iv) Self-evaluation. The management of the human and material resources and the control over the budget appear to be decisive for the development of this autonomy-based model. The results were very positive. Activity and care indicators improved, and savings were invested back in human resources, making it possible to staff the new intermediate care unit.

Although this initiative is no longer running, there is no doubt that clinical governance offers good possibilities for the efficient use of effective and good quality biosimilars by prioritizing health outcomes, motivation, quality of care processes and efficient use of resources. Actually, we might be talking about one of the first gainshare agreements in Spain. This precedent seems significant enough to support a pilot gainshare agreement in Spain like those successfully implemented in the United Kingdom [34].

It is now time to ask what are the barriers and difficulties that incentives to prescribe biosimilars encounter in Spain.

3. Barriers According to Their Nature

As we are particularly interested in barriers to incentives in the framework of a model of clinical governance and both questions are strongly related, we present here different barriers encountered in Spain that we have been found relevant for both concepts.

3.1. Payment System

The current payment system is also a barrier primarily for incentives but also for clinical governance. Its regulation, tradition, and the culture it has generated are very much in opposition to the incentives and flexibility required by efficient organisations. The 2006 report on Spain by the European Observatory on Health Systems and Policies noted that after having completed the healthcare transfer process to the Autonomous Communities in 2002 "the most concerning issue was that most of the pay increases affected the fixed components ... compared with income related with performance" [39] (p. 110). Several sources suggest that remuneration based on results and effort is motivating and that a variable remuneration based on targets should be increased in relation to fixed payments [40–42].

3.2. Rigid and Bureaucratic Budgetary and Economic Management Legislation and Procedures

In Spain, bureaucratic control has traditionally prevailed over the evaluation of outcomes, at all governmental levels. "The budgetary system has long suffered from being excessive rigid" [43] (p. 278). These rigid legislation and budgetary and financial management procedures involve major difficulties and delays and are a significant impediment when implementing incentives and clinical governance. The production of health services requires agility and flexibility to manage personnel and material resources to improve health outcomes. Furthermore, as suggested by Zornoza Pérez [43] (p. 295), "flexibility and control must be properly combined with accountability to induce managers to behave in accordance with the principles of efficiency and economy in the management of public expenditure." This need remains outstanding. In 2016, Esteban and Arias [44] (p. 98) state that "one of the main challenges for the NHS is to progress towards the de-bureaucratisation of the system by leaving the current public law regime in the field of human resources."

3.3. Spanish NHS Labour Relations Model

The employment relationship of physicians and other health professionals with the services that make up the Spanish NHS (so called "statutory personnel") follows the civil service model. The rigidity and the difficulties it entails to achieve efficient management have often been criticised [45]. One of its main problems is the inflexibility in adapting to care needs and the limitations in differentiating individual and collective merit [46]. It hinders decisively the introduction of incentives and clinical governance. The elimination of this model and the establishment of a modern, flexible, and efficient labour relations system, particularly for physicians, is considered one of the basic structural reforms to be addressed in the NHS. That would mean to eliminate civil-service-like regulations and reintroduce professionalism and evolve towards forms of market labour relations [40,46,47].

3.4. Clinical and Health Service Disintegration

The disintegration of health care in the NHS is an especially important barrier to implementing clinical governance and promoting biosimilars through incentives. Disintegration implies gaps and borderlines, multiplicity of providers, uncoordinated services, neglect of patient preferences, poor measurement of relevant outcomes, and lack of incentives oriented towards the provision of comprehensive care [48]. Clinical integration is the basic goal of reform plans for the health services to respond to current needs, mainly determined by chronic and degenerative diseases [45,48]. Sometimes integration is accompanied by financing schemes that cover all health services and generate incentives for efficiency. Excessively rigid boundaries between specialties also prevent cross-sectional and team work, organisation of services according to care processes and patient orientation [47]. This is a key difficulty that opposes the development of incentives for individual and collective merit within the framework of clinical governance.

3.5. Absence of General Legislation on Clinical Governance

In Spain, clinical governance is not regulated by law. The draft Royal Decree RD /2015 laying down the basis for the implementation of Clinical Management Units in the Health Services [49] was an interesting initiative. In the interests of a high-quality, safe, and integrated healthcare, the draft suggested providing professionals in the NHS with greater levels of autonomy and responsibility in their clinical decision-making. It included governance-related terms such as planning, incorporation of new technologies and knowledge management, all from a perspective of "decentralisation of the organisation" as well as continuous evaluation of results. Although promising in terms of progress, it was finally rejected by the Council of State because it had to be passed as a law by Parliament. The opposition from trade unions and certain professional spheres, the lack of sufficient support from the Autonomous Communities and the political instability of the past years made it difficult for the draft Royal Decree to become a Law. However, in view of the impact of Covid-19 pandemic, some proposals of the Commission for Social and Economic Reconstruction of the Congress of Deputies suggest that progress could be expected in this regard. "The professionalisation of the governance of health services must be guaranteed and health professionals must be encouraged to perform managerial roles. The executive directors of health services should follow epidemiological, public health and clinical governance approaches" [13] (pp. 3–4).

3.6. Governance-Related Barriers: Lack of Professionalisation of Health Services Managers and Absence of Governing Boards

In Spain, healthcare managers, such as hospital general managers and others, do not always have the appropriate professional profile and appointments are generally based on discretionary decisions. Open and competitive recruitment and selection processes and periodic performance evaluations are not always the rule. Collective and independent boards of directors controlling the micro-management of elementary organisations such as hospitals and health areas in a decentralised and transparent manner [47] are scarce. Only some Autonomous Communities, such as the Comunidad de Madrid [50], have adopted legislation that reflects these principles. In this scenario, major organisational reforms, such as clinical governance and the establishment of incentives, seem unlikely.

The second Amphos Report [51], prepared with the contribution of 80 managers and clinicians, provides an interesting overview of the barriers that delay the implementation of clinical governance units. Fifteen were identified and classified according to their nature into: political, economic, legal, technological, and human or cultural (Table 2). Some of them match those highlighted above. We also find it interesting to highlight the difficulty in making an organisational change that generates medium-term results when policies are focused on the short term and lack of evidence on objective and reliable results that show the benefits of clinical governance units. These barriers were also classified according to priority. To this end a group of 72 health professionals and managers with previous experience in clinical governance was asked to grade each of the barriers on a scale of 0 to 5 (being 5 the highest) not in absolute values but in comparison with others. The highest barrier was the labour framework, followed by the lack of political will and the regulatory framework.

The potential savings due to biosimilar competition expected in Spain for the period 2020–2022 (€2800 million) [9] may become the pretext to put in place mechanisms to overcome these barriers, provided, of course, that all parties benefit from these savings. Again, gainshare agreements emerge as a powerful tool for that.

Table 2. Barriers to clinical governance and score according to priority [51,52].

Nature of the Barrier	Score
Political	
1. Institutional support: lack of political will to promote decentralised and autonomous management models.	4.6
2. Centralising trends: management oriented towards control, production of rules and regulations, and concentration of activities.	4.0
Economic	
3. Short-term results: Clinical governance units (CGU) generate long-term results.	4.0
4. Insufficient budgets: increased demand for care and scarce resources.	4.0
5. Economies of scale: GCU require a minimum critical mass.	3.2
6. Investment in innovation: lack of resources for innovation and improvements.	3.5
Legal	
7. Regulatory framework: regulations that hinder organisational change and lack of regulations for CGUs.	4.5
8. Labour framework: regulations that limit the HR policies needed by CGUs.	5.0
Technological	
9. Evidence on outcomes: lack of objective and reliable outcomes demonstrating the benefits of CGUs.	3.6
10. Information systems: lack of coverage of information systems and technologies.	4.0
Human/cultural	
11. Managers trust: reluctance to delegate responsibilities and risks.	4.3
12. Culture of innovation: the environment does not encourage change or the search for excellence.	4.1
13. Involvement of relevant groups: reluctance to teamwork from different professionals.	4.2
14. Involvement of clinicians: reluctance to taking risks and co-responsibility.	3.9
15. Leadership skills: poor training of future CGU leaders.	4.3

4. Barriers According to Stakeholders

4.1. Physicians with Limited Information and Distrust of Biosimilars

As biosimilars are biological medicines, they must be prescribed by their brand name [53]. In addition, in Spain the pharmacist cannot dispense a brand other than that prescribed, without authorisation of the prescribing physician according to Order SCO/2874/2007 [54]. Therefore, the physician is the key actor for the market entry of biosimilars. The physician's trust and preference for prescribing biosimilars is critical.

However, as previously pointed out by Acha and Mestre-Ferrándiz (2017) [55] (p. 263) the biosimilar market faces "the second translational gap" once concerns about the guarantees of the regulatory framework have been dispelled. The authors recognise that "Despite many efforts by regulators to reach out to clinicians, there remains a translational gap for biosimilars which need to be incorporated in healthcare pathways and understood by clinicians and patients. Only by bridging this gap will biosimilars fully play their role in healthcare for Europe".

Weise et al. (2012) [56] listed the main uncertainties of physicians about biosimilar medicines: (i) doubts about their quality and manufacturing process; (ii) the "similar but not identical" paradigm; (iii) immunogenicity; (iv) possible gaps in post-marketing pharmacovigilance; and (v) extrapolation of efficacy and safety data without clinical trials in certain indications. A recent systematic review conducted on physicians' perceptions about the uptake of biosimilars suggests that little has changed since then [57]. Physicians still have doubts related to the safety, efficacy, and immunogenicity of biosimilars and consider that cost savings is the main advantages of biosimilars. In addition, most of the physicians had negative perceptions of pharmacist-led substitution of biological medicines.

Another review aimed at identifying the barriers to the use of biosimilar medicines in Europe medicines points out that physicians act as a barrier to biosimilars in several ways [58]. Firstly, their concerns about true similarity between originator and biosimilars. Second, the absence of incentives or benefits for prescribing lower-cost medicines that would compensate the effort they make when explaining to the patient the switch to a biosimilar medicine. Finally, the strong ties between physicians and the originator pharmaceutical companies, which often support clinical research and continuous education (opposite incentive). Given these scenarios, national policies on biosimilars have focused on improving physicians' trust in biosimilars through a variety of training programs, which are sometimes local and generally relying on prescription guidelines [18].

In Spain, Agustí y Rodriguez (2015) [59] predicted that the success in biosimilar adoption would depend largely on the trust of health professionals and pointed out that the accumulated experience with biosimilars would help overcome reluctant attitudes.

As biosimilar medicines are mainly used into the hospital setting, hospital physicians have been the focus of many educational programmes (funded by the industry, scientific societies, professional associations, and regional governments). This is also observed in the constant review of position papers on biosimilars by scientific societies in most relevant specialties, such as Oncology, Rheumatology, Haematology, or Digestive Pathology [60–64]. Although one might expect that these statements build trust and shape prescription patterns equally among physicians, a high variability is found when comparing biosimilar uptake between hospitals within a single region. For instance, in 2014, several hospitals in the Community of Madrid rarely used biosimilars, while others showed uptake rates between 60% and 70% [65]. This suggests that despite sharing guidelines from the same regional health service or scientific society, the influence of opinion leaders or heads of departments can accelerate or slow the biosimilar access to hospitals. Nor can we overlook the effect of some sort of incentive set internally at the hospital level, although there is no evidence in this respect.

In the case of primary care setting, the arrival of new biosimilars is a new challenge. From a survey with over 700 respondents, it appears that 58% of the respondents do not know the definition of biosimilars and 73% do not know that the handling of biosimilars is not comparable to that of generics, for which in Spain prescription by active ingredient is applied [66]. Moreover, in the primary care setting, a strategy based on education/information, and constant communication with health professionals, succeeds in improving knowledge about biosimilars and changing prescription patterns [67]. By contrast, any initiative to promote biosimilars not agreed upon with physicians is doomed to failure [26].

In short, physicians that are informed through official and reliable sources tend to consider biosimilars as alternatives that are efficient for the health system and effective and safe for their patients and are able to convey the trust needed for preventing the nocebo effect (nocebo effect refers to negative expectations of the patient regarding a treatment that translate into negative side effects or outcomes) and ensuring treatment compliance. However, improving the knowledge about biosimilars and afterwards communicating the information to patients require big efforts by physicians. Therefore, it cannot be overlooked that recognising physicians' efforts through incentives or other formulas aimed at sharing benefits will guarantee their commitment in the medium term.

4.2. Misinformed Patients and Mistrust towards Biosimilars

A major barrier to the spread of biosimilar medicines is misinformation and mistrust from the part of patients. The complexity of the world of medicines and their names, especially if they are biological products, makes it difficult for patients to have timely information and knowledge of their characteristics and guarantees [19]. It may be particularly difficult to know and be aware that all medicines that are authorised for marketing, whether they are original products or biosimilars, offer the same safety, efficacy, and quality guarantees. This limited knowledge impacts on their willingness to accept the prescription of biosimilar treatments [68]. In addition, patient organisations often have close links with the originator industry, which sometimes finances their meetings and educational activities [18].

The difficulty often arises, not for the naïve patients, but for those whose treatment was initiated with the original product and are encouraged to change it for a biosimilar product (switch). There may be differences in the brand name or appearance [69]. In addition, sometimes the inherent variability in the manufacturing processes of biological products can lead to certain characteristics not being totally identical to those of the originator, but this variability is strongly controlled within acceptable limits to ensure there is no relevant clinical impact [70]. Despite that, biosimilars are not well understood by many healthcare professionals and patients, and such a mistrust is exacerbated by negatively biased information disseminated by some parties [71].

A study on policies to promote biosimilars in 24 European countries found that educational initiatives aimed at patients were rare. Patients are informed mainly through their organisations, through brochures and letters to explain the switch from originator to biosimilar. It recognises that biosimilar policies should include all stakeholders, including patients, and recommends strengthening educational initiatives through instruments such as question and answer (Q&A) documents [18].

However, a very recent study by Vandenplas and collaborators (2021) [72] emphasised that over the past few years several surveys among European patients have shown a lack of knowledge and trust in biosimilars. In addition, they performed a web-based screening of European Patients' Forum and International Alliance of Patients' Organisations on publicly available information about biosimilars and found a high variability among correctness, the level of detail, and the tone when providing information.

The physician–patient relationship is absolutely crucial to overcome these information or mistrust issues. There is no doubt that as long as the physician is properly informed and trusts biosimilars, the patient will follow his or her guidelines.

It should be borne in mind that having accurate information and access to medicines are rights that are widely recognised in different jurisdictions. According to the Spanish legislation the physician must inform the patient. Indeed, according to Article 10 of the General Health Services Law 14/1986 [73], patients have the right to be informed on the health services they have access to and the requirements for their use. According to Law 41/2002, Article 4, on patient autonomy and rights and obligations regarding clinical information and documentation [74] patients have the right to know all available information on any action touching their health, including, at least, "the purpose and nature of each intervention, its risks and consequences". In addition, the physician must guarantee the fulfilment of this right to information from the part of patients. Article 10 of the General Health Law (LGS) also states that patients have the right "to obtain medicines and medical devices that are considered necessary to promote, preserve or restore their health".

In Spain, Calleja et al. (2020) [75] identify patient education and involvement in the decision-making process as key points to increase acceptance of biosimilars and counteract the nocebo effect. This is the view of at least eleven patient associations in Spain as embodied in the "Joint statement by physicians and patients on treatments with originator biologics and biosimilars" [76]. Thus, some requests read as follows "Health administrations often lack biosimilars training programmes for physicians", "The debate on originator biological and biosimilar medicines should be open to the participation of physicians and patients", "Policies that would make the cost/efficiency principle a systematic argument would not be acceptable", or "Some administrative decisions could seriously interfere with the normal functioning of the physician-patient relationship". The last two could be an obstacle to the establishment of biosimilar prescribing incentives from the patients' perspective.

4.3. Unions Opposition to Productivity-Based Variable Remuneration

One of the barriers to the establishment of biosimilar prescribing incentives is the opposition of trade unions to variable remuneration based on outcomes, targets, or productivity. This exists not only in Spain but also in other countries, and in any sector, not only in health. The study by García-Olaverri y Huerta (2011) [77] shows that trade unions defend salary standardisation and oppose differentiation according to the different abilities or skills of workers. These objections are found also in the governmental and health sectors.

The disagreement clearly appears in the 2014 document of the State Confederation of Medical Trade Unions (CESM, in its Spanish acronym) on clinical governance: "Under no circumstance may incentives be linked to savings over the agreed budget, but rather to the level of compliance with it, and with the care and quality targets established in accordance with the provisions laid down in the management contract." "This implies that the health service that decides to promote clinical governance must allocate additional funds to pay for these incentives" [78] (p. 10). This position is clearly contrary to the establishment of, for example, gain-sharing programmes which have been successfully established in other countries [34] where part of the savings from increased use of biosimilar medicines revert to the healthcare system itself.

4.4. Professional Corporate Bodies, Clinical Governance and Incentives

Professional corporate bodies, especially those of physicians, react positively to clinical governance insofar as it increases their autonomy, responsibility, and decision-making capacity. Other features such as performance assessment, performance-related incentives and transparency and accountability do not generate the same enthusiasm [79,80]. These corporations may defend based on professionalism and technical criteria organisational and management changes that promote their professional practice and the health of patients. However, they also experience the pressure of electoral cycles. Then, they usually oppose structural reforms advocating the interests of less committed colleagues (as if this behaviour were the rule) to get the most votes in their corporation's elections.

4.5. Physicians and Other Health Professionals Not Aligned with the Objectives of the System

Although it is a very limited group, health professionals not aligned with the goals of the system, poorly committed to the public system, can be a barrier to clinical governance and incentives for good performance in general, and for biosimilar prescribing incentives in particular. Attitudes such as opposition to transparency or to performance assessment leading to differentiated remuneration must be corrected, as they have a very negative effect on the morale of the vast majority of those who are compliant. When it comes to biosimilars, the strong ties that originator companies have with physicians through supporting clinical research or training may influence prescription choices [55]. Additionally, guidelines with an economic rationale intended to deliver benefits at societal level may be badly received by some physicians, who may consider that their professional decisions are challenged [81]. Thus, it seems reasonable that a greater alignment between the medical community and the regulators would help build trust on biosimilar medicines [82].

5. Recommendations for Spain to Overcome the Barriers to Implement Incentives for Biosimilars

According to our review we recommend the following actions to overcome the barriers to implement incentives for biosimilars:

- Efforts to inform and educate physicians on the pharmacological and clinical characteristics of biosimilars should be continued and intensified, always on a scientific basis.
- Patients should be informed about biosimilars to ensure their trust on medicines that are approved by the regulatory authorities.
- We recommend informing all types of unions and professional corporations of the improvements that clinical governance schemes including incentives (especially those

based on gain-sharing programmes) can bring about for the NHS, patients, and professional practice.
- Consensus and support from policy makers is required to implement a growing uptake of biosimilars mainly from the Departments of Health but also from the Department of Finance as its endorsement of financial incentive programs might be necessary.
- In the long run, structural reforms of the Spanish NHS are required to overcome other barriers to biosimilar prescribing incentives in the context of clinical governance. We refer to rigidity and bureaucracy in management; clinical and health services disintegration; NHS labour relations model; payment systems and governance. Nevertheless, we think that in the short run there is room for new limited experiments, particularly with non-monetary incentives and the gain-sharing design, which will incite less opposition.

Author Contributions: Conceptualization, F.L. and I.R.-Á.; methodology, F.L. and I.R.-Á.; investigation, F.L. and I.R.-Á.; resources, F.L. and I.R.-Á.; writing—original draft preparation, F.L. and I.R.-Á.; writing—review and editing, F.L. and I.R.-Á.; supervision, F.L. and I.R.-Á.; project administration, F.L. and I.R.-Á. Both authors have read and agreed to the published version of the manuscript.

Funding: The broader study from which this article is extracted was funded by The Spanish Biosimilar Medicines Association, BioSim.

Conflicts of Interest: I.R.-Á. is employee of the Spanish Biosimilar Medicines Association. F.L. has no conflict of interest.

References

1. BioSim. Biosimilares: Nuevas Formas de Innovar. Position Paper. Coordinado por Gonzalo Calvo. 2017. Available online: https://www.biosim.es/documentos/Biosimilares%20position%20paper.pdf (accessed on 20 December 2020).
2. European Commission. Commission Directive 2003/63/EC of 25 June 2003 amending Directive 2001/83/EC of the European Parliament and of the Council on the Community Code Relating to Medicinal Products for Human Use. Available online: https://eur-lex.europa.eu/legal-content/EN/TXT/HTML/?uri=CELEX:32003L0063&from=ES (accessed on 20 December 2020).
3. European Medicines Agency: Similar Biological Medicinal Products (Overarching Guideline). CHMP/437/04 Rev. 1. Available online: https://www.ema.europa.eu/en/documents/scientific-guideline/guideline-similar-biological-medicinal-products-rev1_en.pdf (accessed on 20 December 2020).
4. European Medicines Agency: Similar Biological Medicinal Products Containing Biotechnology Derived Proteins as Active Substance: Non-Clinical and Clinical Issues. EMEA/CHMP/BMWP/42832/2005 Rev. 1. Available online: http://www.ema.europa.eu/docs/en_GB/document_library/Scientific_guideline/2015/01/WC500180219.pdf (accessed on 20 December 2020).
5. European Medicines Agency: Similar Biological Medicinal Products Containing Biotechnology-Derived Proteins as Active Substance: Quality Issues. EMA/CHMP/BWP/247713/2012 Rev.1. Available online: https://www.ema.europa.eu/en/documents/scientific-guideline/guideline-similar-biological-medicinal-products-containing-biotechnology-derived-proteins-active_en-0.pdf (accessed on 20 December 2020).
6. European Medicines Agency: Immunogenicity Assessment of Biotechnology-Derived Therapeutic Proteins. EMEA/CHMP/BMWP/14327/2006. Available online: https://www.ema.europa.eu/en/documents/scientific-guideline/guideline-immunogenicity-assessment-therapeutic-proteins-revision-1_en.pdf (accessed on 20 December 2020).
7. Centro de Información Online de Medicamentos de la Agencia Española de Medicamentos Sanitarios (CIMA). Available online: https://cima.aemps.es/cima/publico/lista.html (accessed on 10 January 2021).
8. Autoridad Independiente de Responsabilidad Fiscal (AIReF). Evaluación del Gasto Público 2019. Estudio. Gasto hospitalario del Sistema Nacional de Salud: Farmacia e Inversión en Bienes de Equipo. 2020. Available online: https://www.airef.es/wp-content/uploads/2020/10/SANIDAD/PDF-WEB-Gasto-hospitalario-del-SNS.pdf (accessed on 20 December 2020).
9. García-Goñi, M.; Carcedo, D.; Villacampa, A.; Lores, M. Análisis de Impacto Presupuestario de los Medicamentos Biosimilares en el SNS de España 2009–2022. Madrid, Septiembre 2020. Study Commissioned by BioSim. Available online: https://www.biosim.es/analisis-de-impacto-presupuestario-de-los-medicamentos-biosimilares-en-el-sistema-nacional-de-salud-de-espana-2009-2022/ (accessed on 20 December 2020).
10. Ministère des Solidarités et de la Santé 2018. Stratégie Nationale de Santé 2018–2022. Available online: https://solidarites-sante.gouv.fr/IMG/pdf/dossier_sns_2017_vdef.pdf (accessed on 20 December 2020).
11. Ministerio de Sanidad, Consumo y Bienestar Social. Plan de Acción Para Fomentar la Utilización de los Medicamentos Reguladores del Mercado en el Sistema Nacional de Salud: Medicamentos Biosimilares y Medicamentos Genérico. 11 April 2019. Available online: https://www.mscbs.gob.es/profesionales/farmacia/pdf/PlanAccionSNSmedicamentosReguladoresMercado.pdf (accessed on 20 December 2020).

12. Bernal-Delgado, E.; García-Armesto, S.; Oliva, J.; Sánchez Martínez, F.I.; Repullo, J.R.; Peña Longobardo, L.M.; Ridao-López, M.; Hernández-Quevedo, C. Spain: Health System Review. *Health Syst. Transit.* **2018**, *20*, 1–179. Available online: https://www.euro.who.int/__data/assets/pdf_file/0008/378620/hit-spain-eng.pdf (accessed on 12 February 2021).
13. Congreso de los Diputados, 2020. Dictamen de la Comisión para la Reconstrucción social y Económica del Congreso de los Diputados. Available online: http://www.congreso.es/docu/comisiones/reconstruccion/153_1_Dictamen.pdf (accessed on 20 December 2020).
14. Lobo, F.; del Río, I. *Gestión Clínica, Incentivos y Biosimilares*, 1st ed.; Díaz de Santos: Madrid, Spain, 2020; Available online: https://www.biosim.es/documentos/BIOSIM%20-GESTION%20CLINICA%20INCENTIVOS%20Y%20BIOSIMILARES_DEF.pdf (accessed on 20 December 2020).
15. European Commission. Expert Panel on Effective Ways of Investing in Health (EXPH) Competition among Health Care Providers Investigating Policy Options in the European Union. 2015. Available online: https://ec.europa.eu/health/sites/health/files/expert_panel/docs/008_competition_healthcare_providers_en.pdf (accessed on 20 December 2020).
16. Costa Font, J.; Rico, A. Vertical Competition in the Spanish National Health System. *Public Choice* **2006**, *128*, 477–498. Available online: http://link.springer.com/article/10.1007%2Fs11127-005-9011-y#page-1 (accessed on 20 December 2020). [CrossRef]
17. Berdud, M.; Cabasés, J.; Nieto, J. Incentives and intrinsic motivation in healthcare. *Gaceta Sanitaria* **2016**, *30*, 408–414. [CrossRef] [PubMed]
18. Moorkens, E.; Vulto, A.G.; Huys, I.; Dylst, P.; Godman, B.; Keuerleber, S.; Claus, B.; Dimitrova, M.; Petrova, G.; Sović-Brkičić, L.; et al. Policies for biosimilar uptake in Europe: An overview. *PLoS ONE* **2017**, *12*, e0190147. Available online: https://pubmed.ncbi.nlm.nih.gov/29284064/ (accessed on 20 December 2020). [CrossRef] [PubMed]
19. Barbier, L.; Simoens, S.; Vulto, A.G.; Huys, I. European Stakeholder Learnings Regarding Biosimilars: Part II-Improving Biosimilar Use in Clinical Practice. *BioDrugs* **2020**, *34*, 797–808. [CrossRef] [PubMed]
20. Rémuzat, C.; Dorey, J.; Cristeau, O.; Ionescu, D.; Radière, G.; Toumi, M. Key drivers for market penetration of biosimilars in Europe. *J. Mark. Access. Health Policy* **2017**, *5*, 1272308. [CrossRef]
21. Rémuzat, C.; Kapuśniak, A.; Caban, A.; Ionescu, D.; Radière, G.; Mendoza, C.; Toumi, M. Supply-side and demand-side policies for biosimilars: An overview in 10 European member states. *J. Mark. Access. Health Policy* **2017**, *5*, 1307315. [CrossRef]
22. European Commission. Economic Policy Committee. Aging Working Group. Joint Report on Health Care and Long-Term Care Systems and Fiscal Sustainability. Country Documents. European Economy. Institutional Paper 37. Luxembourg: Publications Office of the European Union. October 2016. Volume 2. Available online: http://ec.europa.eu/economy_finance/publications (accessed on 20 December 2020).
23. Autoridad Independiente de Responsabilidad Fiscal (AIReF). Evaluación del Gasto Público 2018. Proyecto 2 (Recetas). Estudio Medicamentos Dispensados a través de Receta médica. 2018. Available online: https://www.airef.es/wp-content/uploads/2019/06/Estudio2-SR/Estudio-Proyecto-2-final.pdf (accessed on 20 December 2020).
24. NHS England. Principles for Sharing the Benefits Associated with more Efficient Use of Medicines not Reimbursed through National Prices. 2014. Available online: https://www.england.nhs.uk/wp-content/uploads/2014/01/princ-shar-benefits.pdf (accessed on 12 February 2021).
25. Mestre-Ferrandiz, J.; Towse, A.; Berdud, M. Biosimilars: How Can Payers Get Long-Term Savings? *PharmacoEconomics* **2016**, *34*, 609–616. [CrossRef]
26. Delgado Sánchez, O.; Terrasa Pons, J.; Ginard Vicens, D.; Sampol Mayol, A. Medicamentos biosimilares: Impacto, oportunidades y estrategias. Doce años de experiencia en Europa. *Med. Clín.* **2019**, *152*, 411–415. [CrossRef]
27. Ministère des Solidarités et de la Santé 2018. DSS/1C/DGOS/PF2/2018/42. Instruction no du 19 Février 2018 Relative à L'incitation à la Prescription Hospitalière de Médicaments Biologiques Similaires Lorsqu'ils sont Délivrés en Ville. Available online: https://solidarites-sante.gouv.fr/fichiers/bo/2018/18-03/ste_20180003_0000_0090.pdf (accessed on 12 February 2021).
28. Luley, C.; Pieloth, K. Biologika: Steuern Selektivverträge die Verordnung? *Monit. Versorgungsforschung* **2018**, 10–11. Available online: http://www.shark-patents.com/sites/default/files/2020-02/MVF06_ZDF.pdf (accessed on 12 February 2021).
29. Simon Kucher. Payers' Price & Market Access Policies Supporting a Sustainable Biosimilar Medicines Market -Final Report, Simon, Kucher & Partners. 2016. Available online: https://www.medicinesforeurope.com/wp-content/uploads/2016/09/Simon-Kucher-2016-Policy-requirements-for-a-sustainable-biosimilar-market-FINAL-report_for-publication2.pdf (accessed on 12 February 2021).
30. Regione Campania. Decreto 66 del 14/07/2016: Misure di Incentivazione dei farmaci a Brevetto Scaduto e dei biosimilari e Monitoraggio delle Prescrizioni Attraverso la piattaforma Sani.ARP. Available online: http://www.medinco.it/medinco/wp-content/uploads/2016/07/DCA-n.-66-del-14.07.2016.pdf (accessed on 12 February 2021).
31. Plevris, N.; Jones, G.R.; Jenkinson, P.W.; Lyons, M.; Chuah, C.S.; Merchant, L.M.; Pattenden, R.J.; Watson, E.F.; Ho, G.-T.; Noble, C.L.; et al. Implementation of CT-P13 via a Managed Switch Programme in Crohn's Disease: 12-Month Real-World Outcomes. *Dig. Dis. Sci.* **2019**, *64*, 1660–1667. [CrossRef]
32. Chan, A.; Kitchen, J.; Scott, A.; Pollock, D.; Marshall, R.; Herdman, L. Implementing and delivering a successful biosimilar switch programme—the Berk- shire West experience. *Future Healthc. J.* **2019**, *6*, 143–145. Available online: https://pubmed.ncbi.nlm.nih.gov/31363522/ (accessed on 12 February 2021). [CrossRef]
33. Chung, L.; Arnold, B.; Johnson, R.; Lockett, M.J. OC-038 Making the Change: Switching to 1 Infliximab Biosimilars for IBD at North Bristol NHS Trust. *Gut* **2016**, *65*, A22–A23. [CrossRef]

34. Razanskaite, V.; Bettey, M.; Downey, L.; Wright, J.; Callaghan, J.; Rush, M.; Whiteoak, S.; Ker, S.; Perry, K.; Underhill, C.; et al. Biosimilar Infliximab in Inflammatory Bowel Disease: Outcomes of a Managed Switching Programme. *J. Crohn's Colitis* **2017**, *11*, 690–696. Available online: https://pubmed.ncbi.nlm.nih.gov/28130330/ (accessed on 12 February 2021). [CrossRef] [PubMed]
35. Commissioning Framework for Biological Medicines (Including Biosimilar Medicines): NHS England. 2017. Available online: https://www.england.nhs.uk/publication/commissioning-framework-for-biological-medicines/ (accessed on 13 March 2021).
36. Best Value Adalimumab Product in the NHS. NHS England. 2018. Available online: https://www.england.nhs.uk/wp-content/uploads/2018/11/08-pb-28-11-2018-best-value-adalimumab-product-in-nhs.pdf (accessed on 13 March 2021).
37. NHS Set to Save Record £300 Million on the NHS's Highest Drug Spend. News. NHS England. 26 November 2018. Available online: https://www.england.nhs.uk/2018/11/nhs-set-to-save-record-300-million-on-the-nhss-highest-drug-spend/ (accessed on 13 March 2021).
38. Castro Beiras, A.; Escudero Pereira, J.L.; Juffe Stein, A.; Sánchez, C.M.; Bouzán, J.C. El "Area del Corazón" del Complejo Hospitalario Juan Canalejo. Una nueva forma de gestión clínica. *Rev. Esp. Cardiol.* **1998**, *51*, 611–619. Available online: http://www.revespcardiol.org/es/el-rea-del-corazon-del/articulo/326/ (accessed on 20 December 2020). [CrossRef]
39. Durán, A.; Lara, J.L.; van Waveren, M. Spain: Health system review. Health Systems in Transition, The European Observatory on Health Systems and Policies. 2006. Available online: www.sespas.es/adminweb/uploads/docs/HIT2010English.pdf (accessed on 20 December 2020).
40. Bernal-Delgado, E.; Campillo, C.; González López-Valcárcel, B. La Sanidad Pública ante la Crisis. Recomendaciones para una actuación pública sensata y responsable. Asociación de Economía de la Salud. Barcelona, España. 2011. Available online: http://aes.es/Publicaciones/DOCUMENTO_DEBATE_SNS_AES.pdf (accessed on 20 December 2020).
41. Asociación de Economía de la Salud (AES). Sistema Nacional de Salud: Diagnóstico y Propuestas de Avance. Edición Electrónica, 2014. Coordinado por Junta Directiva de AES. Available online: http://www.aes.es/Publicaciones/SNS_version_completa.pdf (accessed on 20 December 2020).
42. Beltrán, A.; Forn, R.; Garicano, L. Impulsar un Cambio Posible en el Sistema Sanitario. Madrid: McKinsey & Company y FEDEA. 2009. Available online: http://www.cambioposible.es/documentos/sanidad_cambio_posible.pdf (accessed on 20 December 2020).
43. Zornoza Pérez, J. Formas de Organización y Régimen Económico Financiero de los Servicios Públicos Sanitarios. In *La Organización de los Servicios Públicos Sanitarios: Actas de las Jornadas de Estudio Celebradas en la Universidad Carlos III de Madrid los días 10 y 11 de abril de 2000*; Parejo, L., Lobo, F., Vaquer, Y.M., Eds.; Marcial Pons: Madrid, España, 2001; Available online: https://e-archivo.uc3m.es/handle/10016/3853#preview (accessed on 20 December 2020).
44. Esteban Álvarez, A.I.; Arias Rodríguez, A. 30 años de reforma sanitaria. Situación actual y perspectivas de la gestión clínica en España. In *Revista Española de Control Externo*; Tribunal de Cuentas: Madrid, Spain, 2016; pp. 67–105. Available online: https://antonioariasrodriguez.files.wordpress.com/2018/01/recex-2016-mayo-ai-esteban-a-arias-pp-067-106.pdf (accessed on 20 December 2020).
45. Lobo, F. *La economía, la Innovación y el Futuro del Sistema Nacional de Salud*; FUNCAS: Madrid, Spain, 2017; p. 345. ISBN1 978-84-15722-67-0. ISBN2 978-84-15722-68-7. Available online: https://www.researchgate.net/publication/322421516_LA_ECONOMIA_LA_INNOVACION_Y_EL_FUTURO_DEL_SISTEMA_NACIONAL_DE_SALUD_ESPANOLA/link/5a589af80f7e9b409dc51b4d/download (accessed on 21 March 2021).
46. PwC. Diez temas Candentes de la Sanidad Española Para 2012. Dos Agendas Simultáneas: Recortes y Reformas. Temas Candentes de la Sanidad española. PwC. Madrid. 2012. Available online: https://www.pwc.es/es/.../sector.../diez-temas-candentes-sanidad-2012.pdf (accessed on 20 December 2020).
47. Repullo, J.R. La sostenibilidad de las prestaciones sanitarias públicas. In *Crisis Económica y Atención a las Personas y Grupos Vulnerables*; Presno Linera, M.A., Ed.; Procuradora General del Principado; Universidad de Oviedo: Oviedo, España, 2012.
48. Meneu, R. Experiencias de integración clínica. El equilibrio entre gestión de casos y gestión de enfermedades cuando solo existen enfermos. In *Integración Asistencial: Fundamentos, Experiencias y vías de Avance*; Ibern, P., Ed.; Masson-Elsevier: Barcelona, Spain, 2006; Available online: http://www.axon.es/axon/LibroFicha.asp?Libro=58969&T=INTEGRACION+ASISTENCIAL%3A+FUNDAMENTOS%2C+EXPERIENCIAS+Y+VIAS+DE+AVANCE (accessed on 20 December 2020).
49. Ministerio de Sanidad, Servicios Sociales e Igualdad. Proyecto de Real Decreto por el que se Regulan las Bases para Implantar las Unidades de gestión clínica en el Sistema Nacional de Salud. 10 de abril. 2015. Available online: https://transparencia.gob.es/servicios%20buscador/contenido/normaelaboracion.htm?id=NormaEVR-34525&lang=en&fcAct=2017-06-01T14:13:31.554Z (accessed on 20 December 2020).
50. Ley 11/2017, de 22 de diciembre, de Buen Gobierno y Profesionalización de la Gestión de los Centros y Organizaciones Sanitarias del Servicio Madrileño de Salud (BOCM 3 de enero de 2018). Available online: https://www.boe.es/buscar/pdf/2018/BOE-A-2018-1610-consolidado.pdf (accessed on 20 December 2020).
51. Informe AMPHOS. Avanzando en Gestión Clínica. Reflexiones de gestores y clínicos. IESE. Center for Research in Healthcare, Innovation and Management. Abbvie España. 2013. Available online: https://sedisa.net/wp-content/uploads/2018/11/2.-INFORME-AMPHOS-2014.pdf (accessed on 20 December 2020).
52. Delgado Díez, B. Gestión clínica: Una revisión sistemática. Trabajo fin de Máster del Máster Universitario de Investigación en Ciencias Socio-Sanitarias. *Curso Académico 2015–2016*. Universidad de León. 2016. Available online: https://buleria.unileon.es/bitstream/handle/10612/5674/2016_ANA%20BELEN_DELGADO%20DIEZ_1722.pdf?sequence=1 (accessed on 20 December 2020).

53. European Commission. Directive 2012/52/EU of 20 December 2012 Laying Down Measures to Facilitate the Recognition of Medical Prescriptions Issued in Another Member State Text with EEA Relevance. Available online: https://eur-lex.europa.eu/legal-content/EN/TXT/?uri=celex%3A32012L0052 (accessed on 20 December 2020).
54. Ministerio de Sanidad y Consumo. Orden SCO/2874/2007, de 28 de Septiembre, por la que se Establecen los Medicamentos que Constituyen Excepción a la Posible Sustitución por el Farmacéutico con Arreglo al artículo 86.4 de la Ley 29/2006, de 26 de julio, de Garantías y uso Racional de los Medicamentos y Productos Sanitarios. Available online: https://www.boe.es/boe/dias/2007/10/05/pdfs/A40495-40496.pdf (accessed on 20 December 2020).
55. Acha, V.; Mestre-Ferrandiz, J. Translating European Regulatory Approval into Healthcare Uptake for Biosimilars: The Second Translational Gap. *Technol. Anal. Strat. Manag.* **2017**, *29*, 263–275. Available online: https://www.tandfonline.com/doi/pdf/10.1080/09537325.2017.1285396?needAccess=true (accessed on 20 December 2020). [CrossRef]
56. Weise, M.; Bielsky, M.C.; De Smet, K.; Ehmann, F.; Ekman, N.; Giezen, T.J.; Gravanis, I.; Heim, H.-K.; Heinonen, E.; Ho, K.; et al. Biosimilars: What clinicians should know. *Blood* **2012**, *120*, 5111–5117. Available online: https://ashpublications.org/blood/article/120/26/5111/30935/Biosimilars-what-clinicians-should-know (accessed on 20 December 2020). [CrossRef] [PubMed]
57. Sarnola, K.; Merikoski, M.; Jyrkkä, J.; Hämeen-Anttila, K. Physicians' perceptions of the uptake of biosimilars: A systematic review. *BMJ Open* **2020**, *10*, e034183. [CrossRef] [PubMed]
58. Moorkens, E.; Jonker-Exler, C.; Huys, I.; Declerck, P.; Simoens, S.; Vulto, A.G. Overcoming Barriers to the Market Access of Biosimilars in the European Union: The Case of Biosimilar Monoclonal Antibodies. *Front. Pharmacol.* **2016**, *7*, 193. Available online: https://www.frontiersin.org/articles/10.3389/fphar.2016.00193/full (accessed on 20 December 2020). [CrossRef]
59. Escasany, A.A.; Cumplido, D.R. Biosimilares: Una realidad presente, ¿un futuro prometedor? *Med. Clín.* **2015**, *145*, 18–20.
60. Sociedad Española de Farmacología Clínica (SEFC). Posicionamiento Sobre Identificación, Intercambiabilidad y Sustitución de estos Fármacos Biosimilares. 2015. Available online: https://se-fc.org/wp-content/uploads/2020/10/NdP_PosicionamientoBiosimilares.pdf (accessed on 20 December 2020).
61. Sociedad Española de Hematología y Hemoterapia (SEHH). Documento de Posicionamiento sobre Fármacos Biosimilares de la Sociedad Española de Hematología y Hemoterapia. 2016. Available online: https://www.sehh.es/sala-prensa/notas-prensa/3632-documento-de-posicionamiento-sobre-farmacos-biosimilares-de-la-sociedad-espanola-de-hematologia-y-hemoterapia-sehh (accessed on 20 December 2020).
62. Sociedad Española de Oncología Médica (SEOM) Posicionamiento SEOM sobre los Anticuerpos Biosimilares. 2018. Available online: https://seom.org/seomcms/images/stories/recursos/Posicionamiento_sobre_biosimilares_mayo_2018.pdf (accessed on 20 December 2020).
63. Sociedad Española de Reumatología (SER). La SER Actualiza el Documento de Posicionamiento Sobre Fármacos Biosimilares. 2018. Available online: https://www.ser.es/la-actualiza-documento-posicionamiento-farmacos-biosimilares/ (accessed on 20 December 2020).
64. Argüelles-Arias, F.; Barreiro-de-Acosta, M.; Carballo, F.; Hinojosa, J.; Tejerina, T. Joint position statement by "Sociedad Española de Patología Digestiva" (Spanish Society of Gastroenterology) and "Sociedad Española de Farmacología" (Spanish Society of Pharmacology) on biosimilar therapy for inflammatory bowel disease. *Rev. Esp. Enferm. Dig.* **2013**, *105*, 37–43. Available online: http://www.grupoaran.com/mrmUpdate/lecturaPDFfromXML.asp?IdArt=4620479&TO=RVN&Eng=1 (accessed on 20 December 2020). [CrossRef]
65. González, N.Z.; Domínguez, A.G. El Irresistible Ascenso Del Mercado de Los Biosimilares. *Gest. Clín. Sanit.* **2018**, *20*. Available online: https://www.researchgate.net/publication/328341688_El_irresistible_ascenso_del_mercado_de_los_biosimilares (accessed on 20 December 2020).
66. Micó-Pérez, R.M.; Herrera, M.C.; Palomo-Jiménez, P.I.; Sánchez-Fierro, J.; Avendaño-Solá, C.; Llisterri-Caro, J.L. Conocimiento sobre biosimilares en Atención Primaria: Un estudio de la Sociedad Española de Médicos de Atención Primaria (SEMERGEN). *Med. Fam. Semer.* **2018**, *44*, 380–388. Available online: https://www.elsevier.es/es-revista-medicina-familia-semergen-40-pdf-S1138359318300066 (accessed on 20 December 2020). [CrossRef] [PubMed]
67. Saborido-Cansino, C.; Santos-Ramos, B.; Carmona-Saucedo, C.; Rodríguez-Romero, M.V.; González-Martín, A.; Palma-Amaro, A.; Rojas-Lucena, I.M.; Almeida-González, C.; Sánchez-Fidalgo, S. Efectividad de una estrategia de intervención en el patrón de prescripción del biosimilar glargina en atención primaria. *Aten Primaria* **2019**, *51*, 350–358. Available online: https://www.elsevier.es/es-revista-atencion-primaria-27-pdf-S0212656717305218 (accessed on 20 December 2020). [CrossRef] [PubMed]
68. Jacobs, I.; Singh, E.; Sewell, K.L.; Al-Sabbagh, A.; Shane, L.G. Patient attitudes and understanding about biosimilars: An international cross-sectional survey. *Patient Prefer Adher.* **2016**, *10*, 937–948. Available online: https://www.ncbi.nlm.nih.gov/pmc/articles/PMC4889091/pdf/ppa-10-937.pdf (accessed on 20 December 2020). [CrossRef] [PubMed]
69. Farhat, F.; Torres, A.; Park, W.; de Lima Lopes, G.; Mudad, R.; Ikpeazu, C.; Abi Aad, S. The Concept of Biosimilars: From Characterization to Evolution-A Narrative Review. *Oncologist* **2018**, *23*, 346–352. Available online: https://doi.org/10.1634/theoncologist.2017-0126 (accessed on 12 February 2021). [CrossRef]
70. Cornes, P. Variability of Biologics and its Impact on Biosimilar Development. *EMJ* **2019**, *4*, 22–30. Available online: https://www.emjreviews.com/hematology/symposium/variability-of-biologics-and-its-impact-on-biosimilar-development/ (accessed on 12 February 2021).
71. Cohen, H.P.; McCabe, D. The Importance of Countering Biosimilar Disparagement and Misinformation. *BioDrugs* **2020**, *34*, 407–414. Available online: https://link.springer.com/article/10.1007/s40259-020-00433-y (accessed on 12 February 2021). [CrossRef]

72. Vandenplas, Y.; Simoens, S.; Van Wilder, P.; Vulto, A.G.; Huys, I. Informing Patients about Biosimilar Medicines: The Role of European Patient Associations. *Pharmaceuticals* **2021**, *14*, 117. [CrossRef]
73. Gobierno de España. Ley 14/1986, de 25 de abril, General de Sanidad. 1986. Available online: https://www.boe.es/buscar/pdf/1986/BOE-A-1986-10499-consolidado.pdf (accessed on 20 December 2020).
74. Gobierno de España. Ley 41/2002, de 14 de Noviembre, Básica Reguladora de la Autonomía del Paciente y de Derechos y Obligaciones en Materia de Información y Documentación Clínica. 2002. Available online: https://www.boe.es/buscar/pdf/2002/BOE-A-2002-22188-consolidado.pdf (accessed on 20 December 2020).
75. Calleja-Hernández, M.A.; Martínez-Sesmero, J.M.; Santiago-Josefat, B. Biosimilares de anticuerpos monoclonales en enfermedades inflamatorias y cáncer: Situación actual, retos y oportunidades. *Farm Hosp.* **2020**, *44*, 100–108. Available online: https://revistafarmaciahospitalaria.sefh.es/gdcr/index.php/fh/article/view/11280/11280esp (accessed on 20 December 2020).
76. Declaración conjunta (joint statement) de Médicos y Pacientes sobre los Tratamientos con Medicamentos Biológicos Originales y Biosimilares. Encuentros Entre Médicos y Pacientes sobre Medicamentos Biológicos. Universidad Internacional Menéndez Pelayo (UIMP). Madrid, 29 March and 26 April 2017. Available online: https://www.ser.es/wp-content/uploads/2017/06/Declaraci%C3%B3n_conjunta_UIMP_final.pdf (accessed on 12 February 2021).
77. García Olaverri, C.; Huerta, E. Los sindicatos españoles: Voz e influencia en las empresas. Fundación Alternativas. Documento de trabajo 175/2011. 2011. Available online: https://www.fundacionalternativas.org/public/storage/laboratorio_documentos_archivos/76bdc1ec6a3789e97ae66ae6eabb43a3.pdf (accessed on 20 December 2020).
78. Confederación Estatal de Sindicatos Médicos (CESM). Bases Para la Gestión Clínica en el Sistema Nacional de Salud. Enero. 2014. Available online: http://pruebascesm.es/wp-content/uploads/2016/10/GESTION-CLINICA.-Documento-de-CESM.pdf (accessed on 20 December 2020).
79. Organización Médica Colegial (OMC). La gestión Clínica en el Marco del SNS. Mesa Redonda Con la Participación de Moderador Dr. Juan Manuel Garrote, Coordinador Médico de Comunicación de la OMC. Participantes: Dr. Serafín Romero, secretario general OMC.; Dr. Carlos Macaya, presidente Federación Sociedades Científico-Médicas Españolas (FACME); Dr. Tomás Toranzo, vicesecretario de CESM. Dr. Eduardo García Prieto, gerente del Servicio Castellano y Leonés de Salud (SACYL). OMC. *Rev. Oficial Cons. Gen. Col. Méd. Esp.* **2014**, *29*, 23–27. Available online: https://www.cgcom.es/sites/default/files/publication_marzo_2014.pdf (accessed on 20 December 2020).
80. Rodríguez Sendín, J.J.; Presidente de la Organización Médica Colegial (OMC). Es el momento de la gestión clínica. OMC. *Rev. Oficial Cons. Gen. Col. Méd. Esp.* **2014**, *29*, 3. Available online: https://www.cgcom.es/sites/default/files/publication_marzo_2014.pdf (accessed on 20 December 2020).
81. Inotai, A.; Kaló, Z. How to solve financing gap to ensure patient access to patented pharmaceuticals in CEE countries?—The good, the bad, and the ugly ways. *Expert Rev. Pharm. Outcomes Res.* **2019**, *19*, 627–632. [CrossRef]
82. Ebbers, H.C.; Pieters, T.; Leufkens, H.G.; Schellekens, H. Effective pharmaceutical regulation needs alignment with doctors. *Drug Discov. Today* **2012**, *17*, 100–103. [CrossRef] [PubMed]

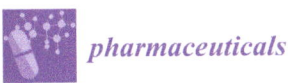

Commentary

The Off-Patent Biological Market in Belgium: Is the Health System Creating a Hurdle to Fair Market Competition?

Philippe Van Wilder

Ecole de Santé Publique, Université Libre de Bruxelles (ULB), Brussels 1050, Belgium; philippe.van.wilder@ulb.be

Abstract: We investigated the off-patent biological market in Belgium from a policy maker's perspective, in light of the Belgian pharmaceutical health system. The main barriers relate to a short-term budgetary focus, to the overwhelming innovator's reach and to a concertation model with assessment and appraisal being mixed which results in poorly effective policy measures.

Keywords: biosimilar; reference biological; competitive market; Belgium

1. Introduction

Biosimilar products have been authorised in the European union in areas such as oncology, inflammatory diseases, diabetes and haematology. As these products are authorised as having no clinically meaningful differences [1] compared to the originator products, the major benefits relate to lower prices for the payer (health insurance), following lower development costs, and in enhanced price competition in theory. The savings may serve as a healthcare budget control tool or may be invested in widening the eligible patient group or in providing access to other innovative but expensive treatments.

Many EU member states have experienced a gradual uptake [2] of biosimilar products with uptake figures [3] in 2019, easily exceeding 30% in big EU-countries while in Belgium [4,5] the uptake is incredibly low with market shares of biosimilar products being three-times lower or less.

Different authors have analysed the limited uptake of biosimilar products in Belgium and identified several factors responsible for this phenomenon. Recently, Moorkens et al. [6] provided a critical overview of these hurdles which include a lack of trust among some stakeholders, a lack of clear, persistent and consistent communication channels, a tremendous innovator's reach and the disturbing impact of a hospital financing system with incentives for high priced medicines.

In this commentary, we aim to consider the impact of the organisation of the pharmaceutical healthcare system. We believe the cumulative impact of distinct policy measures within the Belgian healthcare system is creating a strong hurdle to the access of biosimilar products.

2. Belgian Policy Initiatives to Favour Access to Biosimilar Products

Because of the low use of biosimilar products in Belgium, various policy measures aiming to impact the biosimilar uptake have been implemented. First, there is a simplified and facilitated administrative reimbursement track [7] for biosimilar products if the formal indications and conditions of use are nearly identical between biosimilar and reference biological product. In 2015, a Convention was signed by the competent authority and the main stakeholders [8], to enhance the biosimilar product uptake. This initiative included a regular monitoring of the use of biosimilar products to check this objective. In 2019, financial incentives [9] (between € 750 and € 1500) were provided towards individual prescribers of the biosimilar products of etanercept and adalimumab in the retail market. Finally, a 'best value biological' program management [10] was initiated in 2019, aiming to bring a broader perspective to the use of biological medicinal products [11].

After all of these ad hoc initiatives, the Belgian biosimilar market share evolution illustrates the lack of competition between biosimilar and biological reference product. Clearly, the biosimilar product uptake objectives are not reached at all despite these ad hoc measures.

The relationship between competent authority and pharmaceutical industry is complex and particular. In the BE Healthcare system, decision-making is based on extensive concertation with stakeholders. This allows to capture thoughts from the field and enables the decision-making to hold a balanced view of the expressed legitimate opinions, but it may lack strength because of the weighting of the impact across the stakeholders.

In my opinion, the biosimilar market uptake in Belgium suffers from a short-term narrow budgetary focus, the limits of a concertation model with mixed expert and stakeholder input which (in this field) result in poorly effective policy measures and from the overwhelming innovator's reach.

3. Some Characteristics of the Pharmaceutical Healthcare System
3.1. Short-Term Budgetary Focus

The Belgian healthcare system emphasises the short-term (pharmaceutical) healthcare budget instead of considering the healthcare budget and the longer-term efficiency. To illustrate this, I would refer to the mandatory price decreases that are applicable 12 years after the reimbursement of the reference product or at entrance of the biosimilar product, whichever comes first. These price reductions are applicable to both the reference product and the biosimilar product. The consequence of this policy measure is that there is no or limited additional saving potential between a biosimilar or biological reference product for the healthcare payer. This effect is strengthened by the hospital financing mechanism in which a lower (biosimilar) price would result in less earnings for the hospital, because the discounts offered by a manufacturer are lower if the National Institute of Health and Disability Insurance (NIHDI) list price is lower.

In some cases, the potential for price competition is even further hampered by repeated managed entry agreements (MEAs) for the reference biological product. If such a confidential MEA is still effective at the entrance of the biosimilar product, the type of agreement and the extent of the price–volume compensation is unknown to the applicant of the biosimilar product, making the biosimilar reimbursement submission a blind spot.

Price decreases go beyond 50% resulting in much desired short-term cost savings but without incentives to increase the market share of biosimilar products with the aim to facilitate longer-term competition once biosimilar products achieve substantial market volumes. A mix of off-patent reference biologics, biosimilars, and follow-up treatment alternatives, is considered critical [12] to obtain a competitive and sustainable market for long term access to biological therapy at the lowest cost. The actual regulation is applicable even if the NIHDI is aware of the risks linked to a lack of competition. On its website [13], it expresses the concern of missing future biosimilar products on the Belgian market, which may be a threat to the sustainability and control of the healthcare budget.

The already mentioned simplified reimbursement track for biosimilar products is limited to 90 days (which is half the duration of other reimbursement procedures). It builds on the similarity in the clinical and therapeutic characteristics between biological reference and biosimilar product and will mainly address the budget impact estimates, without any pharmaco-economic assessment. Cost-effectiveness analyses may be of little value in some cases but they are indicated [14] if cost differences exist between these products (administration route and costs, dosing interval, limited price differences, etc.) and if therapeutic alternatives exist on a different anatomic-therapeutic-chemical (ATC)-level, a pharmaco-economic assessment will probably result in a different relative positioning of the available products. The focus should be more directed towards disease strategy and look beyond individual medicinal products.

3.2. Mixing Assessment and Appraisal

The biosimilar market uptake is also affected by the unclear split between assessment and appraisal in the healthcare decision-making. This also affects other medicinal products. The Belgian reimbursement procedure reflects the Transparency Directive [15] requirements and starts with an internal assessment report to be delivered by day 60, followed by appraisal and proposition from the reimbursement commission by day 120 and day 150, prior to the decision of the Minister. However, in my opinion, despite the tremendous support of a dedicated team of NIHDI-experts and pharmacists, assessment and appraisal are sometimes mixed [16] instead of these being clear and distinct activities. This is mainly the consequence of having a commission of stakeholders [17] all along the procedure instead of having distinct expert assessors and stakeholder appraisers. This approach is hampering the scope of the performed assessments, resulting, too often, in limited pharmaco-economic assessments. It is limited because it is not going beyond the individual submitted dossier and because it merely criticises the applicant's submission without making own assumptions and performing own economic analyses. Until now, the impact of the economic assessment as a significant reimbursement factor, could not be demonstrated as opposed to the significant effect of the medical need and the extent of therapeutic value.

The biosimilar conundrum is a topic in which the pharmaco-economic assessment, even from a direct healthcare perspective, should go beyond the individual dossier and include elements of (lack of) future competition (especially if a lifelong time horizon is relevant). A proposal might be to strengthen the possible collaboration between the NIHDI and the formal health technology assessment (HTA) Agency which is the Federal Knowledge Centre for health (KCE). KCE has the expertise for making full HTA-reports. Assessment reports should be 'validated' by expert assessors from NIHDI and KCE and remain unchanged by the reimbursement commission of stakeholders. The Commission members should focus on the appraisal of the assessment report and discuss criteria and weights to provide a documented and informed advice to the competent Minister. Such collaboration would facilitate assessments that go 'beyond the dossier' and include longer-term considerations. Such collaboration may enable the reimbursement commission to prepare for future challenges and develop an adapted framework for oncology biological products.

3.3. Far Reaching Innovator's Reach

The biosimilar market uptake is also affected by the originator's extensive reach [6] and creative off-patent strategy. The innovative pharmaceutical industry is strongly represented in Belgium with R&D centers and/or production facilities of companies such as GlaxoSmith Kline (GSK), Johnson & Johnson, or Pfizer. GSK's site in Rixensart produces various vaccines for world-wide distribution. Pfizer manufactures in Puurs the COVID-19 vaccine Comirnaty® which is distributed across the EU and abroad. The innovative industry [18] represents an export volume of more than € 42 billion in 2018 and invested € 3.6 billion in the development of medicinal products in 2018 (R&D is facilitated by fiscal incentives).

The COVID-19 pandemic offers a marketing opportunity, certainly for the vaccine producing pharma, but also for the whole pharmaceutical sector, if the sector delivers highly valued medicinal products protecting individuals from disease and excessive mortality and making it possible for societies to reopen economic and societal activities.

This innovative industry is particularly creative to manage the off-patent hurdle. Follow-up compounds with claims of added value enter the market prior to the patent expiry and are being promoted to facilitate a shift from the biological product to the follow-up product (e.g., Janus kinase (JAK) inhibitors versus tumor necrosis factor (TNF) blockers).

The biosimilar product manufacturers should consider their own strengths and weaknesses in this 'originator' landscape. They should not only be reactive to the activities of the originator but also develop proactively own strategies, expressing their commitment towards local authorities and stakeholders (including patients), reflecting on product differentiation and investing in a tangible roadmap to achieve the objectives.

The originator is also rapidly reactive to the changing market situation. Initially, as the analysis of Dutch market data [19] illustrates, substantial price differences existed between adalimumab reference product and biosimilar products, which resulted in decreasing market shares for the adalimumab reference product. For etanercept, no or limited price differences exist and market shares of the biological reference product did not dramatically decrease.

A collateral 'benefit' of this tactical approach, is that originator and biosimilar products provide a similar amount of savings, which allows the originator industry to make the (legitimate) claim of facilitating the pharmaceutical healthcare budget control (which budget had an excessive double-digit growth in 2020).

4. The 'Best Value Biologicals' Program 2019–2020

With a less than desirable interest in longer term efficiency in the Belgian healthcare system, the claim by the originator that savings are equally resulting from reference and biosimilar products, yields a considerable threat to any future incentive for biosimilar products.

To illustrate this, the example of the 2019 'best value biologicals' program management is appealing.

The 'best value biologicals' program management, sponsored by the NIHDI and which may be considered as the initiation of a broader and sustained approach towards biological products, ended in April 2020. The program delivered to the competent authority NIHDI, a documented report including recommendations with suggested follow-up measures aiming to create a level playing field for biosimilar and biological reference products in Belgium. Briefly, the report's recommendations referred, among others, to extensive and repeated communication and education channels on biological products to healthcare providers and patients, to smoothen the lengthy and complex tendering process in hospitals, to consider gain sharing mechanisms (sharing the healthcare savings with those enabling them) and a specific recommendation on setting market share quota for biosimilar products.

However, the coronavirus pandemic interfered strongly and obviously modified healthcare priorities.

Still, the report's recommendations were endorsed later, in October 2020, by the General Council of the NIHDI [20] in their approval of the 2021 federal healthcare budget. However, the wording used by the General Council was particular: when it comes to the intention to stimulate the use of biosimilar products, a condition is set and the wording ends with 'with non-discriminatory incentives'.

The General Council inserted the 'no discrimination' condition, prior to any concrete policy measure being written. For initiatives relating to biosimilar product uptake, an a priori condition is already 'adopted', prior to making clear how the policy measure should be conceived and implemented. No other healthcare initiative in the text of the General Council is linked to a non-discriminatory criterion.

Maybe, the proposal to use quota for uptake of biosimilar products is perceived as 'discriminatory' by some General Council members. However, quota is used by other EU Member States. At the EC-workshop of October 2019 on biosimilar products [21], various Member States shared their experience on the effectiveness of local policy measures. France [22] explained their positive pilot experience with quota for biosimilar products which resulted in increased biosimilar market shares. This enabled them to reach a competitive level playing field between original and biosimilar biological products. The French experience was acceptable for the EC, because the economic rationale was clear and unambiguous and the quota policy was limited in time under strict conditions.

5. Conclusions

By having the 'with no discriminatory incentives' written in the General Council document, any forthcoming policy measure creating incentives for the uptake of biosimilar products will be challenged on this condition. The perception of discrimination is made and any initiative having a purpose to enhance uptake of biosimilar products will not only need to be valid for that purpose, but also reverse the created perception. The formulation of the various recommendations and the implementation of concrete measures will probably be an uphill battle, with opportunity for the originators to have lengthy discussions on the compliance of each measure with the non-discrimination condition. In my understanding, some of the proposed recommendations giving incentives to biosimilar products may be differential but not discriminatory, because they are limited in time and are proposed to create a level playing field for both type of biological products, which is hardly the case at patent expiry of the reference biological product. It will be important to refer to the international examples to reverse the perception of discrimination already linked to upcoming incentives.

At stake are the availability of the next biosimilar products in Belgium and the shift towards a real competitive market. The expected future savings in oncology and rare diseases, to be triggered by the local availability of biosimilar products, may be reduced and/or delayed. Non-differential mandatory price decreases do and will not resolve the conundrum of the biosimilar market uptake. Policy makers in Belgium should focus on the longer-term health economic assessment and strengthen the economic assessment capacity and scope (i.e., going broader and beyond the individual dossier). This is much needed to achieve a level playing field for biosimilar products in Belgium, 15 years after the first introduction in the EU.

Funding: This research received no external funding.

Institutional Review Board Statement: Not applicable.

Informed Consent Statement: Not applicable.

Data Availability Statement: Not applicable.

Conflicts of Interest: The thoughts and opinions expressed in this article reflect the personal work experience of the author as healthcare consultant for private pharmaceutical companies and for public institutions. The expressed thoughts, opinions and policy proposals are given at personal title, with no responsibility for the private companies and the public institutions, nor for the actual or former employers of the author.

References

1. European Medicine Agency. Biosimilar Medicines: Overview. Available online: https://www.ema.europa.eu/en/human-regulatory/overview/biosimilar-medicines-overview#biosimilar-development-and-approval-in-the-eu-section (accessed on 25 March 2021).
2. IQVIA. 2019 IQVIA Report—The Impact of Biosimilar Competition in Europe. 2019. Available online: https://ec.europa.eu/docsroom/documents/38461 (accessed on 25 March 2021).
3. Medaxes. Medaxes Verwelkomt Taskforce Biosimilars. Actualiteit 07/02. Available online: https://www.medaxes.be/nl/actualiteit/medaxes-verwelkomt-taskforce-biosimilars (accessed on 25 March 2021).
4. Vandenplas, Y.; Simoens, S.; Van Wilder, P.; Vulto, A.G.; Huys, I. Off-Patent Biological and Biosimilar Medicines in Belgium: A Market Landscape Analysis. Available online: https://www.frontiersin.org/articles/10.3389/fphar.2021.644187/abstract (accessed on 26 March 2021).
5. Van Haecht, K.; Lebbe, C.; Ntahonganyira, R.M. Analyse van het Gebruik van Biosimilars bij CM-Leden in 2019. Available online: https://www.cm.be/media/CM-Info-Geneesmiddelen_tcm47-69788.pdf (accessed on 31 March 2021).
6. Moorkens, E.; Vulto, A.G.; Huys, I. Biosimilars in Belgium: A proposal for a more competitive market. *Acta Clin. Belg.* **2020**. [CrossRef] [PubMed]
7. NIHDI. Richtlijnen Aanvraag tot Opname in de Terugbetaling van een Biosimilaire Specialiteit. Available online: https://www.inami.fgov.be/nl/professionals/andere-professionals/farmaceutische-industrie/Paginas/default.aspx#Richtlijnen_voor_het_indienen_van_CTG_dossiers (accessed on 25 March 2021).
8. NIHDI. Convenant "Doorstart voor Biosimilaire Geneesmiddelen in België". Available online: https://www.inami.fgov.be/nl/themas/kost-terugbetaling/door-ziekenfonds/geneesmiddel-gezondheidsproduct/geneesmiddel-voorschrijven/Paginas/biosimilaire-geneesmiddelen.aspx (accessed on 25 March 2021).
9. NIHDI. Biosimilaire Geneesmiddelen: Incentive Voor het Voorschrijven van Biosimilaire Geneesmiddelen Buiten het Ziekenhuis. Available online: https://www.inami.fgov.be/nl/themas/kost-terugbetaling/door-ziekenfonds/geneesmiddel-

gezondheidsproduct/geneesmiddel-voorschrijven/Paginas/biosimilaire-geneesmiddelen-buiten-ziekenhuis.aspx (accessed on 25 March 2021).
10. NIHDI. Best Value Biologicals Program Management. Report. Available online: https://gbiomed.kuleuven.be/english/research/50000715/52577001/research/publications (accessed on 31 March 2021).
11. NIHDI. Biosimilaire Geneesmiddelen: Aanzienlijke Besparingen voor het Gezondheidszorgsysteem. Available online: https://www.inami.fgov.be/nl/themas/kost-terugbetaling/door-ziekenfonds/geneesmiddel-gezondheidsproduct/geneesmiddel-voorschrijven/Paginas/biosimilaire-geneesmiddelen-belangrijk-besparingen.aspx (accessed on 25 March 2021).
12. Simoens, S.; Vulto, A.G. A health economic guide to market access of biosimilars. *Expert Opin. Biol. Ther.* **2021**, *21*, 9–17. [CrossRef] [PubMed]
13. NIHDI. Available online: https://www.inami.fgov.be/nl/themas/kost-terugbetaling/door-ziekenfonds/geneesmiddel-gezondheidsproduct/geneesmiddel-voorschrijven/Paginas/biosimilaire-geneesmiddelen.aspx (accessed on 25 March 2021).
14. Moorkens, E.; Broux, H.; Huys, I.; Vulto, A.G.; Simoens, S. Economic evaluation of biosimilars for reimbursement purposes—What, when, how? *J. Mark. Access Health Policy* **2020**, *8*, 1739509. [CrossRef] [PubMed]
15. Council Transparency Directive 89/105/EEC. Available online: https://eur-lex.europa.eu/legal-content/EN/TXT/?uri=CELEX%3A31989L0105 (accessed on 26 March 2021).
16. European Parliament, Directorate general for internal policies; Van Wilder, P.; Mabilia, V.; Cavaco, Y.K.; McGuinn, J. Towards a Harmonised EU Assessment of the Added Therapeutic Value of Medicines. Study for the ENVI Committee. 2015. Available online: https://www.europarl.europa.eu/RegData/etudes/STUD/2015/542219/IPOL_STU(2015)542219_EN.pdf (accessed on 25 March 2021).
17. NIHDI. Composition of the Commission on the Reimbursement of Medicines. Available online: https://www.riziv.fgov.be/nl/riziv/organen/Paginas/commissie-tegemoetkoming-geneesmiddelen.aspx#Wat_is_de_samenstelling_van_de_CTG? (accessed on 25 March 2021).
18. Gerkens, S.; Merkur, S. Belgium: Health system review. *Health Syst. Transit.* **2020**, *22*, 1–237. [PubMed]
19. Vulto, A.G.; de Vos Burchart, H. Worden de Biosimilar-Beloften in Nederland Waargemaakt? Een Gedetailleerde 5-Jaar Analyse van de Nederlandse Markt van een Selectie van Biologische Geneesmiddelen (2014–2018). IVM 2019. Available online: https://www.biosimilars-nederland.nl/wp-content/uploads/2020/01/2019_11_24-Biosimilar-beloften-waargemaakt_BOM-rapportage-met-GIP_en_ACM_def_AGV_HdVB.pdf (accessed on 2 April 2021).
20. NIHDI General Council. *Note CGSS 2020/066 Budget des Soins de Santé 2021*; NIHDI: Brussels, Belgium, 2020.
21. European Commission. Directorate-General for Internal Market, Industry, Entrepreneurship and SMEs. Multi-Stakeholder Workshop on Biosimilar Medicinal Products: A Follow-up Event to the Process on Corporate Responsibility in the Field of Pharmaceuticals. Summary. 2019. Available online: https://ec.europa.eu/growth/content/fifth-stakeholder-conference-biosimilar-medicines_en (accessed on 25 March 2021).
22. Ministère des solidarités et de la santé. Ministère de l'action et des Comptes Publics. Directorate of Social Security. Pharmaceuticals and Medical Devices Unit. Promoting the Use of Biosimilars in France. 2019. Available online: https://ec.europa.eu/docsroom/documents/38047 (accessed on 25 March 2021).

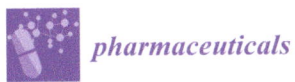 *pharmaceuticals*

Article

Off-Patent Biologicals and Biosimilars Tendering in Europe—A Proposal towards More Sustainable Practices

Liese Barbier [1,*], Steven Simoens [1], Caroline Soontjens [1], Barbara Claus [2], Arnold G. Vulto [1,3] and Isabelle Huys [1]

1. Department of Pharmaceutical and Pharmacological Sciences, KU Leuven, 3000 Leuven, Belgium; steven.simoens@kuleuven.be (S.S.); caroline.soontjens@student.kuleuven.be (C.S.); a.vulto@gmail.com (A.G.V.); isabelle.huys@kuleuven.be (I.H.)
2. Pharmacy Department, Faculty of Pharmaceutical Sciences, UZ Gent, 9000 Gent, Belgium; barbara.claus@uzgent.be
3. Hospital Pharmacy, Erasmus University Medical Center, 3015 CN Rotterdam, The Netherlands
* Correspondence: liese.barbier@kuleuven.be

Abstract: Background: In Europe, off-patent biologicals and biosimilars are largely procured by means of tender procedures. The organization and design of tenders may play a key role in the evolving biosimilar market, and currently, it is not fully elucidated how tenders for off-patent biologicals and biosimilars are designed and if approaches are aligned with sustaining market competition and societal savings for healthcare systems over the long term. This study aims to (i) explore the design and implementation of tender procedures for off-patent biologicals and biosimilars in Europe, (ii) identify learnings for sustainable tender approaches from purchasers and suppliers, and (iii) formulate recommendations in support of competitive and sustainable tender practices in the off-patent biologicals market. Methods: A mixed methods design was applied. A quantitative web-survey was conducted with hospital pharmacists and purchasers (N = 60, of which 47 completed the survey in full), and qualitative expert-interviews with purchasers and suppliers (N = 28) were carried out. Results: The web survey results showed that the organization and design of tenders for off-patent biologicals and biosimilars, and the experience of hospital pharmacists and purchasers with this, considerably varies on several elements across European countries. From the qualitative interviews, signals emerged across the board that some of the current tender approaches might negatively affect market dynamics for off-patent biologicals and biosimilars. The focus on generating short-term savings and existence of originator favouring tender practices were identified as elements that may limit timely competition from and market opportunity for biosimilar suppliers. The need to optimize tender processes, considering a more long-term strategic and sustainable view, was expressed. In addition, challenges appear to exist with differentiating between products beyond price, showing the need and opportunity to guide stakeholders with the (appropriate) inclusion of award criteria beyond price. Due to the variety in tender organization in Europe, a 'one size fits all' tendering framework is not possible. However, on an overarching level, it was argued that tender procedures must aim to (i) ensure market plurality and (ii) include award criteria beyond price (warranted that criteria are objectively and transparently defined, scored and competitively rewarded). Depending on the market (maturity), additional actions may be needed. Conclusions: Findings suggest the need to adjust tender procedures for off-patent biologicals and biosimilars, considering a more long-term strategic and market sustainable view. Five main avenues for optimization were identified: (i) safeguarding a transparent, equal opportunity setting for all suppliers with an appropriate use of award criteria; (ii) fostering a timely opening of tender procedures, ensuring on-set competition; (iii) ensuring and stimulating adherence to laws on public procurement; (iv) securing an efficient process, improving plannability and ensuring timely product supply and (v) safeguarding long-term sustainable competition by stimulating market plurality.

Citation: Barbier, L.; Simoens, S.; Soontjens, C.; Claus, B.; Vulto, A.G.; Huys, I. Off-Patent Biologicals and Biosimilars Tendering in Europe—A Proposal towards More Sustainable Practices. *Pharmaceuticals* **2021**, *14*, 499. https://doi.org/10.3390/ph14060499

Academic Editor: Jean Jacques Vanden Eynde

Received: 19 March 2021
Accepted: 14 May 2021
Published: 24 May 2021

Publisher's Note: MDPI stays neutral with regard to jurisdictional claims in published maps and institutional affiliations.

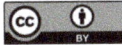

Copyright: © 2021 by the authors. Licensee MDPI, Basel, Switzerland. This article is an open access article distributed under the terms and conditions of the Creative Commons Attribution (CC BY) license (https://creativecommons.org/licenses/by/4.0/).

Keywords: tender; procurement; off-patent; biological; biosimilar; award criteria; switching; interchangeability; sustainability; competition

1. Introduction

Biological medicines represent a growing share of the total pharmaceutical spend, primarily driven by their high prices and increasing use and as such place a growing pressure on healthcare budgets [1]. In Europe, in 2018, over 30% of pharmaceutical expenditure was on biological medicines, totalling approximately EUR 53 billion [2].

With the expiration of patents and other exclusivity rights for numerous block-buster biological medicines, interest in the development and commercialization of biosimilars rose [3]. Biosimilars are products that are similar to an already authorized biological product, the originator product, with regards to quality, safety and efficacy [4]. The EU has the most mature biosimilar market at present, with 57 biosimilars approved for 16 distinct molecules across various therapeutic areas such as rheumatology, gastroenterology and oncology [5]. The biosimilar market is rapidly evolving and the number of approved biosimilars is expected to grow over the following years [6]. Biosimilars pose an opportunity for healthcare systems to foster competition following the originator's loss of market exclusivity and lower spending on biological medicines while safeguarding safe and effective treatment. Of the total spend on biological medicines in the EU, 21% is now exposed to biosimilar competition (EUR 12 billion yearly) [2]. Biosimilar market entry has shown to lead to significant price reductions and increased patient access to biological therapies [3,7]. The 2020 IQVIA *The Impact of Biosimilar Competition in Europe* report showed that, based on list-price changes, biosimilar market entry has led to an overall 5% reduction in the total EU drug budget spending since 2014 [8].

On a pan-European level, moderate biosimilar uptake and considerable price reductions have been achieved. The experience of individual countries, regions and hospitals with biosimilars differs however considerably, which might be partly explained by the differences in biosimilar policies between and within countries [3,9].

To face budgetary pressures, cost-containment measures have been introduced by European payers to reduce pharmaceutical spending [10]. Tender practices are of specific interest as cost-containment measure in the context of off-patent biological and biosimilar procurement as they make use of supplier competition. Tendering is defined as a formal and predefined procedure in which multiple suppliers enter a contract competition, with the aim to select a best value for money medicine or medicines [10–12]. A tender procedure is generally applied to procure medicines when alternatives or equivalents for a specific medicine are available, which is the case for off-patent (originator) biological medicines and biosimilars. Hospital medicines, including most biologicals, should generally be procured by means of tenders in Europe. Public hospitals or non-public hospitals that are considered as bodies governed by public law should in principle organise tenders according to the harmonised EU rules on public procurement [13]. The EU rules are transposed into national legislation and apply to tenders whose monetary value exceeds a certain amount [14,15]. In tender procedures, price reductions beyond (mandatory) decreases at list-price level can be achieved. Together, these allow healthcare systems to optimize spending on off-patent biologicals and biosimilars. In addition to stimulating price competition, tenders may incentivize suppliers to compete on product or service differentiation, creating additional value for the patient and/or the care process.

When organized and applied in an appropriate way, tendering can be an efficient procurement mechanism, providing equal access to the different suppliers on the market and fostering competition between them, creating an opportunity for healthcare systems to contain expenditure and/or achieve savings that can be invested in other areas of care while possibly creating additional value for patients and care processes [12]. However, questions exist around the effective organization and application of tender procedures and significant variation exists in the organization of such tenders across European Member States, regions and purchasing groups [10,16–19]. The way how tender procedures are designed may have important implications on pharmaceutical market competition over the longer term [12,20–22]. Tender design elements such as the level on which tenders are organized, the number of winners, the tender duration and selection-and award criteria are important in this.

The importance of effective biosimilar competition for healthcare systems, together with emerging questions regarding the sustainability of tender approaches, the application of award criteria beyond price and the long-term viability of biosimilar commercialization [2,23], poses a timely opportunity to assess current tender practices for off-patent biologics and biosimilars and considerations regarding its possible influence on dynamics in the off-patent biologics market in Europe.

This study aims to (i) explore the design and implementation of tender procedures by contracting authorities for off-patent biologicals and biosimilars and (ii) identify stakeholders' learnings and components for sustainable tender approaches, to in the end (iii) formulate proposals in support of competitive and sustainable tendering practices, supporting long-term presence of different competitors and accompanying benefits for healthcare systems. Table 1 provides manuscript highlights.

Table 1. Highlights.

What is already known about the topic?
• The organization and implementation of tendering of off-patent biologicals and biosimilars varies across European Member States, regions and purchasing groups.
• The organization and design of tenders may play a key role in the evolving biosimilar market. It is not fully elucidated how tenders for off-patent biologicals and biosimilars are designed, and if approaches are aligned with sustaining market competition and societal savings for healthcare systems over the long term.
What does the paper add to existing knowledge?
• This mixed methods study reports quantitative results derived from a survey among purchasers and hospital pharmacists regarding the application of tenders and qualitative insights from expert-interviews with suppliers and purchasers.
• This paper puts forth an actionable framework with proposals that could contribute towards a more sustainable organization and application of tenders for off-patent biological medicines and biosimilars in Europe.
What insights does the paper provide for informing health care-related decision-making
• Findings may inform and support purchasers, suppliers and policymakers regarding the organization and optimization of tender procedures for off-patent biologicals and biosimilars.
• Tender procedures must aim to (i) ensure market plurality and (ii) include award criteria beyond price (warranted that criteria are objectively and transparently defined, scored and competitively rewarded). Depending on the market (maturity), additional actions are considered needed.

In this manuscript, the term "off-patent biologicals" refers to reference biologicals that lost patent protection and are exposed to competition from biosimilar alternatives.

2. Results

2.1. Survey Results—Organization and Design of Tenders for Off-Patent Biologicals and Biosimilars

In total, 60 hospital pharmacists and purchasers participated in the web-survey. The number of participants varied throughout the survey due to survey logic and participant drop-out. Forty-seven respondents completed the survey in full. Survey participants' characteristics are shown in Table S1 in Supplementary Materials. In general, survey results showed that the implementation and design of tenders for off-patent biologicals varied on several elements.

2.1.1. Perceptions about the Tender Organization

The majority of participants (61%) indicated their organisation to have moderate to extensive *experience* with tendering for biological medicines. Hospital pharmacists (88%), physicians (68%) and a procurement office (67%) were indicated to generally participate in formulating the tender conditions and subsequent product selection. A similar proportion of participants mentioned that differences (44%) and no differences (46%) exist between tender procedures applied for biologicals and small molecule medicines.

When tendering for biological medicines, 60% of participants identified *questions* about interchangeability and switching between biological reference products and biosimilars as challenging. Participants also identified the formulation of appropriate award criteria (25%), supply chain reliability (23%) and the formulation of criteria to select viable suppliers (19%) as challenges when tendering for biologicals. About one fifth of participants indicated to not identify specific challenges with tendering for biological medicines, different from those experienced with tendering for medicines in general. Full survey results are shown in Table S2 in Supplementary Materials.

2.1.2. The Tender Design

The reported *average tender duration* varied substantially. Over one quarter of participants (27%) indicated that tender agreements are made for one up to two years. Approximately 20% of participants indicated that tender agreements last between six months and one year, and a similar number indicated tenders to last between two and three years. Tenders shorter than 6 months (12.5%) or longer, between 3 and 4 years (12.5%) appear less common. Approximately half of participants (55%) indicated that contracts can be *reopened after loss of exclusivity* of the tendered originator product.

Almost half of participants (46%) indicated that tenders are generally awarded to a single *winner*. The same proportion of participants indicated that both single and multiple winner constructs are possible. Only 9% indicated to organize tenders with multiple winning suppliers.

Over half of participants (56%) indicated that the *physician's voice* is incorporated in the tender procedure as being part of the tendering committee. According to 68% of participants, physicians can request a motivated exception to prescribe a different product than the tendered product. Only 10.5% indicated that physicians *maintain therapeutic freedom* to prescribe a different product than the tendered product. Full survey results are shown in Table S3 in Supplementary Materials.

2.1.3. Application of Selection and Award Criteria

According to 68% of participants, no meaningful *differences* exist in the selection criteria applied in tender procedures for small molecule and biological medicines. Similarly, 60% of participants indicated that there are no differences in the award criteria for biological medicines and those for small molecule medicines while 33% made a distinction.

In terms of applied *selection criteria* (when applicable), 27% indicated to consider the financial viability of the supplier. One fifth of participants indicated to consider the supplier's reputation and the supplier's production capacity. To a lesser extent, participants indicated to consider the supplier's track record of previous tenders (16%), previous collaboration (12%), the duration that the supplier already markets the product (8%), the market share of the product (6%) and the supplier's investment in academic research (4%).

In terms of applied *award criteria besides price*, the product's registered indications (49%), the product's stability/shelf life (45%), the product's delivery device (35%) and the packaging (35%) were indicated to be generally considered. In terms of award criteria related to supply, 41% of participants indicated to consider the supply conditions and 29% the emergency delivery and 24/7 reachability of the supplier. Almost a quarter (22%) of participants indicated to award on additional efficacy and/or safety data (in addition to the data required for regulatory approval, such as clinical data in an additional patient population, or switching data). Value added services (e.g., supporting educational activities, product training programs, information brochures for HCPs or patients about the product, support with switching from the medicinal product previously used) (18%), customer support (14%) and expenses incurred from switching from the previous winner (6%) were considered to a lesser extent.

The *relative weight given to price* when awarding the tender varied among participants. The majority of participants indicated that a certain weight was given to award criteria besides price (predominately awarded on price (38%), a 50/50 distribution between price and other criteria (19%), predominately on other criteria besides price (19%)). Approximately 20% of participants indicated tenders to be awarded entirely on price.

When formulating *award criteria*, a large number of participants indicated to do so in collaboration with or advice from experts within their own organization (70%). Over half of participants indicated to base themselves on previous experience and almost half to base themselves on national or European guidelines. Thirteen percent of participants indicated to formulate award criteria in collaboration with or advice from (one of) the suppliers. Full survey results are shown in Table S4 in Supplementary Materials.

2.1.4. Interchangeability and Switching Considerations in the Context of Tenders

For the formulation of the tender, over half of participants deemed biosimilars interchangeable with their reference product, while 28% believed this depends on the product class and 13% indicated that biosimilars and their reference product are not interchangeable. The majority of participants (68%) indicated that biosimilars and the reference product are grouped in the same lot. According to 43% of participants, no *difference* is made between bio-naïve patients and patients already under treatment with the biological medicine when tendering for biological medicines, with 36% indicating that a difference is made. When the patient already undergoes treatment with the previous winner, approximately half of participants indicated that the option is foreseen to keep patients on therapy with the previous winner. This was indicated to be realized via a multiple winner tender, i.e., there are multiple winners, and one of them is the previous winner (29%), direct procurement of the previous winner (42%) or via an existing contract with the previous winner (21%). Full survey results are shown in Table S5 in Supplementary Materials.

2.2. *Interview Results—Considerations Regarding the Design and Organisation of Tender Procedures*

In total, 28 expert-interviews were conducted. Tables S6 and S7 in Supplementary Materials provide an overview of interview participants' characteristics.

2.2.1. Considerations Regarding Tender Design Elements
Dividing Product Volume among Suppliers—Ensuring Market Plurality

Presently, tenders are often organised on a single-winner basis, in which the total tendered volume is awarded to one supplier. A *single-winner tender design* generally leads to significant discounts, certainly if the product volume is significant such as in national single-winner tenders. The generated initial price pressure has proven advantageous for healthcare systems to realize immediate large savings. However, awarding total market volume to a single winner excludes non-winning competitors from the market for the duration of the tender contract. While price-driven, single winner tenders generally translate in welcomed large initial savings for healthcare systems, these might decrease supplier plurality in the market. A proliferation and continuation of the single winner-takes-all approach may as such lead to reduced levels of competition. In addition, relying on a single or limited number of suppliers may impact the continuity of patientcare in case of product shortages. Large volume, single-winner tenders may in addition imply a potentially large time and product write-off for contenders who did not win.

Dividing the market among multiple suppliers, providing a commercial opportunity for several suppliers and ensuring *plurality in the market*, was the single most recommended intervention by interviewees towards creating more sustainable tender practices. Some hesitations were expressed by purchasers, as the organization of multiple winner tenders increases the complexity of tenders and product management in the hospital. Healthcare systems and purchaser authorities need to be equipped to accommodate and effectively organize such a multi-winner tender structure. Besides this remark, both purchasers and suppliers broadly voiced their support. Awarding tenders to multiple winners may also contribute to lower price pressure due to the smaller product volumes. In addition, it provides price reductions on all tendered products and may possibly increase the physician's therapeutic freedom to choose between different products, as such avoiding physicians using a higher-priced non-tendered product. The availability of multiple commercial products on the market may further help to mitigate supply chain issues.

Various scenarios could be explored and applied to ensure market plurality, depending on the market size and product volume. Multi-winner tenders (i.e., the tender is awarded to multiple bidders) can be organized or markets can be divided into multiple commercial single-winner opportunities (e.g., on hospital network or regional level).

To effectively organize a multi-winner tender, interviewees argued that some *conditions* need to be fulfilled. First, the tendered volume on purchaser level needs be large enough to be divided among multiple bidders. Second, from the perspective of the purchaser, purchasing capacity would need to be consolidated to increase the feasibility of organizing multi-winner tenders, as this may add to complexity and workload. Third, suppliers should be provided with a guarantee regarding the allocation of volume per supplier. A clear volume estimation per winner is needed to allow them to manage their supply chain and formulate a competitive bid. Multi-winner scenarios in which the first winner is the utilized product and other winners serve as back-up in case supply issues would occur with the first-ranked winner are to be avoided.

In countries where tendering takes place on hospital (group) level (typified by small volumes and generally small procurement teams), single-winner tender structures may be a more efficient route while still stimulating competition as multiple opportunities to win volume exist across the market.

Dividing the market volume among multiple winners on a central or regional purchasing level should not necessarily translate in the availability of multiple products on an individual hospital level. The different winners may be allocated to certain regions or hospitals, which is for example the case in England.

The advantages and conditions related to the organization of multi-winner tenders are outlined in Table 2.

Table 2. Organizing multi-winner tenders—considerations.

Advantages	Conditions
• Stimulating market presence of multiple suppliers over the longer term	• Volume at purchaser level needs to be sufficiently large to be divided among different suppliers. Alternatively, multiple single-winner opportunities can be organized in a given market to ensure supplier plurality (i.e., the approach and number of winners should be adjusted to market purchasing characteristics.)
• Offering commercial opportunity to multiple suppliers	• The purchaser's capacity needs to be sufficiently consolidated to accommodate the increased complexity and workload
• Lowering immediate steep price pressure (avoid one winner takes all), which may lead to more sustainable price dynamics over the longer term	• The allocation of volume between suppliers needs to be clear and guaranteed
• Providing price reductions on all tendered products	
• Possibly increasing physician's product choice	
• The availability of multiple commercial products on the market may help to mitigate supply issues in case shortages would occur	

Tender Award Criteria—Ensuring a Fair Design and Application

Purchasers are encouraged to award a tender based on the Economically Most Advantageous Tender (MEAT) principle, including qualitative elements linked to the tender-subject beyond price, as outlined in the EU Procurement Directive 2014/24/EU [13,24,25]. Tender procedures that solely or mainly focus on price, while delivering savings in the short term, may lead to price erosion and lower the number of competitors over the longer term. Interviewees cautioned that this could ultimately result in de novo market consolidation and increased prices in a given market.

Lowest bid procedures should be avoided, and suppliers should aim to compete sustainably *on additional elements*. Multiple European trade organizations (both originator and biosimilar oriented associations) and also the European Association of Hospital Pharmacists (EAHP) underwrite the practice to include criteria beyond price in tender procedures [20,21,26–28], as such awarding the best-value biological(s). An overview of position statements of these organizations is made available in Table S8 in Supplementary Materials. The inclusion of award criteria beyond price can lead to benefits for the patient (e.g., less painful injection) or the broader organization of care (e.g., facilitating efficient handling by means of ready-to-use preparation or pre-filled syringes). Including additional criteria besides price can furthermore contribute to countering steep price erosion identified in price-only tenders, as this would stimulate to suppliers to innovate and sustainably compete on value-adding criteria.

Four main *challenges* related to including additional award criteria emerged from the interviews. First, the inclusion of award criteria besides price appears not to be routinely included in tenders for off-patent biologicals and biosimilars. According to interviewees, price remains often the sole or dominant differentiator in tender decisions.

Second, stakeholders appear to have questions on how to exactly formulate and apply these criteria. Both purchasers and suppliers mentioned difficulties with translating the MEAT principle to applicable award criteria for off-patent biologicals and biosimilars. As stipulated in the EU Public Procurement Directive, criteria should be compliant with the principles of transparency, non-discrimination and equal treatment to allow an objective comparative assessment [13]. Any criteria that could be perceived as anti-competitive or introduce bias should be excluded from inclusion. Further, only criteria that are related and proportionate to the subject matter of the tender should be included. Caution should be exerted regarding requesting or offering additional services or benefits. In case these are not directly related to the subject matter, these should be strictly avoided. Some interviewees mentioned for example the offering or requesting of research funding. This leads to the third identified challenge related to the application of award criteria.

It appears that in some cases where additional criteria are included; these may *a priori* favour the reference product or disadvantage the biosimilar. For example, including an award criterion on the length of product market presence would structurally disadvantage recently launched products, i.e., biosimilar alternatives, compared to the reference product. Including such an award criterion could therefore be considered as an unreasonable expulsion of competition. Moreover, criteria that are not directly related to the subject-matter can steer the decision-making on non-product related factors and especially when these are disproportionally weighted in the decision. Additional product-related services are mentioned to be interpreted broadly in some instances. Requesting or offering bonuses or benefits beyond the scope of the product, such as research grants and conference support, should be strictly excluded. In Table 3, an overview of the types of criteria that should be avoided is shown. In Belgium, it was mentioned by stakeholders that the possibility to provide free goods via medical need programs might also disadvantage biosimilars, as these cannot be applied for if already been granted for the reference product.

Table 3. A selection of criteria to consider and avoid in tender procedures.

A Selection of Possible Criteria to Consider beyond Price
1. **Quality and technical related criteria** • Presentation: vial size, available concentrations/dosages strengths, vial protection, etc. • Packaging: labelling, storage volume, etc. • Storage conditions: shelf life, stability pre-post-reconstitution, stability in/out of refrigeration, etc. • Reconstitution and product administration: reconstitution time, efficient use/handling, e.g., ready to use formulation, pre-filled syringe, etc. • Indications: authorization and reimbursement status
2. **Service-related criteria** • Supply: (number of) manufacturing, packing and storage location(s), logistics arrangements, urgent delivery modalities, customer support, policy on returns/expired products, policy on strategic stocks • Value added services related to the subject matter: home delivery, nurse service at home, therapeutic drug monitoring support, training and educational support for HCPs, etc. • Environmental and sustainability criteria: sustainability/environmental company policy (production, transport), sustainability/environmental policy of subcontractors, packaging material
3. **Patient related criteria** • Product administration: (easiness of use of) device, injection pain (needle size, buffer, volume, etc.) • Patient-driven services related to the subject matter: patient support program (online disease education, device training, adherence program, etc.), patient information material
A Selection of Less Desirable Criteria to Consider
Only criteria that drive actual benefits (meaningful product differentiation, advantage for purchaser and/or patient) and are related to the subject matter should be included. The below criteria may be considered to impact the level playing field between products, to be misaligned with the biosimilarity principle and/or to be of limited value. 1. Criteria that require the product **to be already on the market for a certain period of time**, as these would naturally advantage products with longer market presence, i.e., the originator product, and disadvantage recently launched biosimilars • E.g., requiring product sales references of the previous 3 years 2. **Broad application of benefits or extra services** that are **not directly related to the subject matter** • E.g., financial resources/grants for research or financial support to attend conferences or trainings 3. Award criteria related to the **efficacy, safety or quality profile of the biosimilar product** • EMA evaluates the biosimilar candidate, once licensed there is no need to reassess the work of the regulator. Criteria should be formulated based on a full understanding of the biosimilarity principle (e.g., rewards on the extensiveness of the clinical development, although these might be convincing for clinicians, are less desirable). 4. Request for **clinical switch data** or financial support to conduct a **switch study** • This would generate an additional evidence generation hurdle beyond biosimilar licensing requirements • The national competent authority provides guidance in this regard 5. **Contract linkage** via **conditional discount offerings** or other price structuring beyond product price could limit competition • E.g., between linkage between SC and IV products, where only the IV segment is open to biosimilar competition

EMA: European Medicines Agency, HCPs: healthcare professionals, IV: intravenous, SC: subcutaneous. Consulted reference materials, besides interview transcripts: tender contracts, [29,30].

Fourth, suppliers expressed difficulty in terms of determining award criteria that would allow to truly differentiate and compete on. It was mentioned that the applied award criteria beyond price often can be relatively easily fulfilled by all suppliers. In such case, including additional criteria increases the effort and cost for the supplier, without playing a differentiating role in the allotment. Interviewees also mentioned that most criteria only temporarily offer a certain differentiation. With the increasing experience with biosimilars, the need for services in terms of educational switch support may for example wane. Moreover, competitors will prepare to meet differentiating additional award criteria in the subsequent tender rounds. Due to the comparable nature of reference biologicals and biosimilars, it may prove challenging to develop criteria on a product level that could offer differentiation over a longer term. Purchasers also alluded to the fact that the inclusion of additional award criteria should serve to drive actual added value rather than complicating interchangeability of products. To allow for appropriate evaluation of possible differentiating elements such as injection pain of the product, appropriate supporting data are needed.

From both the supplier and purchaser perspective, there is a strong request for a *framework* with general principles regarding the structuring and application of award criteria. In order to stimulate the inclusion of criteria besides price and ensure a correct application, guidance should be drafted to support involved stakeholders, especially purchasers with formulating their tenders. The EU Public Procurement Directive has set out a frame in which Member States and purchasers can operate. Further action may be needed to ensure proper translation and application of MEAT in practice on Member State and purchaser level. Relevant experts should be integrated to identify appropriate award criteria. In countries where procurement is organized on a local or individual hospital level, it may be useful for governments to provide such guidance to purchasers. Here, a flexible or semi-structured tender template could be designed to guide purchasers. Room for flexibility should be foreseen, to allow tailoring based on product-specific considerations and strategic differentiation. Such an award criteria template could be piloted with collaboration from tender authorities and governments.

Only additional criteria that drive *meaningful product differentiation*, leading to an advantage for the organization of care and/or the patient should be included. Criteria could include considerations related to various elements such as supply, packaging, product presentation, storage, reconstitution and easiness of use, licensing and product-related services. To give an example, several purchasers deemed data from stability studies a possible important differentiator for products that require reconstitution. An overview of criteria that can be taken into account is shown in Table 3. Award criteria besides price should also be *proportionally rewarded* based on the additional value created. This should enable criteria besides price to truly play a role in the allotment. Suppliers mentioned that actions are needed to include these additional criteria in the tender, otherwise potential differentiation strategies could be done in vain from the supplier perspective.

Finally, award criteria need to be *transparently formulated*, and it must be clear to participants how these will be evaluated, i.e., which weight will be given to the criteria in the decision-making, and how will they be scored.

Arguments were made that a shift to the inclusion of additional decision-making criteria may gain more attention in future tenders. As first tenders focussed on steep discounts, further discounting opportunities are finite. Including other award criteria may increasingly help differentiate between products.

Tender Frequency and (Re-)Opening of Contracts—Ensuring Timely Competition

The time between the first possible use of a biosimilar after loss of exclusivity of the corresponding originator product and its actual use should be minimized. In addition to streamlining pricing and reimbursement procedures, a *timely opening* of tender procedures is essential to avoid delays in competition and ensure swift market opportunity for biosimilar alternatives. In addition to ensuring commercial opportunity, a timely opening of tenders should be stimulated to generate savings for healthcare systems as soon as possible.

Several interviewees mentioned that in some cases tenders are opened with a *significant and unnecessary delay*. Contracts with the supplier of the reference product that still apply at the time of biosimilar market entry could possibly explain a delayed tender opening. It was hypothesized that in some cases these contracts were strategically agreed prior to biosimilar market entry to as such extend the originator's market exclusivity artificially. Another possible explanation, which was also mentioned by purchasers, links to the fact that an overview of upcoming loss of exclusivities of reference products and biosimilar market entry dates on governmental and/or purchasing level lacks.

To ensure timely competition, healthcare systems and purchasers should *anticipate and prepare* for biosimilar market entry well in advance. Horizon scanning should be performed to identify the upcoming loss of exclusivity of reference products and anticipated biosimilar market entry dates. In addition to early preparation for the opening of tenders upon loss of exclusivity of the reference product, purchasers should coordinate contracts with the originator prior to its loss of exclusivity, taking the future entry of biosimilars into account. The length of the contract with the originator prior to biosimilar market entry should thus be set accordingly and preferably/compulsory include a clause that allows reopening if a biosimilar alternative enters the market, to avoid such blocking contracts at the time of biosimilar market entry.

In essence, competition should be realized as soon as possible, providing commercial opportunity, onset savings and possibly additional benefits. Below, different *approaches* are suggested that could be suitable to translate the timely opening of tenders into practice. First, healthcare systems and purchasers could set a certain term in which for existing public contracts a new tender procedure would need to be organised. This term could be included in legislation and made mandatory, such as is the case in Italy [31]. Here, regional authorities are obliged to re-open supply agreements within 60 days after entrance of the biosimilar medicine to the market [31]. A few interviewees mentioned that it should be made (more) clear if reopening is expected with every new entrant. Opening a tender upon market entry of the first biosimilar(s) could challenge market opportunity for subsequent biosimilar entrants for the same product. On the other hand, launching a new tender upon market entry of each subsequent biosimilar should be avoided as a reopening would increase workload, possibly involve repeated switching and increase uncertainty related to the product volume. The latter may prove especially challenging for suppliers. Installing a shorter-term tender (e.g., 6 months) immediately upon market entry of the first biosimilar competitor(s), combined with a longer subsequent tender duration agreement (12–24 months) once the market has further matured in the number of competitors, could be an appropriate alternative when multiple biosimilars are expected to arrive to market in a staggered way. The combination of an on-set short term tender with a subsequent longer one, would allow direct competition, leading to immediate savings for the payer and commercial opportunity for the first biosimilar supplier(s), while avoiding a closed market for subsequent suppliers for a considerable length of time. Once the market has further crystalized in terms of number of available products (e.g., in 6 months or a year depending on estimated market entry dates), tenders for existing public contracts could be reopened. Such a combined approach is for example applied by the central purchasing body Amgros in Denmark.

The appropriate approach in terms of tender timing and frequency could be determined based on the *market-specific circumstances of the product*, such as the expected number of competitors and their anticipated dates of market entry. Tenders that are organized on a quarterly basis might create a high administrative burden for both purchasers and suppliers in addition to being undesirable from the switch perspective. On the other hand, tenders with a duration beyond two years may restrict competition from other suppliers over the longer term. Generally, a tender duration between 12 and 24 months is considered desirable in terms of stimulating market dynamics, while considering feasibility and avoiding a regular switch of patients by interviewees.

In countries where tendering is organized on a regional, purchasing group or hospital level, tender procedures could open up at varying times throughout the year, to spread commercial opportunity for suppliers and accommodate manufacturing capacity. Such a *rolling system* is in place in England, with the Tranche frameworks opening every six months in another one of the four regions [32]. A *specialist procurement office* can play an important role in organizing and coordinating the timing and duration of tender procedures for products with biosimilar competition.

A *financial stimulus* (positive or negative) could also be considered to motivate purchasing bodies/hospitals to timely organize tenders, aligning the incentives of the purchaser with these of the overall healthcare system (savings for healthcare budgets, and/or premium payers/patients). For example, in Belgium the reimbursement agency lowered the reimbursement for biologicals for which a biosimilar alternative exists with 15% to hospitals [33,34]. As margins on the negotiated price difference between the tendered price and reimbursement limit can be retained by hospitals, hospitals are motivated to organize competitive tenders to procure medicines at low net prices [35]. A similar construct exists in the Netherlands, where health insurers reimburse hospitals the list price of biologics with biosimilar competition only in part, anticipating savings based on discounts that hospitals negotiate in tender procedures [36].

Supply Conditions—Increasing Volume and Predictability to Ensure Continuity of Supply

Tender procedures need to be *efficiently managed*, to increase predictability and plannability for the supplier, which can in turn guarantee timely product supply for the purchaser. Special attention needs to be paid to the setting of product volume, lead time and supply agreements.

First, *increasing predictability* regarding the tendered volume is of benefit for both the purchaser and the supplier. It provides suppliers the ability to accurately assess the economies of scale in their bid, increase the ability of suppliers to participate in tender bidding and manage production. The latter may help to avoid undue pressures on the supply chain.

This includes *setting of reliable estimates of the volume* to be supplied, with guaranteeing a minimum volume and defining a maximum cap. Moreover, in the context of multi-winner tender structures, a clear and guaranteed (division of) volume was considered a prerequisite to allow participating bidders to plan accordingly. In addition, *clinical use guidelines* should be reviewed and revised, if needed in this context, following introduction of biosimilars to allow purchasers to correctly estimate (potentially increased) volumes for tenders. Covering an unexpected increase in demand may be difficult, as it is complex and lengthy to increase the production scale due to the complex manufacturing process of biologicals. In case no minimum volumes would be guaranteed, tenders could lead to a risk of unused stock and issues with scaling [37]. Suppliers with overstock may go for highly competitive offers in pending or subsequent tender procedures, which may lead to unsustainable market dynamics.

Second, the time between the announcement of the winner(s) and the start of the contract (first delivery), also called *lead time*, is in some instances (deemed too) short, making the first supply deadline challenging. Lead times between minimum three to six months should be respected to support the supplier's supply chain management (taking into account that decisions regarding for example packaging cannot be easily re-allocated to other markets), as such reducing the risk of delayed deliveries and shortages. In general, *early communication* regarding the timing of tender procedures and expected volumes should be promoted.

Third, although fortunately no interviewees reported supply inabilities having occurred (yet) in the context of off-patent biologicals and biosimilars, the *hedging agreements for possible supply problems* are a point of consideration. By contract, suppliers are generally obliged to compensate the difference between the tendered price and the price at which the alternative product is offered by a competing supplier, often the list price, to remediate the supply issue. Although the burden of securing and financing an alternative product should naturally not be placed on the purchaser, the supply conditions should be set in such a way that they are manageable for suppliers to achieve, i.e., based on early and accurate communication regarding timing and volume of tender. Moreover, penalties should be proportionate to the contract value and the cause of the inability to supply (force majeure/external reasons for which could not be controlled), ensuring a fair balance of risk and reward for the supplier. For example, in France, penalties are based on list price and not net price, which might lead to an unbalanced risk and reward [37]. Suppliers might decide not to participate in tenders where penalties are disproportionate, leading to reduced competition. *Dialogue* between purchasers and industry should be stimulated to establish manageable supply conditions and balanced penalties.

In the case of a supply issue in a single winner tender market, other manufacturers might not be able to cover the sudden demand and remedy a potential shortage as their production may be reduced or discontinued [37]. *Multi-winner tenders* might thus also be preferred in the context of mitigating the risk of possible medicine shortages, increasing the opportunity to source the product with another supplier. Purchasing strategies that result in steep and perhaps over the longer term unsustainable price reductions may also impact supply, as companies might economize on services such as the presence of strategic stocks. It was argued that focussing on price only may impact additional services and as such the quality of the supply chain.

A *joint tendering initiative* was set up between Norway, Iceland and Denmark in 2019 in response to the growing challenges with regard to supply security, especially for older medicines [38]. Such contracts with large volumes are likely to be prioritized by pharmaceutical companies because of the potential large gain. Such evolution may however be less advantageous on a broader level as it further consolidates the market. Cross border procurement should be reserved to situations where purchasing and supply of products can alternatively not be ensured.

2.2.2. Considerations Regarding the Organization of Tenders

Considerations Regarding Transparency about the Tender Procedure and Price

Transparency in tenders should be stimulated *throughout the procedure*. Prior to the start of the procedure, at the time of publishing, the tender format, including the eligibility and award criteria and the relative weight that is awarded to these, should be clearly communicated. Upon awarding the contract, feedback should be foreseen to the participating supplier regarding the allocation decision and their scoring. Moreover, the obligation to publish the contract award notice for contracts for which prior announcement is not needed, e.g., for exclusivity contracts (negotiated procedure without prior call for competition) with the incumbent/patent holder prior to biosimilar market entry, should be complied to increase transparency towards the biosimilar entrants. Managed entry agreements (MEAs) ask for specific attention in this regard. The confidential and opaque nature of MEAs, with also the concealment of the patent expiration date of the reference biological, hampers the market entry of biosimilar alternatives. Confidentiality provisions should be addressed to improve the design and transparency of such agreements [39].

A few interviewees argued that a *Best and Final Offer (BAFO) procedure*, which involves a negotiation or clarification on a first written offer, after which bidders are invited to submit a final offer, or any route that would provide a certain supplier to submit a second (informal) bid to surpass the offer of competitors, should be avoided. This practice may provide leeway for suppliers and purchasers to include offers or request elements that are outside the scope of the tender subject matter, as transparency lacks during the final offer made, and impact the equal opportunity setting.

The size of rebates in tender procedures is noted to vary considerably (depending on market maturity and tender volume), ranging between 10% and 90% of the list price [8]. In terms of *price transparency*, actual contract prices are seldom publicly available, hampering the insight in the size of actual rebates [8]. In Norway, where prices were made public from 1995 until 2017, prices from tender procedures are no longer made public [40]. Industry might be willing to provide larger discounts when tender prices remain confidential and list prices un-impacted. *Providing confidential discounts in tenders* is likely to be preferred over pricing strategies that lower the medicine's list price. List prices are often included in external reference pricing systems, acting as benchmark in terms of list price regulation in other European countries. Confidential tender discounts avoid such leverage in price negotiations in other jurisdictions.

Switching Considerations in the Context of Tenders—Clinical Data, Cost, Physician Freedom and Guidance

Increasingly, guidance statements from EU Member States support that prescribers can safely switch patients from a reference biological to its biosimilar [41]. Requesting *additional switching studies* could create an extra barrier for biosimilar developers and may advantage the incumbent, who does not need to gather such data, in tender procedures.

Similarly, determining and including *a switch fee per patient* in tender procedures would disadvantage the biosimilar competitor, as an additional price lowering of for example 5% would be needed to offset the switch fee. Most purchasers argue that the *cost of switching* is marginal compared to the savings that are generally generated in a tender and will as such not play a decisive role in tender decisions. Originator companies may have however some leverage in the broader procurement context, as the price of the originator product that may needed to be purchased to treat the rest population (patients that remain under treatment with the reference product) can be raised by the company in case they lose the tender contract. This could limit or offset the discount realized in the tender procedure, where the originator competes with its biosimilar (alternatives).

In addition to *guidance* regarding interchangeability and switching by authorities [41], purchasers and hospitals should receive *practical support* regarding the use of biosimilars and switching in clinical practice. Practical barriers associated with biosimilar use and uncertainty among stakeholders should be lowered. For example, in England, the NHS set-up different initiatives to educate stakeholders about biosimilars and provide guidance, with the aim of supporting safe, effective and consistent use of biologicals, including biosimilars [42,43]. In the Netherlands, some health insurers have applied a differential reimbursement, reimbursing hospitals at a premium for using biosimilars, as a benefit share between insurers and hospitals, with the aim of compensating hospitals for the time and cost investment associated with a switch [36].

Collaboration and Communication in the Context of Tenders

Collaboration among stakeholders could be stimulated to ensure the development of more sustainable tender practices. First, early involvement and agreement between the internal stakeholders at the purchasing side (i.e., dialogue between purchasers, hospital pharmacists, physicians, nurses, etc.) regarding the modalities of the tender is believed to be essential. In hospitals, this is generally organized in a Drug and Therapeutics Committee. In countries with a centrally organized procurement such as Denmark and Norway, procurement bodies work together with specialist groups or expert committees. This approach is argued to result in good agreement of physicians to prescribe the tendered medicine.

Second, collaboration *among purchaser(s) (groups)* can increase negotiating strength and add to the consolidation of expertise, professionalism and capacity which is needed to conduct efficient and high-quality tenders. Third, *communication between industry and purchasers* should be stimulated. Increased dialogue could reduce supplier uncertainties and increase efficiency for the different stakeholders involved, establishing a balanced shared risk and reward between suppliers and purchasers. This could be pursued both on the supplier and purchaser level, in the context of specific procedures (preliminary market consultations, with the prerequisite that every supplier is treated equally and receives the same information) and by stimulating dialogue between umbrella industry and purchaser associations. Position statements on the organisation of tenders for off-patent biologicals and biosimilars have been published by these associations. Table S8 in Supplementary Materials provides an overview of the main viewpoints outlined in the position statements.

In terms of optimizing communication in the tender itself, multiple supplier interviewees mentioned that the information requested in a tender procedure should be streamlined. Only information that would be essential to the tender should be included. Continuing the digitalization of tender procedures will contribute towards increasing efficiency in this regard.

Healthcare Professional Involvement and Motivation

Involving physicians in the procurement process, avoiding top-down organized tenders, may help to increase physician adherence to the tender outcome. In Norway, the high adherence among physicians to prescribe the recommended medicine may be explained by the voluntary nature of and the involvement of stakeholders throughout the tender process [44]. Informing and educating healthcare professionals about biosimilar medicines and related concepts can also help to increase acceptance of the tender outcome.

In some countries, *benefit sharing models*—in which savings generated by tender procedures and or biosimilar use are shared between purchasing bodies or payers and the hospital—are applied to incentivize stakeholders. In England, such benefit sharing is in place between the Clinical Commissioning Groups and the trust providers. The example of the University Hospital Southampton NHS, in which a 3-year benefit sharing model was applied, reported significant cost savings and investment in clinical services (such as increasing the capacity of the nurse-led service) while maintaining similar patient-reported outcomes as result of their managed switch programme from infliximab reference product to biosimilar in inflammatory bowel patients [45].

Instead of providing a positive benefit share incentive, other approaches have been reported such as the abovementioned lowering of the reimbursement level for biological medicines for which a biosimilar alternative is available in Belgian hospitals [35].

Interviewees were in favour of organizing stakeholder incentives to increase motivation among stakeholders and support them in their work but cautioned regarding implementing rewards or quota to drive biosimilar uptake in particular. Establishing quota and incentives for the *use of best-value biologicals*, which could be either the originator or one of its biosimilars, was generally deemed more appropriate in terms of establishing a level playing field.

2.2.3. Considerations Regarding the Sustainability of Tender Procedures and Their Impact on Market Dynamics

Several interviewees considered that current tender designs often focus on *maximizing short-term savings*, which they argued resulted in higher than originally anticipated price erosions. Several interviewees mentioned that the publicly reported discounts up to 70% in the Nordics established a certain precedent for subsequent price competition [23,40,46]. Although tender procedures should aim to obtain the most advantageous offer, a race to the bottom should be avoided. The majority of participants indicated that the *sustainability of current practices* should be reconsidered to ensure benefits to society and patients over the longer term.

The steep price erosion was in part attributed to the fact that companies appear to be willing to fiercely *compete on price* due to important advantages associated with winning first product volumes ("first in the market"). This would allow the supplier to gather real-world data and accustom stakeholders with their product. Early winners may also be successful in retaining the market, as the incentive to reopen soon could be low if subsequent additional savings are low and would for example not outweigh the costs (although estimated to be minimal by interviewees) and work associated with a second switch.

Moreover, originator companies appear to apply *strong defensive tactics* to maintain market share by significant price dropping. This was recognized to limit biosimilar market entry in several markets. Originator suppliers may have more leeway for pronounced discounts compared to their biosimilar counterparts due to the different stage in recuperation of development cost in the lifecycle of the product. Where biosimilar developers need to earn back biosimilar development investments upon market entry, investments are generally recouped at this stage for the originator product. Additionally, it was hypothesized that some companies lower prices to such an extent that other suppliers start to drop out. This was believed to have been the case with tender practices for adalimumab, where the originator company offered especially steep discounts in some markets. In cases where the originator swiftly dropped originator prices, originators have mostly been able to maintain a significant portion of the market.

A balance between realizing short-term savings vs. avoiding possible unintended consequences in terms of decreased competition over the mid-long term should be considered. Some markets could be more at risk than others for reduced competition, depending on the commercial opportunity in terms of volume and expected prices in the given market. Multiple suppliers believed that action is essential to prevent this evolution and cautioned that hesitations exist among developers regarding the continuation of their biosimilar programs. As counterargument, it was reasoned that not all suppliers need to remain on the market for some products, as three to four suppliers would suffice for a sustainable market environment.

In markets with high price pressure, suppliers may economize by for example reducing their emergency stock available, which adds vulnerability to the product supply chain. A race to the bottom in terms of price should be avoided. Several interviewees argued that the shortage sensitive dynamics in the off-patent small molecule market should be avoided for off-patent biologicals and biosimilars.

The development of a longer-term vision is argued to be needed, to avoid competition loss and to ensure sustainable dynamics and benefits for the healthcare system over the longer term. It was mentioned that there is a need to act now, to ensure healthcare systems and tender practices are prepared for the anticipated next wave of biosimilars reaching European markets. Collaboration between the public sector and manufacturers (umbrella organizations) is believed needed to establish such common ground and exchange of perspective. Willingness appears to exist from different parties to work towards a more sustainable framework. As several manufacturers invest in both originator and biosimilars products, consideration for sustainable tender approaches may be increasingly supported.

2.2.4. Considerations Regarding Competition Dynamics—Ensuring a Level Playing Field

As noted earlier, some tender processes appear to advantage the reference product over its biosimilar (alternatives). Suppliers can attempt to steer the structuring of the tender in their favour. Competition-limiting elements (such as considering research financing) are also reported to be pro-actively requested by purchasers, which may be explained by loyalty to and (financial) ties with the incumbent. In addition to a possible deliberate steering of tender structures to favour a certain outcome/bidder, purchasers may in some cases introduce unintentional biases due to limited (procurement) expertise, questions around the structuring or hesitations regarding biosimilars.

Examples of dynamics that favour the originator product include the delayed opening of tenders due to ongoing contracts with the originator at the time of biosimilar market entry, the application of originator favouring award criteria or offering of conditional discounts. The latter could be for example linked to the length of the contract, the ranking of the product or the offering of services that are unrelated with the subject matter of the tender, such as research financing. In the Netherlands, 20–50% of contracts were reported to include such a conditional discount structure in 2018 by a sector enquiry of the anti-Tumour Necrosis Factor product market [36,47]. Clauses that stipulate that the discounts of the competitor will be matched or renegotiated, matching the lowest offer or guaranteeing lowest price, can impact biosimilar market entry and also distort price competition, as the originator is likely to match the offer. Adding a Best and Final Offer (BAFO) round may lead to similar distortions. Contract linkage, in which offers or requests are made to provide rebates for previously delivered or contracted medicines or on a related product, in case the tender contract is won, is also reported to occur.

In case the level of price reductions offered would force biosimilar developers to compete with a price below cost of goods due to a dominant position of the originator, these can also be considered anti-competitive.

The existence of anti-competitive procurement practices warrants action. Awareness should be raised about the public procurement integrity rules; a culture of integrity should be promoted, and a better collection and analysis of data should be ensured to improve governance. Fostering the uptake of e-procurement and supporting procurers with the appropriate tools and exchange of best practice can contribute in this regard. The appropriate application of tenders should be monitored by the EU national Competition Authorities and the European Commission must support actions of EU countries in this regard [48].

2.2.5. Future Outlook of Interviewees: Possible Evolutions in Tender Organization

To contain costs, competition could be further opened up by *tendering beyond the international non-proprietary name (INN)* for biologicals, which is already applied in certain cases or settings, such as in some hospital groups in the Netherlands. Including products in a same therapeutic class, which may include in some cases branded medicines, will allow to further increase competition and could be considered as option to contain spending [49].

Tender procedures may also evolve from focussing exclusively on the product's price, to taking a more holistic approach, including the overall cost of treatment, which includes but is not limited to the medicine price. Procurement, which takes total cost of care delivery into account, also called *value-based procurement*, aims to focus on patient outcomes the product should have an impact on. Where traditional procurement may often focus on the technical specifications of the product, price and short-term benefits, value-based procurement focusses on getting a maximum patient outcome against total cost of care [50]. For instance, the total cost of the in-hospital infusion of an intravenous medicine could be compared to the cost of the patient's self-administering of an oral medicine, or to the home-administration of a subcutaneous alternative.

Another possible foreseen development in tender practices includes *subscription-model tendering*, where for well-defined patient profiles, medicine packages focussing on the broader therapeutic needs of the patient could be tendered. Some countries and regions (US, Australia, UK) are testing such subscription-based procurement models, also called the Netflix-model [51,52]. In this type of procurement model, purchasers pay a pre-agreed flat amount to the supplier, irrespective of the volume of medicines used [51]. Such approach could provide substantial benefits as it includes a capping of costs for the payer and 'derisked' revenue for the supplier. It however also increases volume uncertainty for the supplier, which could result in supply chain management challenges [53].

3. Discussion

Tender procedures warrant a careful organization, design, execution, and evaluation and if needed readjustment, to ensure that they are aligned with sustainable outcomes for patients, industry and society at large over the longer term. It is a delicate balancing between ensuring the most efficient use of public financial resources and safeguarding market opportunity for multiple suppliers, as such stimulating competition over the longer term. In addition to optimizing the spending of public funds, public procurement and the effective use of tender criteria beyond price may achieve other benefits for society, healthcare systems and patients [15].

In this mixed methods study, we sought to assess the experience with tendering procedures for off-patent biologicals and biosimilars in Europe and identify learnings from current practices, drawing from a quantitative web-survey in European purchasers and qualitative expert-interviews with both purchasers and suppliers.

3.1. Challenges in the Organization of Tenders for Off-Patent Biologics and Biosimilars

During the qualitative analysis, three main challenges arose with the organization of tenders for off-patent biological medicines and biosimilars. First, current tender practices appear to focus on realizing short-term savings. This may be explained in part by the design of the tender, which often considers only price and rewards to one single winner. Moreover, changing originator competition strategies may play a part. Whereas originator manufacturers originally appeared to protect market shares via the development of second generation or reformulated products (e.g., Humira®'s new formulation launch aimed for less injection pain, or the subcutaneous versions of Herceptin® and MabThera®), strategies have shifted and include increased competition on price [2]. From the payer's perspective, one could argue that cost savings are realized in such a scenario, regardless of any biosimilar uptake. Considering biosimilar market entry as leverage to encourage a price cut from the incumbent (via a mandated list price decrease or discounts in tender procedures) may be a successful strategy in the short-term in terms of realizing savings. However, over the mid-long term, this is likely to lead to opposite effects due to market impoverishment.

The second main identified challenge pertains to the fact that tender processes were in some cases argued to advantage the reference product over its biosimilar (alternatives). This could be both deliberately or unintentionally driven, possibly because of stakeholder preference to continue with the reference product due to brand loyalty and/or additional benefits and/or issues with the design of the tender due to limited expertise with procurement of off-patent biologicals and biosimilars. While including additional award criteria provides the opportunity to compete more sustainably on value-adding elements besides price, it also gives room for possible steering.

Third, including award criteria beyond price appears to be challenging in practice. Purchasers expressed difficulties to find the right balance between award criteria which allow to differentiate and which are non-discriminatory. From both the survey and expert-interviews, guidance appears to be needed on how to design tenders for off-patent biologicals and biosimilars and especially how to formulate appropriate award criteria. Only when truly differentiating and value-adding criteria are identified, included, objectively assessed and proportionally rewarded in the tender, the concept of MEAT can be successfully implemented and play a role in the allotment.

3.2. Five Main Avenues for Optimization

Based on the stakeholder insights from this study, we conclude with proposals on five identified main avenues for optimization of public procurement processes for off-patent biologicals and biosimilars: (i) safeguarding a transparent, equal opportunity setting for all suppliers; (ii) fostering a timely opening of tender procedures, ensuring on-set competition; (iii) ensuring and stimulating adherence to laws on public procurement; (iv) securing an efficient process, improving plannability and ensuring timely product supply and (v) safeguarding long-term sustainable competition. Table 4 outlines these avenues for tender optimization.

Generally, stimulating market plurality, enabling market opportunity for multiple products, is considered to be the cornerstone towards creating a more sustainable and competitive tender market by stakeholders. This is in line with the findings of the KPMG cross-country analysis into the delivery of healthcare in hospitals by optimized utilization of medicines [37] and is supported by position statements of various industry umbrella organizations (Table S8). To realize the objective of sustained product plurality, several Member States and regions have been actively pursuing new approaches from which best practices can be derived, such as the Commissioning Framework for biological medicines in England and the changes in the Italian legal framework related to biosimilars [31,54,55].

Overall, a combined action of all actors; suppliers, pharmaceutical industry associations, purchasers, payers, governments and competition authorities, is required to promote and strengthen the competition between off-patent biological medicines and biosimilars via tenders, and by extension establishing effective, healthy market dynamics. This requires a combination of practical and policy changes, involving alterations at purchaser level but also in the policy framework. Policymakers should set out a tender policy strategy, with appropriate organizational structures and stakeholder management to ensure adherence to public procurement rules. In addition to changes to the policy framework, any perverse incentives in the financing structure of purchaser bodies should be revised to ensure a level playing field. A combination of guidance (with initiatives such as horizon scanning, a tender template, award criteria framework and feedback systems), transparent reporting on the structuring and evaluation of tender procedures and monitoring and feedback from governments or competition authorities will be necessary to sensitize stakeholders in this regard.

In general, monitoring the application of the tendering policy and subsequent changes in market dynamics is warranted, together with adapting its design if needed. National authorities should actively support purchasers with the appropriate application of tender procedures and introduction of award criteria, by providing the necessary guidance and feedback. Policy makers, purchasers and pharmaceutical industry associations should take action to collaboratively develop tender frameworks that include award criteria beyond price. For example, medical devices industry associations were successful in stimulating dialogue and collaborating with contracting authorities in order to develop a methodology to encourage the uptake of value-based procurement throughout the EU [56,57].

Moreover, guidelines for biosimilar use to increase confidence and lower hurdles with the use of biosimilars [58] and an active promotion of best-value biological use by developing proper stakeholder incentivization schemes are warranted [9,55,59,60].

As exemplified by both the survey and interview data, the design and execution of tenders for off-patent biologicals and biosimilars varies across European countries, regions and hospitals. As the tender landscape is variable across Europe, measures need to be adapted to country, region and setting specific needs. The results from the expert-interviews suggest that countries in which procurement is organized on a more local or hospital individual level, where there is more flexibility and individual purchaser freedom in the design and structuring of the tender, would especially benefit from increased guidance on tender and award criteria design. European regions, where tenders are organized with a central or regionally coordinated approach, such as for example England, were generally considered to have a well thought out procurement strategy and high level of tender expertise by interviewees. In addition to a consolidation of expertise, a more central or coordinated organization of tenders aggregates purchasing needs, as such freeing up resources and time while increasing buying power.

The diverse approaches and outcomes with relation to the market entry of adalimumab biosimilars in the European countries included in the study illustrates again the diversity in healthcare systems and procurement practices across Europe. For example, NHS England and Amgros (the Danish procurement body) sought strategies to ensure rapid biosimilar adoption and generate immediate savings [54,61]. In Norway and the Netherlands, the originator manufacturer was able to retain market share by offering steep discounts [62]. Although the biosimilar market entry of adalimumab biosimilars may have been a unique casus, as a multitude of competitors were lined up to enter simultaneously the market to compete with the number one blockbuster drug worldwide, lessons can be derived, such as the importance of well in advance preparing and planning for biosimilar market entry [54,55].

3.3. Strengths and Limitations

The organisation of tenders for off-patent biologicals and biosimilars has been previously investigated in the context of a KPMG study on improving healthcare delivery in hospitals [37]. Here, authors identify the following elements to foster biosimilar utilization in the hospital environment: swiftly reopening of tenders, organizing multi-winner tenders, implementing benefit sharing methods and switching towards MEAT criteria. These elements are considered relatively easy to implement with a potential high impact on the system [37]. Also, the law firm Baker McKenzie performed a multi-jurisdictional European study, identifying key legal and practical aspects of the biosimilars market, in particular with regard to public tendering [63]. To the knowledge of the authors, this paper is the first scientific publication to assess in-depth stakeholder experiences with tender practices for off-patent biologicals and biosimilars and explore the sustainability of current practices.

The study presents both quantitative and qualitative data and is based on both purchaser and supplier experience. The qualitative survey data provide a snapshot of the heterogeneity of procurement practices and experiences of purchasers with the procurement of off-patent biologicals and biosimilars, across European countries. Participants from 23 different European countries, with varying levels of procurement organization (central, regional, local level) were queried. Overall, the quantitative data exemplify varying experiences across countries and provide a general overview of attitudes and challenges towards procurement of off-patent biologicals and biosimilars.

For the qualitative study part, interviews were conducted with experts in a selection of European countries that represent different tender structures, which enabled gathering information from various European contexts. In addition, interviews on a pan-European level were conducted to strengthen both country-specific and European-broad insights. Interviews were conducted with both purchaser- and supply (industry)-side participants, reflecting the insights of the two principal stakeholder groups in the tender process. The choice of qualitative interviews permitted to gain detailed insight in current practices and gather proposals for improvement from experts in the field. Experts from a purposive sample of European countries were invited, to capture a broad range of insights from countries with varying practices. However, no interview insights were obtained from Eastern-European countries. It may be useful for future research to expand on in-depth country analyses, assess perspectives of policy makers on proposed measures and conduct a systematic analysis on tenders in the EU database on tenders.

The general set of principles and proposals as outlined in Table 4, based on pan-European and country specific expert insights, could be applied mutatis mutandis to specific countries and settings. It is important to note that not all findings are generalizable to the whole off-patent biologicals segment across Europe, as some are product, country, setting or time related. Depending on the tender organization and maturity of the respective country or setting, measures on different levels may be needed and these should be tailored to country context. Some of the proposed recommendations are based on existing best practices. Several countries, regions or hospitals implement at present one or multiple of the proposed practices as outlined in Table 4. Some learnings may not be limited to tender practices for originator biologicals and biosimilar and might apply to tender practices in general. The fact that discounts in tender procedures are generally confidential prevents to properly mirror the gathered qualitative insights on price competition with actual price data beyond list-price level. As estimated by IQVIA, confidential discounts range between 10% and 90% on list price and could offer a 5–10% saving to the overall drug budget [8].

Table 4. Proposals on how to optimize tender procedures for off-patent biologicals and biosimilars, ensuring sustainable competition and associated savings in the long-term in the off-patent biologicals segment—five main avenues for optimization.

Tender practices should abide with the European Union and Member State rules on tendering. The involved actors, suppliers, purchaser bodies, payers, government and competition authorities, have a role to fulfil to ensure efficient, fair and transparent tender procedures for off-patent biologics and biosimilars.
- Purchasers (hospital or procurement body): securing a transparent and efficiently managed process
- Industry/suppliers: ensuring timely, non-disrupted and high-quality supply
- Payers: establishing adequate incentives and resolving any counterproductive motivational schemes Government: enabling sustainable market competition, by implementing policies and tender structures with a long-term perspective. Stimulating market plurality and providing guidance to purchasers
- Competition Authority: monitoring the correct application of tenders, by performing audits and following up purchaser adherence with laws on public procurement

The proposals outlined below can be considered as a general set of principles that can inform the different actors involved on possible improvements. Depending on the tender organization and maturity of the respective country or setting, measures should be selected and tailored to the country's context. Some of the proposed recommendations are based on existing best practices. Several countries, regions or hospitals have implemented already one or multiple of the proposed practices as outlined here.

Table 4. *Cont.*

1. Safeguarding a transparent, equal opportunity setting for all suppliers, with an appropriate use of award criteria
The tender procedure needs to be **transparent** and **non-discriminatory** with **predefined rules and pathway**, which are **adhered to** throughout the process

- Contracts should be awarded on the basis of **objective criteria that are compliant with the principles of transparency, non-discrimination and equal treatment** (as stipulated in the EU Directive (§ 90)) [13], allowing an objective comparative assessment.
- **Other award criteria besides price** that add value to the contract should be included, **applying the Most Economically Advantageous Tender (MEAT)** procedure as stimulated in the EU Public Procurement Directive [13], avoiding lowest bid procedures and stimulating suppliers to compete sustainably on more criteria
- **A clear framework regarding selection—and award criteria** should be implemented and adhered to:
   ○ Selection and award criteria should be carefully formulated, to avoid that participants are excluded a priori or certain products are disadvantaged on improper grounds. **Criteria for which longer market presence is required or would be advantageous should be avoided,** as these could lead to unreasonable competition expulsion, disadvantaging recently launched products.
   ○ Only criteria that are **related and proportionate** to the subject matter should be included. Any criteria that could unreasonably limit competition or introduce bias should be excluded. The link with the subject matter should be clear. Caution should be exerted regarding requesting or offering additional services or benefits, and this should be strictly avoided if not directly related to the subject matter.
   ○ Only additional criteria that **drive actual benefits** (meaningful product differentiation, advantage for purchaser and/or patient) should be included.
   ○ Award criteria besides price should be **proportionally rewarded** based on the additional value created, as the provision of additional services increases investment for suppliers. This will also enable these criteria to truly play a role in the allotment.
   ○ **Relevant experts** should be integrated to identify appropriate award criteria. In countries where procurement is organized on a local or individual hospital level, **governments** should provide **guidance** to purchasers regarding the structuring of the tender and application of selection and award criteria. Here, a **flexible/semi-structured tender template** could be designed to guide purchasers but also allowing room for tailoring based on product—specific considerations and strategic differentiation.
- Contracting authorities should **timely and transparently inform** possible competitors about the criteria that will be applied in the contract, by **specifying the award criteria** as well as **the relative weight or the allocation of points** given to each of those criteria in advance.
- **Linkage between contracts** (e.g., offer of or request to supplier to provide rebates for previously delivered or contracted medicines or rebates on a related product, in case the tender contract is won) can impact the equal opportunity setting and limit competition. Offering extensive conditional rebates with dominant position of the originator can be considered as anti-competitive exclusion.
- Avenues that provide **anonymity throughout the procedure**, such as requesting that bids are filed anonymously with coding identifier, should be applied where possible to avoid incumbent advantages [64].
- In the case of **preliminary market consultations,** these should guarantee that every supplier is **treated equally** and receives the **same information.** Although dialogue between purchasers and suppliers should generally be fostered to improve understanding of each other's needs on an overarching level, no direct input should be sought on the structuring of the tender from a supplier, as this could introduce steering of the structure of the tender.

2. Fostering a timely opening of tender procedures, ensuring on-set competition
Tender procedures should be **opened as soon as possible**, to avoid delays in competition and market opportunity for biosimilar competitors:

- Tender procedures should be prepared to **timely open:**
   ○ Systems should be prepared to organize tenders upon biosimilar market entry to reduce barriers to entry. A continuous re-opening of procedures with every new competitor entering the market should however be avoided, as this could introduce uncertainty in terms of volume and tender duration for the first tender winner(s) (lowering volume predictability) and also be burdensome for contracting authorities and industry.
   ○ Installing a shorter-term tender (e.g., 6 months) immediately upon market entry of the first biosimilar competitor(s), combined with a longer subsequent tender agreement, would allow immediate competition and market opportunity for the different competitors once the market has further crystalized in terms of number of available products.
   ○ Alternatively, a differentiated, product—specific approach in determining the appropriate term for opening a tender, taking into account the number of expected competitors, could be appropriate.

Table 4. *Cont.*

- A **specialist procurement office** involving the appropriate expertise fields could play an important role in organizing and coordinating the timing and duration of tender procedures for products with biosimilar competition. Moreover, such expert coordination office, should apply a long-term view, taking future biosimilar market entry into account to advice on negotiated contract duration, avoiding **blocking contracts** at the time of biosimilar market entry. Such an expert procurement office should perform **horizon scanning** to identify the upcoming loss of exclusivity of reference products and anticipated biosimilar market entry dates. (cfr. infra, bullet D). Such expert procurement office or payers could also strategically set out incentive schemes to stimulate a timely opening of procedures, as needed.
- A **financial stimulus** should be put in place to stimulate purchasing bodies/hospitals to organize tenders, aligning the incentives of the purchaser with these of the overall healthcare system (savings for healthcare budgets).
- A tender **duration between 12 and maximum 24 months** would be desirable to stimulate market dynamics, while considering feasibility and avoiding frequent switching.

3. Ensuring and stimulating adherence to laws on public procurement

The rules on public procurement should be correctly applied:

- **Competition authorities should monitor and audit** the correct, timely and transparent implementation of and adherence to the laws on public procurement by purchasers and **investigate signals of anti-competitive conduct** (e.g., conditional rebates). If needed, they should take **appropriate measures**, ensuring a timely opening of tenders and the application of appropriate award criteria.
- Governments should provide **feedback** to purchasing bodies **on performance** and apply **steering measures** where needed.
- For decentralized purchasing systems, the route of establishing a dedicated, independent and centrally coordinated expert panel (involving lawyers, physicians, pharmacists), to conduct the assessment, could be explored. The transferring of assessment to an independent central organ could improve objectivity of and ensure the appropriate expertise in the evaluation.
- Stakeholders should be stimulated to **actively report** any signals of anti-competitive conduct to the competition authority.
- **Financing streams/structures** of purchaser bodies and involved stakeholders should be **reviewed, removing existing disincentives** and **introducing new incentives** that are aligned with the overall healthcare system
    - Disincentives to organize competitive tenders or **incentives that favour a specific product/preference for the originator/more expensive product** should be removed.
    - **Financial incentives schemes or other policies** should be put in place:
        - Top-down: such as **lowering the reimbursement level** of products that are open to competition to stimulate purchasers to timely organize competitive tender procedures.
        - Stakeholder-involved: Savings from tender procedures could be allocated in part to remunerate HCPs for their time investment in switching, as part of a **gain-sharing model**. Such a gain-sharing model could motivate and involve stakeholders, increasing adherence to the tendered winner(s) and countering possible financial incentives and preferences to use the originator product.
- In addition to motivating stakeholders via above mentioned incentive schemes, **multi-winner tenders** or tenders with a ranking of preferred products can help to increase physician adherence to the tender outcome (avoiding physicians' use of the higher priced non-preferred product), as it may increase **physicians' freedom** to choose between available products. **Involving physicians in the tender procedures**, e.g., in the Drug & Therapeutic committee is also considered important in this regard.
- Authorities and governments should also support stakeholders with **up-to-date guidelines for biosimilar use** (e.g., on (multiple) switching) and develop **policies and information campaigns to improve stakeholder confidence** in biosimilars and **increase awareness on their benefits**. This may help lowering practical barriers associated with biosimilar use and uncertainty among stakeholders.

4. Securing an efficient process, improving plannability and ensuring timely product supply

The tender procedure needs to be efficiently managed, optimizing and reducing the administrative and time burden for both suppliers and purchasers, as well as increasing predictability and plannability for the supplier—supporting timely product supply.

- The **predictability and plannability of tender procedures and** associated **volumes** to be supplied should be **improved** towards suppliers:
    - This includes setting of **reliable estimates of volume to be supplied** (with guaranteeing minimum volumes and a maximum cap), **timely communication regarding** the **timing** of tender procedures and making use of **acceptable lead times** to support suppliers to better forecast and anticipate on demand, as such reducing the risk of shortages.
    - In case of supply issues, **penalties** should be **proportionate** to the contract value and the cause of the inability to supply (force majeure/external reasons for which could not be controlled), ensuring a fair balance of risk and reward. In case of inability to supply volumes that are higher than estimated (e.g., not specified in procurement contract), the supplier should bear no (disproportionate) financial risk.
    - In some cases, a good strategy could be that tender procedures **open up throughout the year**, to spread commercial opportunity for suppliers and accommodate manufacturing capacity.

Table 4. *Cont.*

-	**Expertise on procurement** should be **consolidated** to actively **guide purchasers** in **timely and efficiently** setting up tender procedures
	○ A **dedicated, expert procurement office** that consolidates knowledge, skill and experience with tender procedures should be available **to support purchasers/procurement bodies with the timely planning and efficient organization** of tender procedures.
	○ Such a specialized procurement office should **set out strategy, coordinate** purchasers and tender procedures, **perform horizon scanning** to inform stakeholders on the upcoming loss of exclusivity of reference products and anticipated biosimilar market entry dates, **prepare stakeholder guidance** documents and **monitor** the number of competitors on the market.
	○ Beyond coordinating the procurement strategy for products with anticipated biosimilar competition, the expert office should apply a long-term view and advice on contract length of new contracts, **considering future market entries**, avoiding "**blocking**" contracts at the time of biosimilar market entry, which would delay market competition.
	○ **Specific measures** or a **tailored approach** could be applied to prepare for biosimilar market entry of a specific product (or product category) (as was done in several countries to prepare for adalimumab biosimilar market entry) or could be adjusted based on specific market dynamics.
	○ Such an overarching expert office would also be beneficial in terms of **consolidating efforts, avoiding duplication** and **professionalising** the processes, as required by the increasingly complex structure of tender procedures.
	○ Depending on the country, such expert centre could be established **at national or regional level**.
-	**Tender procedures and documentation requests should be harmonized, simplified and made leaner** to mitigate the administrative workload and increase efficiency, as such reducing the possible sunk cost of participating suppliers. E-procurement should be wider used to allow information to be easily accessible throughout the tender procedure for both purchasers and suppliers. Beyond reducing the administrative burden, this will allow a higher traceability and transparency of procedures [24]. The process should also be streamlined in terms of the **information** which is believed to be **essential**. **Operating on a larger scale** by grouping purchaser bodies and the existence of an **expert procurement office** guiding procedures could benefit purchasers and suppliers in this regard.
5. Safeguarding long-term sustainable competition by stimulating market plurality	
The tender procedures and overall procurement strategy need to take a long-term view into account, tailored to supporting long-term sustainability, providing commercial opportunity for multiple suppliers	
-	**Stimulating market plurality and multiple commercial opportunities for suppliers**
	○ Single-winner tenders can exclude non-winning competitors from the market for the duration for the tender contract, and long-term lead to reduced levels of competition. **Ensuring market plurality is a cornerstone for a sustainable and competitive tender market and should be part of tendering strategy.** Depending on market size and specific context (product volume), different scenarios can be appropriate and applied. **Multi-winner tender** can be organized on national level or regional level (if there is a **sufficiently large scale**), or markets could be divided into **multiple commercial single-winner opportunities** (e.g., on hospital network or regional level).
	○ In the case of the scenario of multiple single or multi-winner opportunities across the market, a **rotating system** between regions or hospitals could be set up to increase dynamics and opening of commercial opportunities for suppliers over time.
	○ Multi-winner tenders also provide price reductions on all tendered products and may increase the physician's **therapeutic freedom** to choose between different products, as such avoiding physicians using a higher-priced non-preferred product.
	○ The availability of multiple commercial products on the market may also help to mitigate possible **supply issues**.
-	**Regular evaluation of the market situation and if needed revision of procurement and tendering mechanisms**
	○ Market dynamics such as the numbers of competitors and associated manufacturers should be reviewed on an annual basis and tendering policies should be reviewed in this context, avoiding market concentration and de novo monopolies

3.4. Balancing Short and Long Term Benefits

It is clear from this study that it is a delicate balance between optimizing efficient spending of public funds, addressing patient needs and preserving competition over the longer term. When designed efficiently and conducted appropriately, tenders can stimulate competition and as such form a cornerstone for sustainable market dynamics. As ensuring the most efficient use of public resources and broad access to medicines is a common societal goal, actions to ensure that tender processes are effective and motivate suppliers to participate over the longer-term are essential. Starting in the next five years, the number of biologic loss of exclusivities will increase substantially [8]. Healthcare systems across

Europe need to be prepared to facilitate and optimize market access for and competition from the next wave of biosimilar market entries, drawing from earlier experiences. This will allow healthcare systems to maximize the benefit of biological competition efficiently over the long term.

4. Materials and Methods

The study follows a mixed methods design, consisting of a survey and semi-structured interviews, gathering both quantitative and qualitative data. The study concentrates on tender procedures organised by contracting authorities. Tenders that are organized by private entities are not bound to organise public procurement procedures and are therefore out of scope. Ethics approval of the study was granted by the Research Ethics Committee UZ/KU Leuven (MP006498, Belgium).

4.1. Quantitative Web-Survey

4.1.1. Recruitment

A quantitative, anonymous web-questionnaire was developed to survey purchasers and hospital pharmacists about the organisation of tenders for off-patent biologicals and biosimilars. The survey was disseminated to hospital pharmacists and purchasers across Europe, via professional associations such as the European Association of Hospital Pharmacists, by contacting procurement entities and the network of the research group.

4.1.2. Survey Development

The survey was developed based on a study of the literature and consisted of questions about (i) the experience of participants with tender procedures for off-patent biologicals and biosimilars and perceived challenges, (ii) the design of tender procedures (number of winners, average tender duration, reopening of tenders, physician involvement), (iii) the application of selection-and award criteria and (iv) considerations about interchangeability and switching, as tenders may result in an exchange of products. The survey questions were refined based on comments from both a hospital pharmacist and a supplier. The survey was developed online in the KU Leuven Websurvey-server and gathered anonymous data. The survey consisted of closed multiple choice, ranking or Likert-scale questions. Participants were given the possibility to add additional information in an open text field for certain questions and answer options such as "Other". The first window of the web survey provided participants with information about the study, the voluntary nature of participation and a statement regarding agreement to participate. The survey was anonymous, and no personal data were collected.

4.1.3. Analysis

Responses were gathered between October 2018 and February 2019. The survey answers were analysed descriptively on an overall group level.

4.2. Qualitative Semi-Structured Interviews

4.2.1. Recruitment

To gather qualitative, in-depth expert insights regarding the organization of tenders for off-patent biologicals and biosimilars, semi-structured interviews were conducted with hospital pharmacists, purchasers and pharmaceutical industry employees. The sampling was purposeful to obtain a range of experiences and perspectives, reflecting both the purchaser and supply side perspective, from individuals that are knowledgeable about and experienced with tender processes for off-patent biologicals and biosimilars.

Eligible participants worked currently or formerly as (i) medicine purchaser or hospital pharmacist, (ii) in, or as consultant to, a pharmaceutical company with at least one EMA-approved originator biological or biosimilar (or having both originator and biosimilar products) or for a pharmaceutical industry trade organization. Employees from both legacy originator and legacy generic companies were recruited. Participants were selected for their experience with and knowledge about tender practices for off-patent biologics and biosimilars [65].

To capture diverse and comprehensive insights, both participants with insights on a pan-European level (e.g., from European professional associations, European pharmaceutical company headquarters or trade organizations) and participants with country specific insights were invited. For the latter, participants were recruited from a purposive selection of seven European countries, representing different tender organizational systems (central purchasing: Denmark and Norway, regional purchasing: England and Italy, buying group/hospital individual purchasing: France, the Netherlands and Belgium). The choice to capture the insights of both purchaser- and supply (industry)-side participants was made to obtain views from the two principal stakeholder groups in the tender process.

Participant recruitment was carried out by screening relevant websites, scientific and professional stakeholder associations, relevant conferences and publications and the network of the research group for eligible participants.

While different sampling strategies were applied for the survey and the interviews (broad vs. purposeful sampling), a certain overlap in participants may theoretically have been possible. The impact of having a respondent possibly participating in the survey and a subsequent interview is considered negligible on interview results since the survey and interviews served distinct purposes.

4.2.2. Interview Guide and Interviews

Interviews were carried out in English, with the exception of a few interviews in Dutch, in person, via telephone or teleconference between March 2019 and February 2020. All participants provided written informed consent prior to the start of their interview. Consent was given by all participants for using the encoded and anonymized data from their interview for scientific publication. Interviews were conducted using an interview guide based on topics identified from scientific literature, policy documents, position statements related to the procurement of off-patent biologics and biosimilars and the quantitative survey results. Interviewees were asked to share their insights on challenges, best practices and learnings regarding tender practices for off-patent biologicals and biosimilars, as well as proposals towards long-term sustainable tender practices. An overview of discussed topics is shown in Supplementary Materials Table S9. All interviews were audio-recorded and transcribed verbatim. Interviews were carried out until saturation of the data [65].

4.2.3. Analysis

Interview transcripts were pseudonymised and analysed according to the thematic framework method, using Nvivo® data analysis software [66].

5. Conclusions

This study found that opportunity exists to improve tender practices for off-patent biologicals and biosimilars in Europe. In order to realise the competition potential of biosimilars and benefits from appropriate tender procedures for healthcare systems and patients, concerted actions by policymakers and purchasers, in dialogue with industry associations, with a long-term strategic view are needed to optimize tender frameworks. Depending on the country's policy environment and the maturity of the procurement body, different sets of policy and practical measures are needed. In general, measures should aim to ensure supplier market plurality, establish a transparent and objective process, and include award criteria beyond price. This may contribute to creating a sustainable climate, with long-term competition in the off-patent biologicals market.

Supplementary Materials: The following are available online at https://www.mdpi.com/article/10.3390/ph14060499/s1, Table S1: Survey participants' characteristics, Table S2: Experience with and perceptions about tenders for off-patent biologicals and biosimilars, Table S3: Structuring of tenders for off-patent biologicals and biosimilars, Table S4: Application of selection and award criteria in tenders for off-patent biologicals and biosimilars, Table S5: Interchangeability and switching considerations in tender design, Table S6: Interview participants' characteristics, Table S7: Interview participants' characteristics, Table S8: Recommendations extracted from position/white papers on tender procedures (for off-patent biological medicines and biosimilars) in Europe, Table S9: Main topics addressed during the interviews.

Author Contributions: A.G.V., I.H., S.S. and L.B. developed the idea of this study and were involved in its design. B.C. provided feedback at different stages of the study. L.B. and C.S. collected and analysed the survey data. L.B. collected and analysed the interview data. L.B. prepared the first draft of the manuscript. All authors critically reviewed the manuscript. All authors have read and agreed to the published version of the manuscript.

Funding: This work is supported by KU Leuven and the KU Leuven Fund on Market Analysis of Biologics and Biosimilars following Loss of Exclusivity (MABEL Fund).

Institutional Review Board Statement: Ethics approval was granted by the Research Ethics Committee UZ/KU Leuven (MP006498, Belgium).

Informed Consent Statement: Written informed consent was obtained from all interviewees involved in the study. All interviewees provided consent for using the encoded and anonymized data from their interview for publication in scientific journals.

Data Availability Statement: The survey data presented in this study are available on reasonable request from the corresponding author. The interview data are not available upon request as they contain information that could compromise interviewees' privacy and consent.

Acknowledgments: First, the authors thank all participants who shared their insights in the survey and/or in an interview. The authors thank T. De Rijdt (UZ Leuven) and A. Abouzid (IQVIA) for their review of the survey. The authors would like to thank A. Baeyens (DG GROW, European Commission), B. Boone (Apollegis) and F. Turk (University of Paderborn) for their valuable comments on the manuscript. The authors also express their thanks to the European Association of Hospital Pharmacists (EAHP) and the organizers of the Biosimilars Educational Masterclass for Pharmacists (BEAM) for disseminating the survey among hospital pharmacists.

Conflicts of Interest: I.H., S.S. and A.G.V. are founders of the KU Leuven Fund on Market Analysis of Biologics and Biosimilars following Loss of Exclusivity (MABEL Fund). A.G.V. is involved in consulting, advisory work and speaking engagements for a number of companies, i.e., AbbVie, Accord, Amgen, Biogen, Medicines for Europe, Pfizer/Hospira, Mundipharma, Roche, Novartis, Sandoz, Boehringer Ingelheim. S.S. was involved in a stakeholder roundtable on biologics and biosimilars sponsored by Amgen, Pfizer and MSD; he has participated in advisory board meetings for Sandoz, Pfizer and Amgen; he has contributed to studies on biologics and biosimilars for Hospira, Celltrion, Mundipharma and Pfizer; and he has had speaking engagements for Amgen, Celltrion and Sandoz. L.B., I.H., C.S. and B.C. declare no conflicts of interest that are directly relevant to the content of this article. Authors declare that the research was conducted in the absence of any commercial or financial relationship that could be perceived as a potential conflict of interest.

References

1. IMS Institute for Healthcare Informatics. *Delivering on the Potential of Biosimilar Medicines: The Role of Functioning Competitive Markets Introduction*; IMS Institute for Healthcare Informatics: Parsippany, NJ, USA, 2016.
2. IQVIA. *The Impact of Biosimilar Competition in Europe*; IQVIA: Durham, NC, USA, 2019.
3. IQVIA. *Advancing Biosimilar Sustainability in Europe—A Multi-Stakeholder Assessment*; IQVIA: Durham, NC, USA, 2018.
4. European Medicines Agency. *Guideline on Similar Biological Medicinal Products*; European Medicines Agency: Amsterdam, The Netherlands, 2014.
5. European Medicines Agency. Biosimilar Medicines. Available online: https://www.ema.europa.eu/en/medicines/field_ema_web_categories%253Aname_field/Human/ema_group_types/ema_medicine/field_ema_med_status/authorised-6/ema_medicine_types/field_ema_med_biosimilar/search_api_aggregation_ema_medicine_types/field_ema_med_biosim (accessed on 23 January 2021).
6. European Medicines Agency. *Applications for New Human Medicines under Evaluation by the Committee for Medicinal Products for Human Use*; European Medicines Agency: Amsterdam, The Netherlands, 2020.
7. IQVIA. *The Impact of Biosimilar Competition in Europe*; IQVIA: Durham, NC, USA, 2018.
8. IQVIA. *The Impact of Biosimilar Competition in Europe*; IQVIA: Durham, NC, USA, 2020.
9. Rémuzat, C.; Kapuśniak, A.; Caban, A.; Ionescu, D.; Mendoza, C.; Toumi, M. Supply-side and demand-side policies for biosimilars: An overview in 10 European member states. *J. Mark. Access Health Policy* **2017**, *5*, 1307315. [CrossRef] [PubMed]

10. Vogler, S.; Gombocz, M.; Zimmermann, N. Tendering for off-patent outpatient medicines: Lessons learned from experiences in Belgium, Denmark and the Netherlands. *J. Pharm. Health Serv. Res.* **2017**, *8*, 147–158. [CrossRef]
11. Simoens, S.; Cheung, R. Tendering and biosimilars: What role for value-added services? *J. Mark. Access. Health Policy* **2020**, *8*, 1705120. [CrossRef] [PubMed]
12. Dranitsaris, G.; Jacobs, I.; Kirchhoff, C.; Popovian, R.; Shane, L.G. Drug tendering: Drug supply and shortage implications for the uptake of biosimilars. *Clin. Outcomes Res.* **2017**, *9*, 573–584. [CrossRef] [PubMed]
13. European Union. *Directive 2014/24/EU of The European Parliament and of The Council of 26 February 2014 on Public Procurement and Repealing Directive 2004/18/EC*; Off. J. Eur. Union: Luxembourg, 2014.
14. European Commission. Public Procurement. Available online: https://ec.europa.eu/growth/single-market/public-procurement_en (accessed on 24 February 2021).
15. European Commission. Public Procurement: Legal Rules and Implementation. Available online: https://ec.europa.eu/growth/single-market/public-procurement/rules-implementation_en (accessed on 24 February 2021).
16. Simon-Kucher & Partners. *Payers' Price & Market Access Policies Supporting a Sustainable Biosimilar Medicines Market*; Simon-Kucher & Partners: Bonn, Germany, 2016.
17. Reiland, J.-B.; Freischem, B.; Roediger, A. What pricing and reimbursement policies to use for off-patent biologicals in Europe?—Results from the second EBE biological medicines policy survey. *Gabi. J. Generics Biosimilars Initiat. J.* **2017**, *6*, 61–78. [CrossRef]
18. Medicines for Europe. *Market Review—European Biosimilar Medicines Markets*; Medicines for Europe: Brussels, Belgium, 2017.
19. Bird&Bird. *Public Procurement of Medicinal Products White Paper—Common Legislation But Diverging Implementation Approaches Throughout the EU*; Bird&Bird: London, UK, 2014.
20. Medicines for Europe. *Position Paper on Best Procurement Practices*; Medicines for Europe: Brussels, Belgium, 2018.
21. European Association of Hospital Pharmacists. *EAHP Position Paper on Procurement*; EAHP: Brussels, Belgium, 2018.
22. Sammarco, C. Competition in Public Bidding Exercises for Pharmaceutical Products. *Opinio Juris Compratione* **2010**, *2*, 4.
23. Schoonveld, E. *The Price of Global Health: Drug Pricing Strategies to Balance Patient Access and the Funding of Innovation*; Taylor and Francis: London, UK, 2020.
24. European Commission. *EU Public Procurement Reform: Less Bureaucracy, Higher Efficiency*; European Commission: Brussels, Belgium, 2015.
25. O'Mahony, B. *Guide to National Tenders for the Purchase of Clotting Factor Concentrates*; World Federation of Hemophilia: Montréal, QC, Canada, 2015.
26. European Biopharmaceutical Enterprises. *EBE Position Paper on Tendering of Biosimilars/Biologicals*; EBE: Brussels, Belgium, 2011.
27. EuropaBio. *Public Procurement of Biological Medicines*; EuropaBio: Brussels, Belgium, 2015.
28. EuropaBio. *"Buying Innovative" in the Healthcare Biotech Market in Europe*; EuropaBio: Brussels, Belgium, 2017.
29. Vulto, A.; Cheesman, S.; Stuart, P. Tender-criteria biosimilars 'beyond price'. In Proceedings of the Amgen BEAM Workshop, Zurich, Switzerland, 5–6 September 2019.
30. Alhola, K. *Environmental Criteria in Public Procurement Focus on Tender Documents*; Finnish Environment Institute: Helsinki, Finland, 2012.
31. Raffaelli, E.A.; Massimino, F. Biosimilars: Considerations in light of the Italian legal framework. *Generics Biosimilars Initiat. J.* **2019**, *8*, 5–23. [CrossRef]
32. NHS. *An Overview of NHS Procurement of Medicines and Pharmaceutical Products and Services for Acute Care in the United Kingdom Executive Summary*; NHS: London, UK, 2018.
33. Minister of Social Affairs and Health. *Omzendbrief Actieplan Biosimilars*; Minister of Social Affairs and Health: Brussels, Belgium, 2016.
34. Vandenplas, Y.; Huys, I.; Van Wilder, P.; Vulto, A.G.; Simoens, S. *Probleemstelling en Voorstellen tot Maatregelen Voor Af-Patent Biologische en Biosimilaire Geneesmiddelen in België*; KU Leuven: Leuven, Belgium, 2020.
35. RIZIV/INAMI. Terugbetaling van Geneesmiddelen: Wat Is Gewijzigd Sinds 1 April 2019—RIZIV. Available online: https://www.inami.fgov.be/nl/professionals/andere-professionals/farmaceutische-industrie/Paginas/terugbetaling-geneesmiddelen-01042019.aspx#Daling_tot_85%25_voor_de_facturatie_van_bepaalde_geneesmiddelen_in_het_ziekenhuis (accessed on 13 October 2020).
36. Akker, I.; Sauter, W.A. Cure for All Ills? The Effectiveness of Therapeutic and Biosimilar Pharmaceutical Competition in the Netherlands. *Eur. Pharm. Law. Rev.* **2020**, *4*, 57–66. [CrossRef]
37. KMPG. *Improving Healthcare Delivery in Hospitals by Optimized Utilization of Medicines: A Study into 8 European Countries*; KMPG: Amstelveen, The Netherlands, 2019.
38. Amgros. All the Agreements in the First Joint Nordic Tendering Procedure Are in Place. Available online: https://amgros.dk/en/knowledge-and-analyses/articles/all-the-agreements-in-the-first-joint-nordic-tendering-procedure-are-in-place/ (accessed on 11 June 2020).
39. European Commission. *Expert Panel on Effective Ways of Investing in Health—European Commission. Opinion on Public Procurement in Healthcare Systems*; European Commission: Brussels, Belgium, 2021.
40. Madsen, S. Regulation of Biosimilars and Success Factors for Uptake in Clinical Practice. In Proceedings of the 'Biological Medicines in Belgium' Symposium of the Belgian Federal Agency of Medicinal Products and Health, FAMHP, Brussels, Belgium, 8 February 2018.

41. Medicines for Europe. *Positioning Statements on Physician-Led Switching for Biosimilar Medicines*; Medicines for Europe: Brussels, Belgium, 2019.
42. The Cancer Vanguard. *Project Evaluation Report: Biosimilars Getting It Right 1st Time*; NHS: London, UK, 2018.
43. The Cancer Vanguard. Biosimilars—Getting It Right First Time. Available online: https://cancervanguard.nhs.uk/biosimilars-getting-it-right-first-time/ (accessed on 9 November 2020).
44. OECD. *Tackling Wasteful Spending on Health*; OECD: Paris, France, 2017.
45. Razanskaite, V.; Bettey, M.; Downey, L.; Wright, J.; Callaghan, J.; Rush, M.; Cummings, F. Biosimilar Infliximab in Inflammatory Bowel Disease: Outcomes of a Managed Switching Programme. *J. Crohns. Colitis.* **2017**, *11*, 690–696. [CrossRef] [PubMed]
46. Welch, A.R. *Biosimilars: Regulatory, Clinical, and Biopharmaceutical Development—Chapter: Biosimilars 101: An Introduction to Biosimilars*; Springer: Berlin/Heidelberg, Germany, 2018.
47. Autoriteit Consument & Markt. *Sectoronderzoek Concurrentie voor en na Toetreding van Biosimilars*; Autoriteit Consument & Markt: Den Haag, The Netherlands, 2019.
48. European Commission. Limiting the Temptation for Corruption in Public Procurement. Available online: https://ec.europa.eu/growth/content/limiting-temptation-corruption-public-procurement_en (accessed on 24 February 2021).
49. Kanavos, P.; Ferrario, A.; Nicod, E.; Sandberg, D. *Tender Systems for Outpatient Pharmaceuticals in the European Union: Evidence from the Netherlands and Germany*; London School of Economics: London, UK, 2012.
50. Bax, H. *Value-Based Procurement: The Unexpected Driver of Patient- Centric and Sustainable Healthcare*; VBP CoP: Brussels, Belgium, 2020.
51. Plackett, B. No money for new drugs. *Nature* **2020**, *586*, S50–S52. [CrossRef]
52. Cherla, A.; Howard, N.; Mossialos, E. The 'Netflix plus model': Can subscription financing improve access to medicines in low- and middle-income countries? *Health Econ. Policy Law* **2020**, *16*, 113–123. [CrossRef]
53. Macaulay, R.; Miller, P.; Turkstra, E. Subscription model for reimbursement: A fad or the future? In Proceedings of the ISPOR Europe 2019, Copenhagen, Denmark, 2–6 November 2019.
54. NHS. *Regional Medicines Optimisation Committee Briefing Best Value Biologicals: Adalimumab Update 6*; NHS: London, UK, 2019.
55. NHS England. *Commissioning Framework for Biological Medicines (Including Biosimilar Medicines)*; NHS England: Leeds, UK, 2017.
56. Verboven, Y. *MedTech Europe View—Value Based Procurement & Most Economic Advantageous Tendering (MEAT)*; MedTech Europe: Brussels, Belgium, 2018.
57. Gerecke, G.; Clawson, J.; Verboven, Y. *Procurement: The Unexpected Driver of Value-Based Health Care*; MedTech Europe: Brussels, Belgium, 2015.
58. Barbier, L.; Simoens, S.; Vulto, A.G.; Huys, I. European Stakeholder Learnings Regarding Biosimilars: Part I—Improving Biosimilar Understanding and Adoption. *BioDrugs* **2020**, *34*, 783–796. [CrossRef] [PubMed]
59. Barbier, L.; Simoens, S.; Vulto, A.G.; Huys, I. European Stakeholder Learnings Regarding Biosimilars: Part II—Improving Biosimilar Use in Clinical Practice. *BioDrugs* **2020**, *34*, 797–808. [CrossRef] [PubMed]
60. Duggan, B.; Smith, A.; Barry, M. Uptake of biosimilars for TNF-α inhibitors adalimumab and etanercept following the best-value biological medicine initiative in Ireland. *Int. J. Clin. Pharm.* **2021**. [CrossRef] [PubMed]
61. Amgros. New International Record for Switch to Biosimilar. Available online: https://amgros.dk/en/knowledge-and-analyses/articles/new-international-record-for-switch-to-biosimilar/ (accessed on 11 June 2020).
62. Moorkens, E.; Godman, B.; Huys, I.; Hoxha, I.; Malaj, A.; Keuerleber, S.; Vulto, A.G. The expiry of Humira® market exclusivity and the entry of adalimumab biosimilars in Europe: An overview of pricing and national policy measures. *Front Pharm.* **2021**, *11*. [CrossRef] [PubMed]
63. Gabriel, M. Public Procurement Laws and Tendering of Biological Pharmaceuticals and Biosimilars in the EU. In Proceedings of the EU Commission Stakeholder Event on Biosimilar Medicinal Products, Brussels, Belgium, 14 September 2018.
64. OECD. *Recommendation of the OECD Council on Fighting Bid Rigging in Public Procurement*; OECD: Paris, France, 2012.
65. Palinkas, L.A.; Horwits, S.M.; Green, C.A.; Wisdom, J.P.; Duan, N.; Hoagwood, K. Purposeful sampling for qualitative data collection and analysis in mixed method implementation research. *Adm. Policy Ment. Health* **2015**, *42*, 533–544. [CrossRef] [PubMed]
66. Lacey, A.; Luff, D. *Qualitative Data Analysis*; The NIHR RDS: Nottingham/Sheffield, UK, 2007.

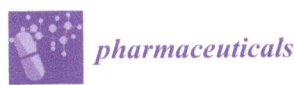

Review

Sustainability of Biosimilars in Europe: A Delphi Panel Consensus with Systematic Literature Review

Arnold G. Vulto [1,2], Jackie Vanderpuye-Orgle [3,*], Martin van der Graaff [4], Steven R. A. Simoens [2], Lorenzo Dagna [5], Richard Macaulay [6], Beenish Majeed [6], Jeffrey Lemay [7], Jane Hippenmeyer [8] and Sebastian Gonzalez-McQuire [8]

1. Hospital Pharmacy, Erasmus University Medical Center, NL-3015 CN Rotterdam, The Netherlands; a.vulto@gmail.com
2. Department of Pharmaceutical and Pharmacological Sciences, KU Leuven, 3000 Leuven, Belgium; steven.simoens@kuleuven.be
3. Access Consulting, Parexel International, Billerica, MA 01821, USA
4. Ex-National Health Care Institute, Zorginstituut Nederland (ZIN), NL-1110 AH Diemen, The Netherlands; m.vandergraaff@ziggo.nl
5. IRCCS San Raffaele Scientific Institute, Universita Vita-Salute San Raffaele, 20132 Milan, Italy; dagna.lorenzo@unisr.it
6. Access Consulting, Parexel International, Uxbridge UB8 1LZ, UK; Richard.Macaulay@parexel.com (R.M.); Beenish.Majeed@parexel.com (B.M.)
7. Amgen Inc., Thousand Oaks, CA 91320, USA; jlemay@amgen.com
8. Amgen Inc. Europe GmbH, CH-6343 Rotkreuz, Switzerland; jhippenm@amgen.com (J.H.); sebgonza@amgen.com (S.G.-M.)
* Correspondence: Jackie.Vanderpuye-Orgle@parexel.com; Tel.: +1-978-495-4024

Received: 7 August 2020; Accepted: 31 October 2020; Published: 17 November 2020

Abstract: Introduction: Biosimilars have the potential to enhance the sustainability of evolving health care systems. A sustainable biosimilars market requires all stakeholders to balance competition and supply chain security. However, there is significant variation in the policies for pricing, procurement, and use of biosimilars in the European Union. A modified Delphi process was conducted to achieve expert consensus on biosimilar market sustainability in Europe. Methods: The priorities of 11 stakeholders were explored in three stages: a brainstorming stage supported by a systematic literature review (SLR) and key materials identified by the participants; development and review of statements derived during brainstorming; and a facilitated roundtable discussion. Results: Participants argued that a sustainable biosimilar market must deliver tangible and transparent benefits to the health care system, while meeting the needs of all stakeholders. Key drivers of biosimilar market sustainability included: (i) competition is more effective than regulation; (ii) there should be incentives to ensure industry investment in biosimilar development and innovation; (iii) procurement processes must avoid monopolies and minimize market disruption; and (iv) principles for procurement should be defined by all stakeholders. However, findings from the SLR were limited, with significant gaps on the impact of different tender models on supply risks, savings, and sustainability. Conclusions: A sustainable biosimilar market means that all stakeholders benefit from appropriate and reliable access to biological therapies. Failure to care for biosimilar market sustainability may impoverish biosimilar development and offerings, eventually leading to increased cost for health care systems and patients, with fewer resources for innovation.

Keywords: biosimilar market; biosimilar/supply and distribution; biosimilar sustainability; Delphi technique

1. Introduction

The global biosimilars market was valued at $4.5 billion in 2019 and is expected to reach $23.6 billion by 2024; this is an estimated growth rate of 39.4%, with most of this growth occurring in Europe [1,2]. Such a rapid acceleration in the biosimilars market may result in numerous challenges, and it is important to support a thoughtful deployment of biosimilars. This will provide an opportunity for sustainability of global health care budgets and evolving health care systems [3,4].

At present, the European Medicines Agency (EMA) defines a "biosimilar" as "a biological medicinal product that contains a version of the active substance of an already authorized original biological medicinal product (reference medicinal product)" for which "similarity to the reference medicinal product in terms of quality characteristics, biological activity, safety, and efficacy based on a comprehensive comparability exercise needs to be established" [5,6]. Manufacturers in both the United States and Europe are required to demonstrate that the proposed biosimilar and its reference product are highly similar and have no clinically meaningful differences [5,7].

Thus, biosimilars are manufactured following the same strict standards of quality, safety, and efficacy observed for the reference product [5,7]; this is reflected in the development cost, which ranges from $100 to 300 million [8]. Biosimilars can broaden product choice and have the potential to reduce prices, whilst continuing to support a high standard of patient care [9]. In the United States, potential cost saving from switching from originator biologics to biosimilars is projected to be between $40 and 250 billion by 2025, and in Europe, cost savings are already estimated to be more than €10 billion [2,10–12].

Many organizations representing physicians, pharmacists, and patients across Europe support the use of biosimilars [3,4,13–15], and have issued position papers outlining best practices for their use. However, biosimilar markets are still evolving, and there are marked differences between policies and practices across European countries [16–18]. For example, some payer bodies have implemented single winner tender-based systems. While this can secure significant short-term payer savings, such systems risk locking out many biosimilar manufacturers, and may limit the number of competing manufacturers in the medium term. In addition, single-manufacturer tenders can place a lot of risk on the supply chain and, potentially, on patient access. Therefore, systems need to be set up to ensure that long-term savings are realized for payers and sufficient manufacturer incentives are in place to sustain multiplayer competition. Further, the notion of biosimilar sustainability is currently inconsistently and poorly defined, and there is a lack of awareness on the vulnerability of the current system. Previous analyses of the biosimilars market have concluded that there is a need to improve sustainability, and several areas have been identified for further research to develop a coherent long-term vision of sustainability. These include safeguarding the interests of patients, maintaining physician autonomy and patient choice, effective purchasing/pricing and reimbursement strategies, good pharmacovigilance practices, and healthy levels of competition to ensure consistent supply of a range of high-quality products [11,19,20].

To consider these issues and examine biosimilar market sustainability in more detail, we conducted a systematic literature review (SLR) and Delphi panel discussion to: (i) establish a multistakeholder definition of biosimilar market sustainability; (ii) further identify components of a sustainable biosimilar market; and (iii) identify drivers and risks of a sustainable biosimilar market.

2. Methods

2.1. Design

The modified Delphi process is a commonly published approach to generate discussion around topics without consensus and is an effective way to start dealing with complex multifactorial challenges [21]. A modified Delphi process, involving 11 key opinion leaders representing various sectors of the health care system in Europe, was conducted between September and November 2019. Participating stakeholders comprised one patient advocate, two physicians, two hospital pharmacists, two procurement pharmacists, one national payer, two policy advisors, and one manufacturer from across Europe. The modified Delphi process was based on a published approach, [22] and consisted of brainstorming, structured feedback, and a facilitated roundtable discussion (Figure 1).

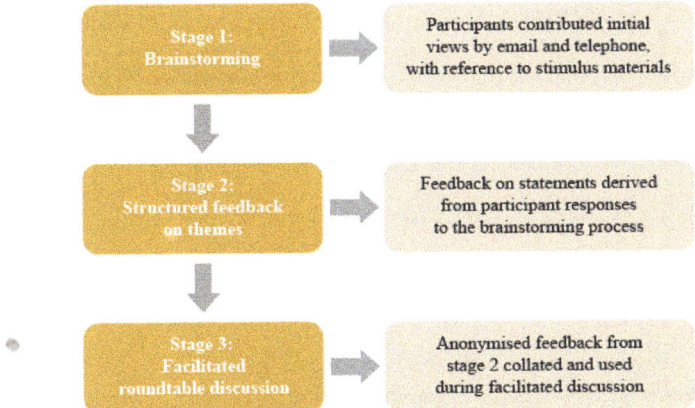

Figure 1. Modified Delphi process.

2.2. Procedure

The Delphi process was initiated by multiple stages of brainstorming, in which participants contributed their initial views by email and telephone using the questionnaire shown in Appendix A. Participants were provided with stimulus materials identified by an SLR and they were also asked to identify any key papers to support their feedback. The SLR is briefly described in this paper, but it is published elsewhere [18].

The SLR was conducted using EMBASE, MEDLINE, and grey literature searches. The searches were conducted using recent evidence (from 2008 to 2019) to capture all key biosimilar publications after their introduction in Europe in 2006. Only publications in English were included. Search methods were based on recommendations from the Cochrane Handbook [23] and the Centre for Reviews and Dissemination [24]. The SLR identified materials relating to major economies in Europe and answered three predefined key questions on the: (Q1) frequency, causes, and consequences of shortages of reference product biologics and biosimilars; (Q2) costs (direct and indirect costs, resource utilization, and external costs) and impacts resulting from switching patients between biosimilar products; and (Q3) causation between tendering, market concentration, drug shortages, and achievement of savings, and the implications of tender models for supply risk (reliability) and sustainability of competitive biosimilar markets.

In an initial screening phase, one reviewer identified relevant titles and abstracts from among all retrieved records; in a second screening stage, one reviewer re-evaluated each selected publication in a full-text review. In both stages, a second reviewer was consulted in cases of uncertainty, and consensus between the two was reached. Data extraction was performed by two reviewers, with one extracting the data and the second checking the data against the original publication. Any discrepancies were resolved through discussion or through the intervention of a third reviewer. The SLR flow chart is shown in Appendix B. The findings of the SLR were provided to the panel during the brainstorming stage; participants reviewed the material (amendments were allowed) and provided their ideas. The feedback was discussed with each participant via telephone to ensure that it was interpreted correctly, and the finalized brainstorming responses were collected via email. The amended stimulus material is shown in Appendix C [3,4,16–18,25–27]. These references and the brainstorming responses were used to develop the themes and statements for the second stage.

In the second stage of the Delphi process, the brainstorming responses and evidence extracted from the stimulus materials were converted into themes and statements (Appendix D), using standard primary research methodology. Feedback was sought on: (i) the components for a definition of biosimilar market sustainability and (ii) drivers and risks to achieving sustainability. Participants were asked to indicate on a Likert scale (from "strongly disagree" to "strongly agree") their level of agreement with each theme and statement, and how strongly they felt the evidence supported each theme and statement. Each participant had 1 week to provide their responses.

Stage 3 was a facilitated roundtable discussion that aimed to derive a multistakeholder definition of sustainability and achieve consensus on the components of a sustainable biosimilar market. First, the participants were presented with a definition of sustainability (derived from feedback supplied in stage 2) and were then asked to provide feedback on the definition, stating their level of agreement ("strongly disagree" to "strongly agree"), and providing any revisions they wished to make in free text. Based on the responses, the initial definition was revised and presented to participants for comment and final agreement at the end of the roundtable discussion. Participants were then presented with eight statements on the components of a sustainable biosimilar market and on drivers and risks to sustainability (derived from feedback supplied in stage 2). Participants were asked to provide individual feedback regarding how much they agreed with each statement, how important each statement was to them, and free-text suggestions on how to rephrase each statement so that it would align better with their views. The purpose of the discussions on each statement was to explore areas of agreement and disagreement between stakeholder groups. Where groups agreed, consensus was noted; however, the process could cease if stakeholder views remained divergent.

3. Results

3.1. Delphi Panel Consensus

3.1.1. A Multistakeholder Definition of Biosimilar Market Sustainability

The multistakeholder consensus definition of a sustainable biosimilars market is provided in Box 1. After much deliberation, this definition was agreed upon by all participants; however, different stakeholder groups emphasized different priorities within this definition. Patients wanted to be well-informed, physicians wanted biosimilar-related savings reinvested, pharmacists/manufacturers emphasized quality, and payers/policy advisers focused on mechanisms (e.g., competition) to lower prices. These differing priorities were not considered to be mutually exclusive, and all participants considered it important to incorporate the perspectives of all stakeholders into the definition of a sustainable biosimilar market in Europe.

Box 1. A multistakeholder consensus definition of a sustainable biosimilar market.

- A sustainable biosimilar market means that ... "All stakeholders, including patients, benefit from appropriate and reliable access to biological therapies. Competition leads to a long-term predictable price level, without compromising quality, while delivering savings that may be reinvested."

3.1.2. Components of a Sustainable Biosimilar Market

Participants agreed that a sustainable biosimilar market: (i) must deliver tangible and transparent benefits to the health care system; (ii) must address the needs of all stakeholders; and (iii) requires collaboration between stakeholders. The level of consensus achieved on these key points is summarized in Box 2 and Table 1.

Table 1. Consensus on components of a sustainable biosimilar market.

I.	**A sustainable biosimilar market must deliver tangible and transparent benefits to the health care system**
Biosimilars have the potential to reduce the cost of treatment; this, in turn, strengthens the sustainability of health care expenditure	CONSENSUS
Biosimilar-related savings must be tangible and transparent and should be reinvested efficiently; this may include addressing deficits, and funding innovative therapies, health care or other public services. Biosimilars have the potential to expand access	CONSENSUS
Providers (physicians and pharmacists) incur real costs when transitioning to a new biosimilar; transition should only occur if savings substantially exceed these transition costs and a portion of the savings are used to meet these costs	PHYSICIAN PHARMACIST
II.	**A sustainable biosimilar market must address the needs of all stakeholders**
Transitioning between biosimilars causes disruption to patient care and health care services. Unnecessary disruptions (i.e., frequent transitions and/or transitions that do not deliver tangible savings) should be minimized	CONSENSUS
Disruption caused by biosimilar transition may be unavoidable in some therapeutic areas (e.g., acute vs. chronic conditions); however, switch is not advisable if treatment duration is short	PATIENT PHYSICIAN PHARMACIST
Disruption and transition costs occur in both hospital and out-of-hospital (including retail and home care) settings; these differences may need to be considered	PHYSICIAN PHARMACIST

Table 1. Cont.

III. A sustainable biosimilar market requires collaboration between stakeholders	
Policies and practices must encourage trust in biosimilar use among patients through effective communication between stakeholders	CONSENSUS
Language and messaging should be consistent among stakeholders and coordinated nationally	CONSENSUS
Clear guidance from regulators and clinical organisations at European and national levels is required to motivate multiple switches (i.e., following the initial transition from original biological to biosimilar)	PATIENT PHYSICIAN
• This guidance may benefit from real-world studies (e.g., registry studies)—although not all stakeholders agree that this would be sufficient evidence	PHYSICIAN PHARMACIST PAYER
• Research would need to be led by providers (pharmacists and physicians), as there are limited incentives for manufacturers to invest in this research	MANUFACTURER PHARMACIST PAYER

Note: icons shown on the right represent level of agreement between the stakeholders. The 'consensus' icon indicates that all stakeholders (physicians, payers, policy advisors, manufacturers, pharmacists, and patients) agreed on that point. Benefits, such as expanded access, have also been noted in the literature [9].

Box 2. Consensus on components of a sustainable biosimilar market.

A sustainable biosimilar market must:
• Deliver tangible and transparent benefits to the health care system, while
• Addressing the needs of all stakeholders
This requires collaboration between stakeholders.

In brief, participants strongly agreed that biosimilars have the potential to promote competition among biologic options and reduce treatment costs. However, there was a need to identify and minimize transition and disruption costs when switching to a biosimilar or between biosimilars to improve savings associated with these products further. These savings should be tangible (i.e., measurable) and reinvested in health care or other public services where possible. This could include budget deficits and funding of innovative therapies; biosimilars have the potential to expand access [8]. Transparency regarding reinvestment was regarded as another important motivator for physicians and patients to use biosimilars. Minimizing transition costs could be achieved by identifying key differences between therapeutic areas and clinical settings. For example, oncology treatments usually follow a short, defined treatment course reducing the need for switch, whereas rheumatoid arthritis treatments may be chronic with multiple use of biosimilars and combinations. Clear guidance (policies and practices) from regulators and clinical organizations, such as the EMA, regarding biosimilar transition is warranted with the need for real-world evidence based on biosimilars that physicians can effectively communicate to patients to avoid any negative perceptions. Collaboration between stakeholders would help enable any guidance to be consistent, more comprehensive, and more easily communicated.

3.1.3. Drivers and Risks of a Sustainable Biosimilar Market (Competition and Incentives)

The consensus achieved by participants regarding drivers and risks of a sustainable biosimilar market is summarized in Box 3 and Table 2. Points of consensus were formulated as follows: (i) competition is a more effective mechanism to achieve a long-term predictable price level than regulation; (ii) there needs to be incentives for investment in future biosimilars; and (iii) government and pricing bodies need to drive incentives.

For key market drivers, participants agreed that competition generated by the introduction of biosimilars has been effective in reducing prices for biological therapies in Europe [28,29]. Participants also agreed that the price expectations of decision makers must reflect market opportunity. This was illustrated by the case of adalimumab biosimilars, the entry of which into the market in 2018 triggered almost immediate and substantial discounting. However, adalimumab was used in a large patient population and had achieved extremely high revenues prior to biosimilar entry, making it a very attractive target for biosimilar manufacturers. Consequently, the price levels achieved by adalimumab biosimilars might not be repeated in other biosimilar products, especially those with orphan status. Incentives driven by governments and pricing bodies (such as limits on tender) were also identified as key drivers for future market; these incentives could include procurement design, including contract length, a cap on the number of manufacturers selected, and introduction of geographical divisions (national vs. regional vs. local).

Table 2. Consensus on drivers and risks to biosimilar market sustainability (competition and incentives).

1.	**Competition is a more effective mechanism to achieve a long-term predictable price level than regulation**
Increased competition leads to more rapid price reduction and, if procurement policies contribute to business continuity, a sustained lower price level	CONSENSUS
There is a need to develop better prospective indicators to warn about potential risk of *de facto* monopoly	CONSENSUS
• Existing indicators, such as the number of manufacturers and manufacturing sites for biosimilars, are imperfect and may only indicate a problem that is too late to reverse • Additional indicators that could be explored include procurement design (e.g., contract length), geographic division (national vs. regional) and factors other than cost	POLICY MANUFACTURER
New entrants may bring minor improvements (e.g., administration devices), although competition has been primarily price-focused and has led to a reduction in "value-add" (e.g., patient support programs)	PHARMACIST PAYER
Price-setting regulation, if needed to prevent predatory behaviour, should not aim primarily at the lowest possible prices but at long-term viability of a vibrant and competitive marketplace	PAYER POLICY

Table 2. *Cont.*

II. There needs to be incentives for investment in future biosimilars		
Continued investment in biosimilar development and market entry is important to generate competition for biological therapies for which no biosimilar is currently available and, to a lesser extent, therapies with biosimilars already available	CONSENSUS	
Price expectations of policy and budget holders must reflect market opportunity, e.g., biosimilars of orphan therapies may require lower price discount levels	POLICY	MANUFACTURER
A stable, predictable price level enables manufacturers to make the long-term decisions that are required to invest in biosimilar development	POLICY	MANUFACTURER
III. Governments and pricing bodies need to drive incentives		
These bodies need to supply incentives that enable enough suppliers to survive free market onslaught; this may assure the continuity of long-term competition and sustainable discounts from originator biological therapy price levels	CONSENSUS	
• This could be achieved by varying tender available to manufacturers	POLICY	

Note: icons shown on the right represent level of agreement between the stakeholders. The 'consensus' icon indicates that all stakeholders (physicians, payers, policy advisors, manufacturers, pharmacists, and patients) agreed on that point.

Box 3. Consensus on drivers of and risks to a sustainable biosimilar market.

- Competition is a more effective mechanism to achieve a long-term predictable price level, compared to regulation
- There needs to be incentives for industry investment in future biosimilars
- Government and pricing bodies need to drive incentives
- Procurement processes should avoid monopolies and minimize patient discomfort and disruption to the health care system
- The principles for procurement should be defined by all stakeholders.

For key market risks, there was agreement that there is a need for better indicators than those currently available (e.g., the number of biosimilar manufacturers and manufacturing sites) to warn of potential de facto monopoly [30]. Participants agreed that the emergence of monopolies could lead to higher price levels and/or enhanced supply risks (such as poor quality), or supply shortages (e.g., limited production capabilities and poor distribution channels) for biosimilars. This risk also exists for generics, but it would be greater for biosimilars due to the lengthier development and market entry processes, and the much longer lead time in manufacturing (1 year or more). Participants felt that there was a need for more research to identify prospective indicators of market performance; these should be based on a thorough understanding of the role that procurement level (national vs. subnational (procurement is described below)), market size, number of awarded contracts (and market share awarded), and tender criteria may play in ensuring markets perform well. Unfortunately, published evidence on indicator performance or biosimilar supply risks and shortages are scarce making generalizability difficult, but also highlighting the need for establishing validated approaches to long-term quantification of these frameworks.

3.1.4. Drivers and Risks of a Sustainable Biosimilar Market (Procurement Processes)

Issues surrounding procurement processes are summarized in Box 3 and Table 3. Participants agreed that procurement processes should avoid monopolies and minimize patient and health care system disruption, and the principles for procurement should be agreed by all stakeholders. The participants also identified two main goals of procurement design from a multistakeholder perspective. The first goal was to prevent predatory behavior by considering factors in selection criteria other than price or aggressive price discounting; these could include differentiation based on formulation and quality attributes, or stock and distribution channels. The second goal was to minimize disruptions to patient care based on the needs of individual therapy areas, perhaps by setting a contract duration that is proportional to the duration of treatment. Given the potential implications of procurement policies for all stakeholders, participants agreed that all stakeholders should have a voice in setting procurement policies. Participants agreed that there cannot be a "one size fits all" approach to procurement, as the structure and characteristics of health care systems vary; however, procurement policies should be consistent, guided by a common set of principles, and abide with European Union rules on tendering. Participants also advised that biosimilar procurement must be managed carefully over the product lifecycle to preserve competition and promote new investment in biosimilar development.

Table 3. Consensus on drivers and risks to biosimilar market sustainability (procurement processes).

	Stakeholders
I. Procurement processes should avoid monopolies and minimize patient and health care system disruption	CONSENSUS
The emergence of monopolies may lead to higher price levels and/or enhanced supply risks	
• There are examples of this in generics, although these issues would be more pronounced for biosimilars due to lengthy development and market entry processes	PHARMACIST, POLICY, MANUFACTURER
Procurement design should aim to:	
• Prevent predatory behaviour, e.g., by considering factors other than price to avoid aggressive price discounting	PHARMACIST, PAYER
• Minimize disruption of patient care, based on the needs of individual therapeutic areas, e.g., by setting contract duration that is proportional to duration of treatment	PATIENT, PHYSICIAN
II. The principles for procurement should be agreed by all stakeholders	CONSENSUS
There should be a multistakeholder group that sets principles for policy and practice around biosimilar procurement	
Patients and physicians should have an opportunity for their views to be represented (e.g., in a national forum) and patients should be informed of the rationale behind procurement decisions that impact on their care	PATIENT, PHYSICIAN
There can be no one-size-fits-all approach to procurement, as the structure and characteristics of health care systems vary; however, there should be a consistent approach and a common set of guiding principles	POLICY, MANUFACTURER

Note: icons shown on the right represent level of agreement between the stakeholders. The 'consensus' icon indicates that all stakeholders (physicians, payers, policy advisors, manufacturers, pharmacists, and patients) agreed on that point.

3.2. Key Findings from the SLR

A total of 36 studies were identified in the SLR (Appendix B). Nine publications were identified that discussed (Q1). However, these were too limited to provide any comprehensive evidence and demonstrate the lack of a consistent, comprehensive database of medicine shortages in Europe. Nineteen publications addressed (Q2). None of these reported switching between biosimilars; rather, all considered switches from a reference product to a biosimilar. Nine publications focused on (Q3). These offered insufficient evidence from which to reach generalized conclusions about the effects of different tender models on the outcomes of interest. However, one policy paper concluded that barriers to entry, including the use of single-manufacturer tenders, will limit competition in biosimilars [16]. This paper was considered by the panel, together with additional evidence summarized in Appendix C.

4. Discussion

A Delphi process, involving diverse stakeholders from across Europe, was conducted to achieve a consensus opinion on biosimilar market sustainability in Europe. Divergent views between stakeholder groups, and the reasons for these, were explored through individual, anonymized feedback and facilitated discussion at a roundtable meeting. This important exercise was undertaken to increase our understanding of the current system and to address concerns regarding sustainability, including the unmet need to develop a long-term vision, as highlighted in previous analyses [11,19,20]. Participants agreed that a sustainable biosimilar market must deliver tangible and transparent benefits to the health care system, while meeting the needs of all stakeholders. The definition (as shown in Box 1) was approved by all participants; however, different stakeholder groups emphasized different priorities within this definition, which is consistent with the previous literature on a lack of a unified approach [19,20]. Participants also agreed that, to make this approach work, collaboration between stakeholders is required and a greater awareness of the drivers of and threats to a sustainable market. In brief, strategies around competition, incentives, and procurement policies were identified and discussed with key consensus highlighted in the tables. These areas (notably the need to establish healthy competition, pricing, and market access policies (considering gain sharing and price reductions), government policy and guidance, identification of risks associated with biosimilar drug supply (e.g., quality issues), and patient access to information and education) were highlighted in the previous literature as key areas requiring further improvements [11,19]. Participants in the Delphi process agreed that these key findings should be developed further into a white paper that highlights the need for multistakeholder collaboration on establishing principles for biosimilar procurement in Europe.

Several priorities for future research were identified by stakeholders. First, understanding and measuring the impact of biosimilar transition on hospital and health care services will better enable costs and benefits to be weighed up and help minimize disruption for patients and health care services. Second, there is a need to understand and develop prospective indicators of market sustainability and potential risks to competitive biosimilar markets, particularly the emergence of de facto monopolies and supply risks. Finally, it will also be important to understand the implications of procurement structure and design for biosimilar market sustainability, especially with regard to how the procurement level (national vs. subnational), market size, number of awarded contracts (and market share awarded), and tender criteria affect market sustainability.

There is currently very limited published evidence available to support detailed arguments in the three priority areas described above, largely because there are limited data with which to conduct analyses. Biosimilar markets are still relatively new in Europe, which means that the available data relate to limited time periods and newly emerging trends that may be expected to mature over time. Further, the currently available data (e.g., on supply shortages of biosimilars) are kept at the national level; this allows cross-country comparisons but poses a challenge for pan-European analysis. It is therefore recommended that any further research begins with a scoping phase, in which the available data are reviewed in detail to assess their suitability for the proposed purpose. Further research would also benefit from a more quantifiable approach to the sustainability framework, allowing us to measure the extent to which a biosimilar market in a specific jurisdiction can be effectively maintained.

Collaboration with stakeholders to develop principles for biosimilar procurement may be progressed in tandem with further research. The objective of establishing processes is to ensure that the concerns of all stakeholders—patients, physicians, pharmacists, payers, policy advisers, and manufacturers—are considered in procurement design. In the absence of evidence, open communication and collaboration between stakeholders may provide the necessary information that procurement decision makers need to prevent risks to biosimilar market sustainability from materializing.

This Delphi process involved a limited number of stakeholders and, as with any Delphi exercise, may also be biased by those who chose to participate [31]. For example, a number of issues were not considered such as the evolution of the biosimilar production process over time. However, the process encompassed evidence from a broad review of available literature and covered a broad range of stakeholder perspectives. Despite a rigorous approach, the findings of the SLR indicated that there was an absence of consistent, comprehensive information about drug shortages (specifically biosimilar shortages) and the costs of switching to biosimilars in Europe; these gaps exacerbate a lack of evidence regarding the impact of different tender models for savings, sustainable competition, and supply risk. The panel identified eight key papers (Appendix C), some of which were not identified by the SLR. The consensus reached by the Delphi process provides further direction for future research into, and implementation of, potential strategies to support these different aspects of sustainability.

5. Conclusions

A sustainable biologics market including biosimilars is essential for ensuring that health care savings are maintained into the future, both for existing molecules and those approaching a loss of exclusivity. This Delphi approach resulted in a consensus definition of biosimilar market sustainability in Europe, specified the components of a sustainable biosimilar market, and identified key drivers and risks to sustainability. Crucially, participants in the Delphi process highlighted the need for multistakeholder collaboration in designing policy and practice relating to biosimilars (including procurement). Further research is required alongside stakeholder collaboration to inform biosimilar policy and practice in alignment with the principles identified in this Delphi process. Failure to care for biosimilar market sustainability may impoverish the biosimilar development and offerings, eventually leading to increased cost for health care systems and patients, with fewer resources for innovation.

Author Contributions: Conceptualization, A.G.V. and J.H.; methodology, A.G.V. and J.H.; validation, A.G.V., J.V.-O., M.v.d.G., S.R.A.S. and L.D.; informal analysis, A.G.V., J.V.-O. and B.M.; investigation, A.G.V., M.v.d.G., S.R.A.S. and L.D.; resources, A.G.V. and J.V.-O.; data curation, A.G.V. and J.V.-O.; writing—original draft preparation, J.V.-O. and J.L.; writing—review and editing, All authors; visualization, All authors; supervision, A.G.V. and J.V.-O.; project administration, B.M.; funding acquisition, A.G.V. and J.H. All authors have read and agreed to the published version of the manuscript.

Funding: This research received funding from Amgen.

Acknowledgments: The authors would like to thank the following for their participation in the panel discussions: Nathalie Deparis (patient advocating, rheumatoid arthritis), Hans-Christian Kolberg (physician), Stuart Parkes and Noemi Martinez Lopez De Castro (hospital pharmacists), Jean-Michel Descoutures and Tim Visser (procurement pharmacists), Jorge Mestre Ferrandiz (policy advisers, health economist), and Stephan Rönninger (manufacturer).

Conflicts of Interest: A.G.V. reports personal fees from AbbVie, Accord-Healthcare, Amgen, Biogen Idec, Febelgen, Fresenius-Kabi, Hexal, Medicines for Europe, Mundipharma, Novartis, Pfizer, Samsung, and Sandoz; J.V.-O., R.M., and B.M. are employees of Parexel who were contracted by Amgen; M.v.d.G. reports personal fees from Amgen and BioMarin; L.D. reports personal fees from Abbvie, Amgen, Biogen, BMS, Celltrion, Novartis, Pfizer, Roche, Sanofi-Genzyme, and SOBI; J.L. and J.H. are employees of Amgen; S.G.M. is an Amgen employee and stockholder; S.S. is one of the founders of the KU Leuven Fund on Market Analysis of Biologics and Biosimilars following Loss of Exclusivity (MABEL). He was involved in a European stakeholder roundtable on biologics and biosimilars sponsored by Amgen, Merck Sharp and Dohme, and Pfizer; he has participated in advisory board meetings for Amgen and Pfizer; and he has contributed to studies on biologics and biosimilars for Celltrion,

Hospira, Mundipharma, and Pfizer. S.S. is also member of the leadership team of the International Society for Pharmacoeconomics and Outcomes Research Special Interest Group on Biosimilars.

Appendix A

Table A1. Brainstorming questionnaire (Delphi process stage 1).

I.	Define a sustainable biosimilar market in Europe from your perspective.
	• What does a sustainable biosimilar market look like? • Provide up to five key points
II.	What factors contribute to, or create a risk to, biosimilar market sustainability?
	• How important are each of these factors in achieving sustainability? • Provide up to five key points and indicate how important they are to you (low/moderate/high)
III.	How have biosimilars contributed to the sustainability of health care system(s)?
	• Are you aware of any specific, direct benefits from biosimilars entering the market?

Appendix B

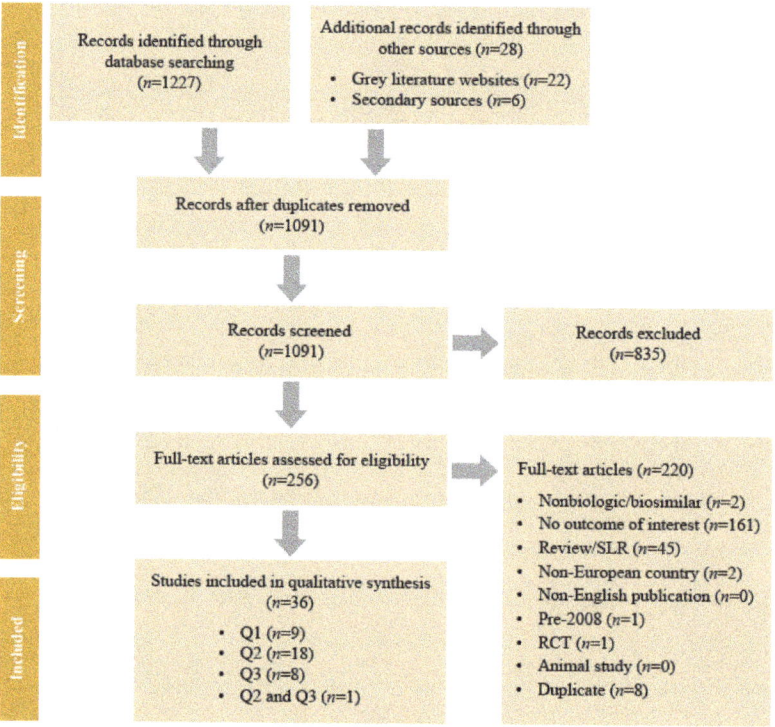

Figure A1. PRISMA Flow Diagram. RCT, randomized controlled trial. SLR, systematic literature review.

Appendix C

Table A2. Key literature identified during brainstorming (Delphi process stage 1).

Topic	Source	References
Savings (implications for health system sustainability)	Systematic literature review/targeted additional search	Vulto A, et al. (2019) [18]
Sustainable competition	Systematic literature review	Mestre-Ferrandiz J, et al. (2016) [16] Dave CV, et al. (2017) [25] Dave CV, et al. (2018) [26]
Access and pricing	Targeted additional search	Moorkens E, et al. (2017) [17] Kawalec P, et al. (2017) [27]
Procurement/purchasing	Review of tender documents (2018)	Vulto A, et al. (2019) [18]
Patient safety/use	Targeted additional search	Tabernero J, et al. (2016) [4] EULAR PARE (2018) [3]

Appendix D

Table A3. Themes and statements (Delphi process stage 2).

Presence of multiple suppliers on an ongoing basis—although there is no "correct" number of suppliers	1.	Biosimilars offer choice and are an important savings opportunity that can benefit the health care system broadly
Competition that is effective in reducing prices for biologics/biosimilars to a sustainable level	2.	The presence of multiple suppliers offers benefits (with some trade-offs)
Shared decision making with payer, pharmacist, physician, and patients around biosimilar use	3.	Competition offers benefits (with some trade-offs)
Reliable supply of biosimilars that meet appropriate standards for quality	4.	Effective implementation is necessary for sustainability
Stability in procurement structure and approach	5.	Excessive levels of competition have potential to be detrimental to the future of competition in biosimilars markets
Avoidance of price erosion that leads to market exit and the emergence of monopolies or the consolidation of suppliers	6.	The level at which procurement happens has consequences for the number of manufacturers in the market—national versus sub-national

References

1. Market Data Forecast. Biosimilars Market. Available online: https://www.marketdataforecast.com/market-reports/biosimilars-market (accessed on 13 May 2020).
2. Technavio. Global Biosimilars Market 2018–2022. Available online: https://www.technavio.com/report/global-biosimilars-market-analysis-share-2018?tnplus (accessed on 13 May 2020).
3. EULAR (European League Against Rheumatism) Standing Committee of People with Arthritis/Rheumatism in Europe (PARE). Biosimilars—Position Paper. Updating Position Statement from the European League against Rheumatism (EULAR) Standing Committee of People with Arthritis/Rheumatism in Europe (PARE). Available online: https://www.eular.org/myUploadData/files/biosimilars_paper_updated_2018_09_14_dw.pdf (accessed on 13 May 2020).

4. Tabernero, J.; Vyas, M.; Giuliani, R.; Arnold, D.; Cardoso, F.; Casali, P.G.; Cervantes, A.; Eggermont, A.M.; Eniu, A.; Jassem, J.; et al. Biosimilars: A position paper of the European Society for Medical Oncology, with particular reference to oncology prescribers. *ESMO Open* **2016**, *1*, e000142. [CrossRef] [PubMed]
5. EMA (European Medicines Agency). European Commission. Biosimilars in the EU. Information Guide for Healthcare Professionals. Available online: https://www.ema.europa.eu/en/documents/leaflet/biosimilars-eu-information-guide-healthcare-professionals_en.pdf (accessed on 13 May 2020).
6. EMA (European Medicines Agency). Guidelines on Similar Biological Medicinal Products. Available online: https://www.ema.europa.eu/en/documents/scientific-guideline/guideline-similar-biological-medicinal-products-rev1_en.pdf (accessed on 13 May 2020).
7. US FDA (Food and Drug Administration). Biosimilar and Interchangeable Products. Available online: https://www.fda.gov/drugs/biosimilars/biosimilar-and-interchangeable-products#generic (accessed on 13 May 2020).
8. IQVIA Institute. The Impact of Biosimilar Competition in Europe. Available online: https://ec.europa.eu/docsroom/documents/38461 (accessed on 13 May 2020).
9. Dutta, B.; Huys, I.; Vulto, A.G.; Simoens, S. Identifying key benefits in European off-patent biologics and biosimilar markets: It is not only about price! *BioDrugs* **2020**, *34*, 159–170. [CrossRef] [PubMed]
10. IQVIA Institute. The Global Use of Medicine in 2019 and Outlook to 2023. Forecasts and Areas to Watch. Institute Report. Available online: https://www.iqvia.com/insights/the-iqvia-institute/reports/the-global-use-of-medicine-in-2019-and-outlook-to-2023 (accessed on 13 May 2020).
11. IQVIA Institute. Advancing Biosimilar Sustainability in Europe. A Multi-Stakeholder Assessment. Institute Report. Available online: https://www.iqvia.com/insights/the-iqvia-institute/reports/advancing-biosimilar-sustainability-in-europe (accessed on 13 May 2020).
12. Deloitte Development LLC. Winning with Biosimilars: Opportunities in Global Markets. Available online: https://www2.deloitte.com/content/dam/Deloitte/us/Documents/life-sciences-health-care/us-lshc-biosimilars-whitepaper-final.pdf (accessed on 13 May 2020).
13. Danese, S.; Fiorino, G.; Raine, T.; Ferrante, M.; Kemp, K.; Kierkus, J.; Lakatos, P.L.; Mantzaris, G.; Van Der Woude, J.; Panes, J.; et al. ECCO position statement on the use of biosimilars for inflammatory bowel disease-an update. *J. Crohns Colitis* **2017**, *11*, 26–34. [CrossRef] [PubMed]
14. Digestive Cancers Europe. Position Paper on the Use of Biosimilar Medicines in Colorectal Cancer. Available online: https://digestivecancers.eu/Documents/Uploaded/468-Document-Positionpaperbiosimilarsfinal.pdf (accessed on 13 May 2020).
15. EAHP (European Association of Hospital Pharmacists). EAHP Position Paper on Biosimilar Medicines. Available online: https://www.eahp.eu/content/position-paper-biosimilar-medicines-0 (accessed on 13 May 2020).
16. Mestre-Ferrandiz, J.; Towse, A.; Berdud, M. Biosimilars: How can payers get long-term savings? *Pharmacoeconomics* **2016**, *34*, 609–616. [CrossRef] [PubMed]
17. Moorkens, E.; Vulto, A.G.; Huys, I.; Dylst, P.; Godman, B.; Keuerleber, S.; Claus, B.; Dimitrova, M.; Petrova, G.; Sović-Brkičić, L.; et al. Policies for biosimilar uptake in Europe: An overview. *PLoS ONE* **2017**, *12*, e0190147. [CrossRef] [PubMed]
18. Vulto, A.; Cheesman, S.; Gonzalez-McQuire, S.; Lebioda, A.; Bech, A.; Hippenmeyer, J.; Lapham, K. Sustainable biosimilar procurement in Europe: A review of current policies and their potential impact. *Value Health* **2019**, *22*, S427. [CrossRef]
19. Simon Kucher & Partners. Payers' Price & Market Access Policies Supporting a Sustainable Biosimilar Medicines Market. Final Report. Available online: https://www.medicinesforeurope.com/wp-content/uploads/2016/09/Simon-Kucher-2016-Policy-requirements-for-a-sustainable-biosimilar-market-FINAL-report_for-publication2.pdf (accessed on 13 May 2020).
20. Pugatch Consilium. Towards a Sustainable European Market for Off-Patent Biologics. Available online: https://www.pugatch-consilium.com/?p=2760 (accessed on 13 May 2020).
21. Eubank, B.H.; Mohtadi, N.G.; Lafave, M.R.; Wiley, J.P.; Bois, A.J.; Boorman, R.S.; Sheps, D.M. Using the modified Delphi method to establish clinical consensus for the diagnosis and treatment of patients with rotator cuff pathology. *BMC Med. Res. Methodol.* **2016**, *16*, 56. [CrossRef] [PubMed]
22. Hirschhorn, F. Reflections on the application of the Delphi method: Lessons from a case in public transport research. *Int. J. Soc. Res. Methodol.* **2019**, *22*, 309–322. [CrossRef]

23. Higgins, J.P.T.; Green, S. (Eds.) The Cochrane Collaboration. Cochrane Handbook for Systematic Reviews of Interventions. Version 5.1.0 (updated March 2011). Available online: https://handbook-5-1.cochrane.org/front_page.htm (accessed on 13 May 2020).
24. Centre for Reviews and Dissemination. Systematic Reviews. CRD's Guidance for Undertaking Reviews in Health Care. Available online: https://www.york.ac.uk/media/crd/Systematic_Reviews.pdf (accessed on 13 May 2020).
25. Dave, C.V.; Kesselheim, A.S.; Fox, E.R.; Qiu, P.; Hartzema, A. High generic drug prices and market competition: A retrospective cohort study. *Ann. Intern. Med.* **2017**, *167*, 145–151. [CrossRef] [PubMed]
26. Dave, C.V.; Pawar, A.; Fox, E.R.; Brill, G.; Kesselheim, A.S. Predictors of drug shortages and association with generic drug prices: A retrospective cohort study. *Value Health* **2018**, *21*, 1286–1290. [CrossRef] [PubMed]
27. Kawalec, P.; Stawowczyk, E.; Tesar, T.; Skoupa, J.; Turcu-Stiolica, A.; Dimitrova, M.; Petrova, G.I.; Rugaja, Z.; Männik, A.; Harsanyi, A.; et al. Pricing and reimbursement of biosimilars in central and eastern European countries. *Front. Pharmacol.* **2017**, *8*, 288. [CrossRef] [PubMed]
28. NHS (National Health Service). NHS Cuts Medicines Costs by Three Quarters of a Billion Pounds. Available online: https://www.england.nhs.uk/2019/08/nhs-cuts-medicines-costs-by-three-quarters-of-a-billion-pounds/ (accessed on 13 May 2020).
29. Zorginstituut Nederland. GIPdatabank.nl. Available online: https://www.gipdatabank.nl/databank (accessed on 13 May 2020).
30. Amgros. Price Negotiations and Effective Competition. Available online: https://amgros.dk/en/pharmaceuticals/price-negotiations-and-effective-competition/ (accessed on 13 May 2020).
31. Strober, B.; Ryan, C.; van de Kerkhof, P.; Van Der Walt, J.; Kimball, A.B.; Barker, J.; Blauvelt, A.; Bourcier, M.; Carvalho, A.; Cohen, A.; et al. Recategorization of psoriasis severity: Delphi consensus from the International Psoriasis Council. *J. Am. Acad. Dermatol.* **2020**, *82*, 117–122. [CrossRef] [PubMed]

Publisher's Note: MDPI stays neutral with regard to jurisdictional claims in published maps and institutional affiliations.

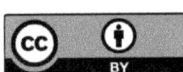

© 2020 by the authors. Licensee MDPI, Basel, Switzerland. This article is an open access article distributed under the terms and conditions of the Creative Commons Attribution (CC BY) license (http://creativecommons.org/licenses/by/4.0/).

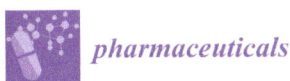

Article

Analysis of the Regulatory Science Applied to a Single Portfolio of Eight Biosimilar Product Approvals by Four Key Regulatory Authorities

Beverly Ingram [1,*], Rebecca S. Lumsden [2], Adriana Radosavljevic [1] and Christine Kobryn [3]

1. Pfizer Inc., Andover, MA 01810, USA; adriana.radosavljevic@gmail.com
2. Pfizer Inc., Walton Oaks, Surrey KT20 7NS, UK; rebecca.s.lumsden@pfizer.com
3. Pfizer Inc., Groton, CT 06340, USA; christine.kobryn@pfizer.com
* Correspondence: bev.ingram@pfizer.com; Tel.: +1-978-247-4558

Abstract: Slow uptake of biosimilars in some regions is often attributed to a lack of knowledge combined with concerns about safety and efficacy. To alleviate physician and patient apprehensions, regulatory reviews from four major regulatory authorities (RAs) (European Medicines Agency, US Food and Drug Administration, Health Canada, and Japan Pharmaceuticals and Medical Devices Authority) across a portfolio of eight biosimilars were analyzed to provide insight into RA review focus and approach. RA queries were evaluated in an unbiased and systematic manner by major classification (Chemistry, Manufacturing and Controls [CMC], nonclinical, clinical or regulatory) and then via detailed sub-classification. There was a consistent, predominant focus on CMC from all RAs. The review focus based on sub-classification of clinical and regulatory queries was influenced by molecular complexity, with significant differences between categories (monoclonal antibody or protein) in the distribution of query topics; specifically, bioanalytical ($p = 0.023$), comparative safety and efficacy ($p = 0.023$), and statutory (including the justification of extrapolation) ($p = 0.00033$). Each biosimilar had a distinct distribution of clinical query topics, tailored to product-specific data. This analysis elucidated areas of heightened RA interest, and validated their application of regulatory science in the evaluation of biosimilar safety and efficacy.

Keywords: biosimilars; regulatory; review; approval; clinical; queries; regulatory science

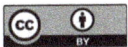

1. Introduction

Biosimilars represent an increasingly important option in the delivery of high-quality treatments for patients and offer the potential to address one of the greatest access constraints to biologics globally, namely price [1–3]. Since the first biosimilar was approved in 2006 by the European Medicines Agency (EMA) a dedicated regulatory framework for such products has spread rapidly across the world, with biosimilar-specific regulatory paradigms currently established in over 20 countries [4].

The requirement to establish dedicated biosimilar-specific regulatory paradigms by regulatory authorities (RAs) is well documented and is necessary since biosimilars cannot be safely regulated by the pathway used for typical 'small molecule' generic drugs [5,6]. The inherent variation of biological systems means that biosimilars cannot be manufactured to be identical to the originator biologic reference product (i.e., reference product) but are instead structurally and functionally "highly similar" [7]. Building and expanding on scientific principles and methodologies established for novel biologics (i.e., concepts outlined in the International Council for Harmonisation Q5E [8]), the EMA issued the first dedicated biosimilar-specific guidance in 2005. This was followed by the World Health Organization (2009), The Japanese Ministry of Health, Labour and Welfare (2009), Health Canada (HC) (2010) and the US Food and Drug Administration (FDA) (2012) (Initial draft overarching guidance was published in 2012; final guidance was published in 2018). Although developed at different times, these guidances share the same fundamental scientific approach to establishing biosimilarity [9,10]. Major regulators such as the FDA, EMA, HC, and the Pharmaceuticals and Medical Devices Authority (PMDA) have leveraged cross-communication, such as health authority cluster meetings, in order to share learning and foster greater consistency, due to the rapid pace at which the regulatory science has evolved [11].

The concept of biosimilar development is underpinned by both established scientific knowledge and the application of regulatory science during the assessment by RAs [11,12]. The extent and type of the data required, and the studies conducted during biosimilar development, to meet the regulatory requirements for biosimilarity differ from those required for novel biologics, both in their design and the relative emphasis of contributing parts (Figure 1) [13–15]. RAs also have discretion, as per their respective regulatory guidelines, to determine whether some nonclinical and clinical studies are not required; for example, animal studies may be conducted if residual uncertainties remain following the analytical assessment that need to be resolved prior to conducting a comparative clinical trial [16–18].

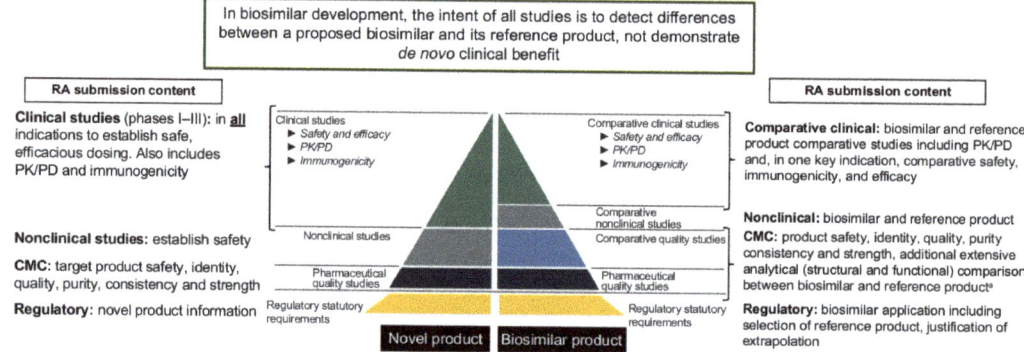

Figure 1. Development Aim and Impact on Regulatory Information for Novel Biologics and Biosimilars (Adapted from Biosimilar Development and Approval in the EU, European Medicines Agency [15]). [a] While CMC information for a novel biologic is focused solely on the target product, the corresponding information for a biosimilar is highly comparative, with additional content required focusing on both the biosimilar and the reference product. CMC, Chemistry, Manufacturing and Controls; EU, European Union; PD, pharmacodynamic; PK, pharmacokinetic(s); RA, Regulatory Agency.

The demonstration of similarity is first and foremost required at a molecular level, by the application of a number of in vitro analytical techniques [19]. These analytical studies are extensive and form the foundation for establishing similarity [13,16,20]. Hence, biosimilar development is focused on the production of a similar molecule to the reference product, analytical (in vitro) assessments that support demonstration of similarity, and manufacturing controls that ensure similarity is maintained [17]. All of these aspects are complemented by a targeted clinical study, sensitive enough with regard to the design, conduct, endpoints and/or population to detect differences should they exist with the reference product [21]. Demonstration of biosimilarity is based on careful consideration of the totality of the information provided [13].

The biosimilar developer can seek approval of their product for other authorized indications of the reference product via extrapolation of similarity. This is a scientific and regulatory principle that is applied without the need to conduct a comparative clinical study in the extrapolated disease indication(s) [22]. Without this facility, biosimilar development would not follow an abbreviated pathway [23]. Extrapolation of efficacy and safety data from one indication to another is not a given; it must be thoroughly scientifically justified, based on data that indicates certain properties of the originator, such as the mechanism of action, PK and immunogenicity, are consistent between the indications [24].

Despite many biosimilars now approved by the EMA [25] and a growing number of biosimilars authorized by the FDA [26], barriers remain to their adoption and use in clinical practice, driven by several issues, including concerns among healthcare providers and patients over their safety and effectiveness [27]. These reservations suggest that gaps may exist between the extent of the evidence required for biosimilars to gain RA approval and the evidence needed to achieve wider acceptance and use by physicians and patients [28]. When the development components and supporting data of a novel biologic and biosimilar are compared (Figure 1), the unique aspects of biosimilar development are revealed as one potential root cause of this gap. The use of an expanded analytical assessment, together with targeted clinical data obtained in a sufficiently sensitive patient population (with justification of extrapolation for additional indications), in place of the more extensive clinical data required for novel biologics, is the foundation of biosimilarity and of the scientific benefit–risk considerations applied by RAs [11].

Pfizer has established a portfolio of biosimilars, which differ in their molecular complexity and span disease indications in inflammation and oncology (including supportive care). Proactive engagement with RAs occurred throughout each product's development (via advice procedures) to ensure alignment with expectations and requirements. The RA advice from multiple agencies was incorporated into the respective product's development to inform a global development strategy. This permitted a global dossier preparation and submission approach, whereby the same data for each biosimilar were used to support all submissions (with the inclusion of additional/alternative data to meet a limited number of country-specific requirements). This strategy, and the breadth and extent of regulatory submissions, provides a unique opportunity to analyze the focus of RA review and gain an understanding of the approaches applied by different regulatory bodies in ensuring the requirements for biosimilarity are met. We conducted an analysis of the queries received from multiple RAs in response to license applications for this portfolio of biosimilars. We aimed to bring a greater awareness and appreciation of the RA approach, scientific consistency, and reviewer focus during biosimilar review, to increase confidence in the safety and effectiveness of biosimilars amongst physicians and patients [29].

2. Results

A total of 2438 queries were received from the FDA, EMA, PMDA, and HC in relation to 21 applications for the eight biosimilars. Except for two queries relating to legal matters received from the PMDA, all other queries were retained and included in the analysis.

CMC was the largest category of query assignments received from the FDA (83%), EMA (66%) and PMDA (58%). For HC, 41% of queries were assigned to CMC, which were comparable in number to those assigned to the regulatory category (Figure 2). CMC queries encompassed data supporting the comprehensive in vitro comparative analysis of the biosimilar and its reference product, as well as manufacturing details and quality control aspects, while those assigned to the regulatory category included those focused on the relevance of the reference product, justification of extrapolation of indications, and labeling topics. Nonclinical queries, which related to the limited in vivo studies required, comprised 0.3% or fewer of the overall number of queries received from each RA.

A main focus on CMC-related information was also reflected in the queries associated with the individual biosimilars received from the FDA, EMA and PMDA, which was maintained throughout the duration of review period covered by the first and most recent biosimilar to be authorized (Figure 3A–C). Emphasis on the regulatory classification by HC was apparent across all four biosimilars (Figure 3D). Closer evaluation of the queries assigned to this category for HC found that the majority (90%) were related solely to labeling, with CMC queries representing 65% of the overall share when labeling queries were not included. In contrast, both the FDA and EMA directed the lowest proportion of queries towards regulatory topics, comprising 5% and 3%, respectively, of the total queries received from each RA (Figure 2), irrespective of the particular biosimilar (Figure 3A,B).

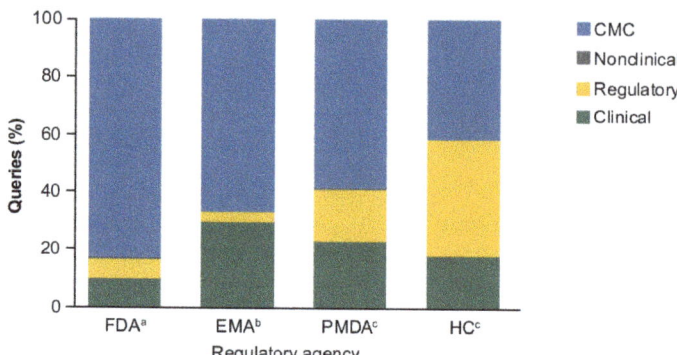

Figure 2. Regulatory Agency Queries Overall (FDA [n = 1397]), EMA [n = 791], PMDA [n = 608], and HC [n = 640]) by Major Classification. CMC, Chemistry, Manufacturing and Controls; EMA, European Medicines Agency; FDA, US Food and Drug Administration; HC, Health Canada; PMDA, Pharmaceuticals and Medical Devices Agency. Number of biosimilars: [a] n = 8, [b] n = 5, [c] n = 4.

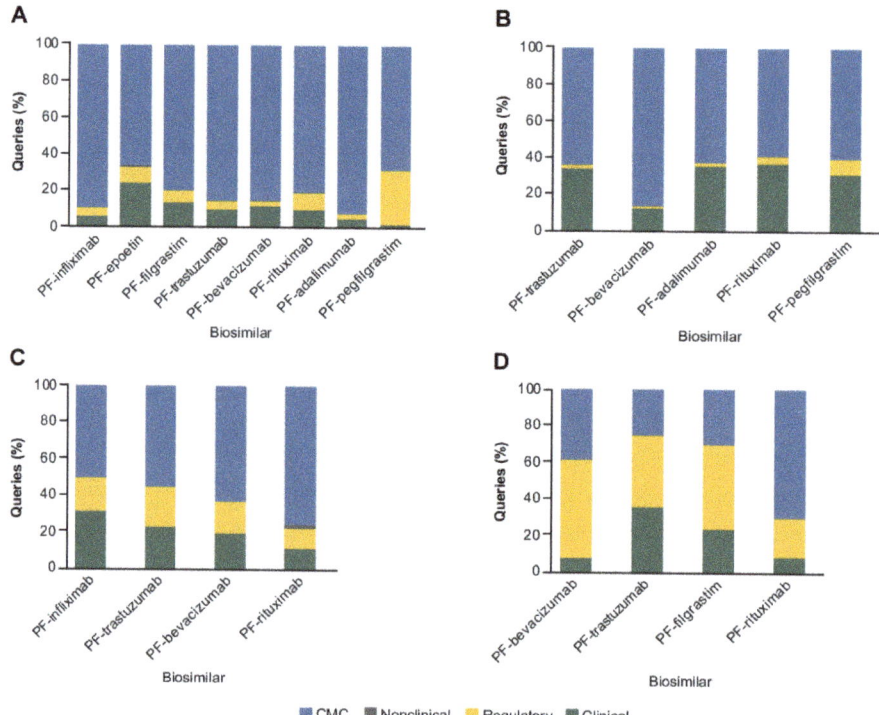

Figure 3. Major Classification Queries by Biosimilar across the (**A**) FDA (n = 1397), (**B**) EMA (n = 791), (**C**) PMDA (n = 608), and (**D**) HC (n = 640). CMC, Chemistry, Manufacturing and Controls; EMA, European Medicines Agency; FDA, US Food and Drug Administration; HC, Health Canada; PMDA, Pharmaceuticals and Medical Devices Agency.

For the three biosimilars that were assessed by all four RAs (Figure 3A–D), the analysis found a high focus on CMC topics (PF-trastuzumab [Trazimera™], 25–86% of queries; PF-bevacizumab [Zirabev™], 38–86%; and PF-rituximab, 59–81%). While the FDA raised the highest number of queries overall for each biosimilar, the proportions of queries assigned to the clinical (1–23%) and regulatory (2–30%) categories were relatively low across products with respect to the proportion of CMC queries (67–92%). CMC also represented the most frequent category of queries received from the EMA, with the proportion overall (Figure 2) and by individual product being relatively lower than that seen for the FDA. Amongst the three biosimilars assessed by both RAs, the proportions of CMC queries for PF-bevacizumab were the same for the FDA and the EMA (86%).

2.1. CMC Category

Analysis of the CMC queries revealed that the RAs showed a consistent focus on specific aspects, irrespective of molecular complexity or therapy area (Figure 4). The FDA and EMA showed a consistently high focus on both drug substance (DS) (31–54% and 37–69%, respectively) and drug product (DP) content (38–51% and 22–47%, respectively) to a greater extent than analytical similarity (aspects regarding manufacturing and testing control were highly consistently in their inclusion). The FDA were uniquely interested in DP shipping validation information as part of their focus on DP control. Queries related to facilities/good manufacturing practices (GMP) represented <10% (0–3% and 1–7%, respectively) of the overall CMC queries for any individual biosimilar across both the FDA and EMA (Figure 4A,B). In contrast, the queries related to facilities/GMP represented a far higher share of the CMC queries arising from PMDA review of four biosimilars (19–36%) (Figure 4C). Neither the EMA nor the PMDA conducted on-site inspections of manufacturing facilities as part of their review process, in contrast to the approach applied by the FDA and HC. Compared with the other RAs a higher proportion of queries related to DP were received from HC (38–80%), with between 23% and 70% of these being related to sample testing questions (namely detailed queries on how to conduct the analytical methods as well as data interpretation) across the biosimilars assessed. Analytical similarity was generally the least frequent CMC category amongst the HC (0–9%) and PMDA queries (2–3%). Extensive in vitro functional data was submitted and categorized under analytical similarity, which always received close attention by all RAs especially when it related to the product mechanism of action.

2.2. Clinical and Regulatory Sub-Classification

On sub-classification of the clinical and regulatory queries by RA assigned in the major classification, queries from the FDA and EMA were more focused on bioanalytical aspects than on PK/PD or immunogenicity. A high proportion of those received from HC were assigned to labeling (62%), compared with 29% and 24% on this topic amongst those received from the PMDA and FDA, respectively (Figure 5). Labeling represented <5% of the clinical and regulatory queries received from the EMA. The apparent focus on labeling queries by HC and PMDA was further assessed to identify the share of queries directed towards the presentation of specific biosimilar data in the product label and monograph, or non-data-related queries (including formatting, use of reference product trade name vs. international nonproprietary name vs. biosimilar trade name, etc.). The majority of HC labeling queries were not related to the presentation of biosimilar-specific data in the product label, but on non-data-related queries, with 89% of labeling queries being focused on formatting (Supplementary Figure S1). Likewise, the PMDA reviews overall had only 1 out of 68 (1.5%) labeling queries directed towards biosimilar-specific content, with that query being editorial in nature.

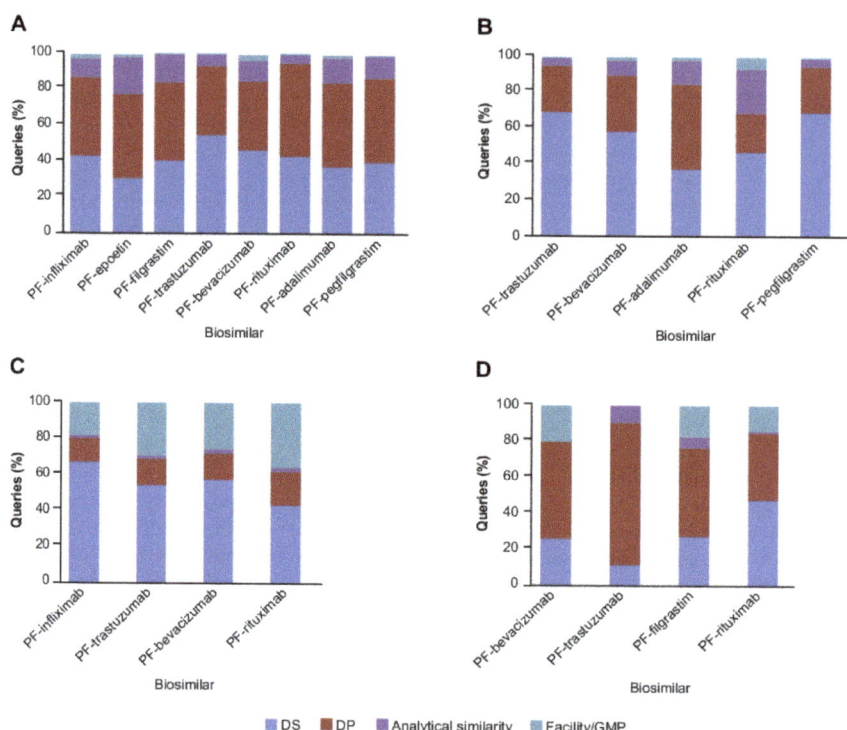

Figure 4. CMC Queries by Biosimilar across the (**A**) FDA (*n* = 2766), (**B**) EMA (*n* = 1134), (**C**) PMDA (*n* = 588), and (**D**) HC (*n* = 318). CMC, Chemistry, Manufacturing and Controls; DP, drug product; DS, drug substance; EMA, European Medicines Agency; FDA, US Food and Drug Administration; GMP, good manufacturing practices; HC, Health Canada; PMDA, Pharmaceuticals and Medical Devices Agency.

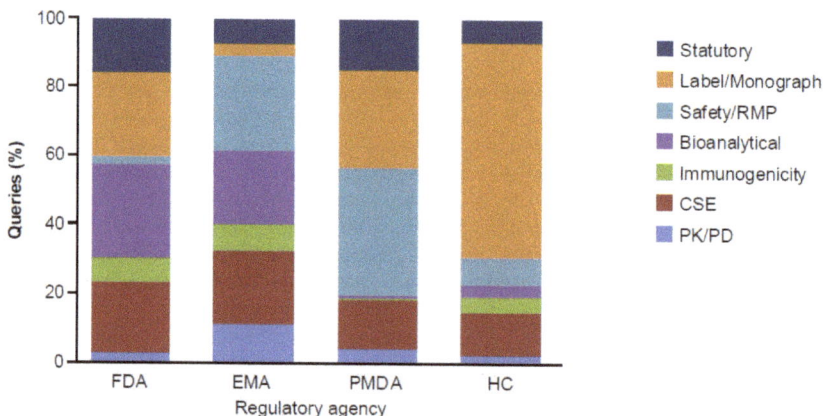

Figure 5. Sub-Classification of Regulatory (Including Labeling) and Clinical Queries by RA (FDA [*n* = 235]), EMA [*n* = 265], PMDA [*n* = 251], and HC [*n* = 377]). CSE, comparative safety and efficacy; EMA, European Medicines Agency; FDA, US Food and Drug Administration; HC, Health Canada; PK, pharmacokinetic; PMDA, Pharmaceuticals and Medical Devices Agency; RMP, risk-management plan.

There was no clear focus on any specific clinical and regulatory sub-category when assessing the queries by biosimilar product for the FDA and EMA (Figure 6A,B). Results of the analysis appeared to reflect that safety/risk management plan (RMP) and labeling topics were of consistent interest to PMDA, with the former category comprising 37% of clinical and regulatory queries overall (Figure 6C). The highest frequency of label queries was observed with HC reviews (Figure 6D) comprising 62% of those received across all biosimilars submitted to this RA. Queries directed towards pharmacokinetic (PK)/pharmacodynamic (PD) data were relatively low across all four RAs (Figure 6A–D) and biosimilar products, ranging from 2% to 11%, while bioanalytical assays used to derive the clinical data, comprised 27% and 22% of the clinical and regulatory queries received from the FDA and EMA, respectively (Figure 6A,B). For the three biosimilars (PF-trastuzumab, PF-bevacizumab and PF-rituximab) assessed by all four RAs, each authority raised a different composition of queries on the clinical and regulatory content when presented with essentially the same data (Figure 6A–D).

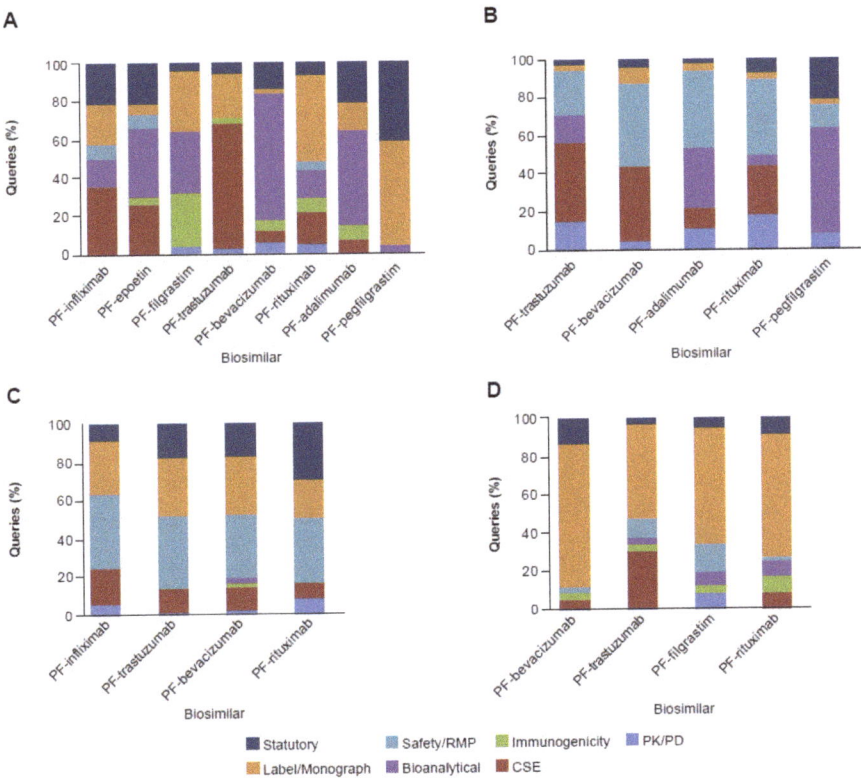

Figure 6. Sub-Classification of Regulatory (Including Labeling) and Clinical Queries by Biosimilar from the (**A**) FDA (*n* = 235), (**B**) EMA (*n* = 265), (**C**) PMDA (*n* = 251), and (**D**) HC (*n* = 377). CSE, comparative safety and efficacy; EMA, European Medicines Agency; FDA, US Food and Drug Administration; HC, Health Canada; PK, pharmacokinetic; PMDA, Pharmaceuticals and Medical Devices Agency; RMP, risk-management plan.

As indicated in Table 1, the eight biosimilars assessed in this analysis differ in their molecular complexity, which is reflected in their distinct development programs and the data accumulated to support their regulatory approval. They are approved for specific indications within oncology (including supportive care) and inflammatory disease. PF-rituximab is approved for disease indications in both therapy areas.

Table 1. Biosimilars and Approval Dates.

Biosimilar		Regulatory Agency, Approval Date				Reference	Molecule Complexity	Therapy Area
Product	INN (Trade Name), US/RoW	FDA	EMA	PMDA	HC	Product, Trade Name (INN)		
PF-filgrastim	filgrastim-aafi (Nivestym®)/ filgrastim (Nivestim) [a]	20 July 2018	8 June 2010 [e]	_ [d]	20 April 2020	Neupogen® (filgrastim)	Protein	Oncology
PF-epoetin	epoetin alfa-epbx (Retacrit®) [b]	15 May 2018	_ [d]	_ [d]	_ [d]	Epogen®/Procrit® [g] (epoetin alfa)	Protein	Oncology
PF-epoetin	epoetin zeta (Retacrit®) [b]	_ [d]	18 December 2007 [e]	_ [d]	_ [d]	Epogen®/Procrit® [g] (epoetin alfa)	Protein	Oncology
PF-rituximab	rituximab-pvvr/ rituximab (Ruxience™)	23 July 2019	1 April 2020	20 September 2019	4 May 2020	Rituxan® (rituximab)	MAb	Oncology, inflammation [h]
PF-trastuzumab	trastuzumab-qyyp/trastuzumab (Trazimera™)	11 March 2019	26 July 2018	21 September 2018	15 August 2019	Herceptin® (trastuzumab)	MAb	Oncology
PF-bevacizumab	bevacizumab-bvzr/bevacizumab (Zirabev™)	28 June 2019	14 February 2019	18 June 2019	14 June 2019	Avastin® (bevacizumab)	MAb	Oncology
PF-pegfilgrastim	pegfilgrastim-apgf/pegfilgrastim (Nyvepria™)	11 June 2020	20 November 2020	_ [d]	_ [d]	Neulasta® (pegfilgrastim)	Protein	Oncology
PF-adalimumab	adalimumab-afzb (Abrilada™)/ adalimumab (Amsparity) [c]	18 November 2019	13 February 2020	_ [d]	_ [d]	Humira® (adalimumab)	MAb	Inflammation
PF-infliximab	infliximab-qbtx/infliximab (Ixifi™)	13 December 2017	Divested [f]	2 July 2018	_ [d]	Remicade® (infliximab)	MAb	Inflammation

[a] Known the US as Nivestym® and in the RoW as Nivestim. [b] Known in the US and in the RoW as Retacrit®, with the products designated by the INNs epoetin alfa-epbx and epoetin zeta, respectively. [c] Known as Abrilada™ in the US and as Amsparity in the EU. [d] Not all biosimilars have been submitted in all domains. Some applications are ongoing. [e] Excluded from the analysis as the reference product was developed to include several different aspects in the US and EU (e.g., strength and presentation). [f] Licensing by the EMA was divested by Pfizer in February 2016. [g] Market authorization for reference epoetin alfa is held by two companies (Epogen®; Amgen Inc., Thousand Oaks, CA, USA and Procrit®; Janssen Products, LP, Horsham, PA, USA). [h] Approved for the inflammatory disease indications of granulomatosis with polyangiitis and microscopic polyangiitis in the US; not approved for rheumatoid arthritis in the US. EMA, European Medicines Agency; FDA, US Food and Drug Administration; HC, Health Canada; INN, international nonproprietary name; MAb, monoclonal antibody; PMDA, Pharmaceuticals and Medical Devices Authority; RoW, Rest of the World.

Across all RAs, neither therapy area [χ^2 (3, n = 1623) = 1.12, p = 0.78] nor molecular complexity [χ^2 (3, n = 3436) = 2.14, p = 0.54] was found to have a significant relationship with major classification category (Supplementary Figure S2A). The relationship between therapy area and clinical and regulatory sub-classification was also found to be not significant [χ^2 (6, n = 277) = 0.31, p = 1.0]. On the other hand, a chi-square test of independence performed to examine the relationship between molecular complexity and clinical and regulatory sub-classification (Supplementary Figure S2B) found the relationship between these variables to be significant [χ^2 (6, n = 1128) = 12.62, p = 0.049]. Assessment of the individual clinical and regulatory sub-classifications confirmed that comparative safety and efficacy (CSE) [χ^2 (1, n = 1128) = 5.13, p = 0.023], bioanalytical [χ^2 (1, n = 1128) = 5.11, p = 0.023], and statutory [χ^2 (1, n = 1128) = 12.88, p = 0.00033] query sub-classifications each demonstrated significant relationships with molecular complexity.

3. Discussion

In line with the foundational role analytical data plays in the biosimilar development pathway, this analysis established there was a consistently high focus by all RAs on CMC information across all biosimilars, irrespective of their molecular complexity or therapy area (Figure 2).

Analysis of the assignment of queries to CMC categories showed RAs were all highly focused on aspects related to the DS and/or DP including manufacturing/testing controls reflecting the interdependence of this content with analytical similarity. The DS and DP content includes the controls upon which analytical similarity is based; the level of interest by RAs may stem from their aim to establish sufficient rigor will be applied by the manufacturer in maintaining analytical similarity throughout product development. The DS and DP content also includes the control measures to be applied to subsequent commercial manufacturing of the approved biosimilar, and again, review focus on this aspect would ensure similarity should be maintained in the future. The content of the DS and DP release specifications was an area of focus for all RAs, although the attributes and expectations were not identical. Despite the different queries received, the RA intent was clearly to ensure analytical similarity was measured and controlled to meet high expectations.

From the sub-classification of the clinical and regulatory queries there was a relatively greater focus on bioanalytical than on PK/PD or immunogenicity aspects by the FDA and EMA compared with the other RAs. This review approach was applied across all submitted products but not at consistent levels, suggesting it may have been influenced by individual reviewer preference. However, it should be noted that interrogation of the bioanalytical methods by reviewers can be considered an indirect assessment of the validity of the clinical (i.e., PK/PD or immunogenicity) data and this approach may be reflected in the findings for the FDA and EMA. During review, HC typically request visibility of FDA and EMA queries, if available, which may allow them to focus their review elsewhere on elements related to national regulatory (labeling) requirements. In the present analysis, based on the CMC categorization, the PMDA and HC both issued a higher proportion of queries related to facilities/GMP, compared with FDA and EMA, which is most likely due to differences in approval procedures rather than fundamental differences in GMP expectations. Both the FDA and HC review procedures can include site inspections; this only occurs during EMA and PMDA application assessments if a site has not previously been inspected within an acceptable time frame. HC was the only RA of the four covered in this analysis that routinely conducted sample testing as part of their review, which required DP samples and information on the analytical testing method to be provided. The high proportion of DP-related queries issued by HC amongst the CMC categorization across biosimilars could be attributed to sample testing activities, including those related to the transfer of analytical testing methods.

One area that received little attention from the RAs was nonclinical information, comprising <0.3% of queries in our analysis, which is consistent with the less significant role such studies play in biosimilar development compared with a novel biologic. It also supports the ongoing regulatory focus on the principle of the 3Rs (Reduce, Replace, Refine) that has been applied in updates to the earlier biosimilar guidance in some regions [16]. The low number of nonclinical queries received from the RAs that require animal studies (i.e., FDA, PMDA) supports the view that little or no nonclinical information should be necessary for demonstrating biosimilarity [30].

The proportion of clinical queries overall was low compared with requests for CMC information. Differences in the distribution of CMC and clinical queries between RAs is not unexpected and may reflect the experience of the RA authority or reviewer with biosimilars, their expectations, and/or discrete approach to reviewing data. Analysis of the query topics within the clinical sub-classification demonstrated alignment in the focus of the reviews and the principles of the scientific guidance for biosimilars across all four RAs (Figure 1). Analysis of the distribution of clinical queries following sub-classification revealed that the RA questions were tailored to individual biosimilars. Moreover, no prescribed review approach was evident from any of the RAs, with a different composition and distribution of queries being received on clinical topics for each biosimilar. Based on sub-classification of the clinical queries, there was no evidence that the tailored RA review approach was influenced by the therapy area (oncology or inflammation) of the biosimilar. However, the molecular complexity of the biosimilar showed significant association with queries sub-classified to bioanalytical, CSE, and statutory topics (which encompassed biosimilar-specific requirements, including the justification of reference product selection and extrapolation of indications).

Amongst the clinical and regulatory queries following sub-classification, a relatively low proportion were directed towards PK/PD data for all four RAs (Figure 6A–D). This finding was somewhat surprising since comparative PK studies are considered a key component of biosimilar development, due to their role in addressing residual uncertainties arising from the analytical assessment and in establishing there will be no clinically meaningful differences between the proposed biosimilar and reference product. They are also key to guiding the requirement for, and nature of, subsequent comparative clinical studies [31]. The proportion of PK/PD queries was unaffected whether the study was conducted in patients (such as for PF-rituximab [32]) or in healthy subjects (PF-infliximab [Ixifi™] [33], PF-epoetin [34,35], PF-filgrastim [36], PF-trastuzumab [37], PF-bevacizumab [38], PF-adalimumab [Abrilada™/Amsparity] [39], PF-pegfilgrastim [Nyvepria™] [40]). The generally low focus on PK information across RAs may reflect the proactive engagement of the applicant with the relevant RA during the study design process, the transparency of the data disclosure and interpretation. The approach to review of the clinical information was often two-pronged; indirect, via queries related to bioanalytical assays that supported the clinical study conclusions (PK/PD, CSE, and immunogenicity), and direct, with questions focused on the clinical data. In particular, the FDA and EMA appeared to favor focusing on bioanalytical assays as an indirect assessment tool to complement assessment of the data generated in clinical studies (PK/PD, CSE, and immunogenicity) (Figure 5). In the case of the FDA this included routinely requesting internal method validation reports and sample management records.

In general, neither the EMA nor the FDA allow inclusion of clinical data for the biosimilar on the product label, but instead use the data already provided in the reference product label [41,42]. In contrast, the PMDA and HC permit certain data for the biosimilar generated in comparative clinical trials to be included in the label [43,44]. It might be expected that these differences between RAs in relation to inclusion of data in the product label would be reflected in the distribution of the labeling and statutory topics following sub-classification of the regulatory and clinical queries. While our analysis found that both HC and the PMDA placed a greater focus on labeling queries compared with the FDA and EMA, in-depth analysis of their labeling questions determined that biosimilar data-related queries comprised only 11% and 2% of the overall labeling queries received from HC and the PMDA, respectively. This suggests that there may be opportunity for RAs to provide more operationally focused labeling guidance for biosimilars to reduce their effort and resources on raising queries on this topic.

The biosimilar guidance and regulatory requirements for the four RAs covered by this analysis were largely aligned, with only minimal divergence to meet country-specific content requirements. This allowed for submission of consistent content across the different RAs. Each RA showed a broadly similar approach in implementing their guidance, which was evident in their high focus on CMC content (ranging, on average from 41–83%), minimal nonclinical queries (<0.3%), and between 17% and 59% of queries directed to clinical and regulatory topics combined. Comparison of the clinical and regulatory sub-classification queries of the three biosimilars assessed by all four RAs suggested a tailored approach to their review, focused on different topics and with varying frequency across RAs for each biosimilar. Despite aligned guidance and shared high-level expectations across RAs on biosimilar development, the differences in the review focus highlighted here may reflect RA-specific guidance implementation approaches with regard to sub-classification content. For the biosimilars assessed by more than one RA, while their review decision was the same, with approval granted for all requested indications via the justification of extrapolation, their approach to data review and assessment of benefit–risk differed. No common review strategy was observed across the four RAs; however, the approach for each RA reflected a robust assessment of data, and the justification of that data to support biosimilarity and extrapolation of indications. Interestingly, while the RAs were equally effective, the level of review of the sub-classification topics may reflect their differing implementation of the biosimilarity concept.

The biosimilars assessed in this analysis formed a single portfolio of products developed following a global strategy, guided by proactive RA engagement, whereby the same data for each biosimilar were used to support all submissions. Our analysis revealed that the RAs do not have a pre-set approach to data review and their focus is influenced by the individual submission data per product. Although we applied the same global development strategies, the data provided was unique to each product. Therefore, it is anticipated that when assessing other biosimilars of the same reference products covered in our analysis, RAs will focus on the same topics (according to the classification and categorization system used here).

Not all biosimilars were submitted to all RAs. The data submitted to the RAs reflected product-specific information and the particular studies conducted during the biosimilar development program (e.g., comparative PK/PD and immunogenicity for PF-filgrastim and PF-pegfilgrastim were derived from studies conducted in healthy volunteers, in lieu of CSE; data for delivery by autoinjector formed part of the submission package for PF-adalimumab).

The volume of queries served solely as a proxy measure of areas of the biosimilar product dossier that received attention by the RAs. It was not possible to weight the queries to reflect the importance of the questions to the regulators or the complexity of the response required.

4. Materials and Methods

From 2017 to November 2020, 21 regulatory submissions for market authorization were undertaken for eight biosimilars in one or more of the major domains comprising the USA, EU, Japan, or Canada, in advance of cascading to further submissions globally. Contemporaneous submissions of the same data content for each biosimilar allows comparison of the review approaches between four RAs: US FDA, EMA, PMDA, and HC. These RAs were selected due to the consistency of their biosimilar guidance and their regulatory requirements, as well as the leading role their guidance has played in shaping regulatory expectations in other countries.

Details of the biosimilars included are provided in Table 1, together with the approval dates in these four RA domains. To ensure comparisons were based on consistent submission content and time frame, EMA approvals of the filgrastim (PF-filgrastim; Nivestim) and epoetin (PF-epoetin: Retacrit®) biosimilars in 2010 and 2007, respectively, were excluded from this analysis. The reference products, Neupogen® and Epogen®/Procrit®, respectively, were developed to include several different aspects in the US and EU (e.g., strength and presentation), and the biosimilars were developed to align with the EMA-approved reference products. As a result, the differences in submission information between EU and US meant that direct comparison could not be made.

Queries received during the course of review of all eight biosimilars by the four RAs were collated and each was categorized retrospectively by the authors using the methods of classification outlined below. Any uncertainties in category assignments were resolved by author calibration meetings. In instances where a query included subsidiary questions (e.g., query X, parts i-v) the main query and subsidiary components were counted separately. In some cases, a query related to a single topic, while others covered multiple topics (e.g., one CMC query could have included aspects that related to both DS and DP). In such instances, a single question could be assigned to more than one sub-classification category.

4.1. Major Classification

Initially, queries were assigned to one of four major categories: CMC, nonclinical, clinical, and regulatory (encompassing all statutory requirements such as labeling and justification of extrapolation of indications) (Table 2). The relative frequencies of each category were determined as a percentage of the overall number of queries received from each RA and for each biosimilar. There were relatively few queries assigned to the nonclinical category. Therefore, queries assigned to this category were not sub-classified further.

Table 2. Query Classification and Category Assignment Criteria.

Classification Level	Category (Assignment Criteria)			
Major	CMC (all aspects of drug substance [DS] and drug product [DP] manufacturing, testing, control and analytical similarity [including in vitro functional analysis])	Nonclinical (in vivo animal studies and comparative toxicokinetics between biosimilar and reference product)	Clinical (all clinical studies including PK/PD studies in healthy volunteers or patients, comparative safety and efficacy, where appropriate, and immunogenicity)	Regulatory (statutory requirements of the submission including prescribing information, selection of reference product, justification of extrapolation, and regulatory procedural topics)
Sub-classification	DS (DS development, manufacture, control, storage, transportation and stability) DP (DP development, manufacture, control, storage, transportation and stability, including queries related to product testing activities [e.g., product sample testing for HC]) Analytical similarity (analytical similarity studies, data, and interpretation [including in vitro functional analysis]) GMP/Facility (GMP status of facilities involved in the development, manufacturing, and testing of the DS and DP, including queries issued following facility inspections conducted as part of an application (e.g., HC On-Site Evaluation and FDA pre-approval inspection)		Bioanalytical (assays used to generate and assess clinical data [all clinical studies]; this included the assay development, validation/qualification, and sample preparation across all clinical studies) PK/PD (data derived from the comparative PK/PD modeling) Immunogenicity (immunogenicity information derived from the clinical studies) Comparative Safety and Efficacy (CSE) (comparative study, generally conducted in only one clinical indication) Safety/RMP (safety, including the RMP where applicable [e.g., EMA, PMDA, HC] and pharmacovigilance) Label/Monograph (product information [e.g., US PI, EU SmPC, including the Canadian-specific product monograph]) [a] Statutory (justification of extrapolation, reference product selection, and general regulatory procedural topics [e.g., trade name approval])	

[a] Queries received from HC and PMDA assigned to labeling/monograph sub-class were further subdivided by assignment to either data (queries related to the presentation of biosimilar data from comparative clinical studies) or to format (queries related to label text and unrelated to biosimilar clinical data). CMC, Chemistry, Manufacturing and Controls; EMA, European Medicines Agency; EU, European Union; FDA, US Food and Drug Administration; GMP, good manufacturing practice(s); HC, Health Canada; PD, pharmacodynamic(s); PK, pharmacokinetic(s); PMDA, Pharmaceuticals and Medical Devices Authority; RMP, risk management plan; SmPC, Summary of Product Characteristics; US PI, United States Prescribing Information.

4.2. CMC Sub-Classification

All queries assigned to the CMC category in the major classification were further assigned to four CMC categories according to the criteria in Table 2. Since individual CMC queries may have not have been related to a single topic they could be assigned to more than one CMC category. Relative frequencies of each topic were determined as a percentage of the total volume of CMC queries by RA and by biosimilar.

4.3. Clinical and Regulatory Sub-Classification

All queries that were assigned to the clinical and regulatory categories in the major classification were further sub-classified to one of seven categories according to the assignment criteria in Table 2. Relative frequencies of each category were determined as a percentage of the total number of queries received from each RA.

Labeling queries received from HC and PMDA were further subdivided by assignment to either 'data' (queries related to the presentation of biosimilar data from comparative clinical studies) or 'format' (queries related to label text and unrelated to biosimilar clinical data).

4.4. Statistical Analysis

Chi-square tests of independence were performed between molecular complexity (monoclonal antibody [MAb] or protein) and therapy area (oncology or inflammation) versus major query classification for each RA. The rituximab biosimilar (PF-rituximab; Ruxience™) was included under inflammation and oncology therapy areas in this analysis since it is approved for disease indications in both.

Chi-square tests of independence were also performed on the basis of molecular complexity and query sub-classification, as well as on the basis of therapy area and query sub-classification.

5. Conclusions

Analysis of the focus of the FDA, EMA, HC, and PMDA review of the biosimilars described here gives an indication of the practical application of the regulatory science underpinning the robust regulatory standards that exist in the countries and region served by these RAs. The distinct distribution of queries received for three biosimilars assessed by all four RAs may reflect a different approach in assessing benefit–risk, while still ultimately reaching the same regulatory decision.

Analysis of the focus of RAs on specific query topics identified areas of heightened interest and gave some insight as to their significance. When provided with essentially the same data, aside from country-specific content, all four RAs focused primarily on CMC-related topics, irrespective of the molecular complexity or therapy area of the biosimilar. The level of focus on CMC information was consistent with the fundamental importance of data in this domain to the demonstration of similarity, as the basis for extrapolation of indications, and to the controls applied to biosimilar manufacturing and testing.

The clinical and regulatory data review was tailored and product-specific, irrespective of therapy area, but the focus of the queries based on their sub-classification was significantly associated with the category of molecular complexity. Nevertheless, the proportion of queries on clinical topics overall was relatively low, confirming that the information from clinical studies is deemed by RAs to be largely supportive in demonstrating biosimilarity. The greatest area of RA focus was consistently placed on the assessment of data that represented the most sensitive information in the demonstration of biosimilarity, namely CMC, and the justification for extrapolation of indications.

Supplementary Materials: The following are available online at https://www.mdpi.com/article/10.3390/ph14040306/s1, Figure S1: Sub-classification of Labeling and Monograph Queries for HC, Figure S2: Major Classification Queries and Sub-classification of Regulatory (Including Labeling) and Clinical Queries by Molecular Complexity for all RAs, Table S1: Relationship of therapy area and molecular complexity with major classification, and clinical and regulatory sub-classification.

Author Contributions: All authors were involved in the conception and design of the study. B.I. and C.K. were involved in the assignment of the queries (except for those received from the PMDA and for sub-classification of the CMC queries). All authors were involved in analysis and interpretation of the data. All authors were involved in the drafting of and revising the manuscript, and approved the final version for submission. All authors have read and agreed to the published version of the manuscript.

Funding: This study was funded by Pfizer.

Institutional Review Board Statement: Not applicable.

Informed Consent Statement: Not applicable.

Data Availability Statement: The data are contained within the article or supplementary material.

Acknowledgments: The authors wish to thank their regulatory colleagues in Japan, Yuko Yao and Ayako Ohno, for supporting the assignment of PMDA queries. The authors also thank Pei-Li Wang for advice on the statistics analysis, and their colleagues Heather Hufnagel, Scott Tennyson, and Lisa LeSueur for assistance in assignment of the CMC queries. Medical writing support was provided by Iain McDonald of Engage Scientific Solutions and was funded by Pfizer.

Conflicts of Interest: Beverly Ingram, Rebecca S. Lumsden, and Christine Kobryn are full-time employees, and hold stock or stock options in Pfizer. Adriana Radosavljevic participated in this work while completing a student internship at Pfizer.

References

1. US Food and Drug Administration. Biologics Price Competition and Innovation Act of 2009. Available online: https://www.fda.gov/media/78946/download (accessed on 13 August 2020).
2. IQVIA. The Impact of Biosimilar Competition in Europe. Available online: https://ec.europa.eu/docsroom/documents/31642 (accessed on 25 November 2020).
3. Ghosh, P.K. Similar Biologics: Global Opportunities and Issues. *J. Pharm. Pharm. Sci.* **2017**, *19*, 552–596. [CrossRef] [PubMed]
4. Kang, H.N.; Thorpe, R.; Knezevic, I. Survey Participants from 19 Countries. The Regulatory Landscape of Biosimilars: WHO Efforts and Progress Made from 2009 to 2019. *Biologicals* **2020**, *65*, 1–9. [CrossRef]
5. Gamez-Belmonte, R.; Hernandez-Chirlaque, C.; Arredondo-Amador, M.; Aranda, C.J.; Gonzalez, R.; Martinez-Augustin, O.; Sanchez de Medina, F. Biosimilars: Concepts and Controversies. *Pharmacol. Res.* **2018**, *133*, 251–264. [CrossRef]
6. Rugo, H.S.; Rifkin, R.M.; Declerck, P.; Bair, A.H.; Morgan, G. Demystifying Biosimilars: Development, Regulation and Clinical use. *Future Oncol.* **2019**, *15*, 777–790. [CrossRef]
7. Wang, J.; Chow, S.C. On the Regulatory Approval Pathway of Biosimilar Products. *Pharmaceuticals* **2012**, *5*, 353–368. [CrossRef]
8. ICH. Q5E Comparability of Biotechnological/Biological Products Subject to Changes in Their Manufacturing Process. Available online: https://www.fda.gov/regulatory-information/search-fda-guidance-documents/q5e-comparability-biotechnologicalbiological-products-subject-changes-their-manufacturing-process (accessed on 13 August 2020).
9. Schiestl, M.; Zabransky, M.; Sorgel, F. Ten Years of Biosimilars in Europe: Development and Evolution of the Regulatory Pathways. *Drug Des. Devel. Ther.* **2017**, *11*, 1509–1515. [CrossRef]
10. Tariman, J.D. Biosimilars: Exploring the History, Science, and Progress. *Clin. J. Oncol. Nurs.* **2018**, *22*, 5–12. [CrossRef] [PubMed]
11. Klein, A.V.; Wang, J.; Feagan, B.G.; Omoto, M. Biosimilars: State of Clinical and Regulatory Science. *J. Pharm. Pharm. Sci.* **2017**, *20*, 332–348. [CrossRef] [PubMed]
12. Daller, J. Biosimilars: A Consideration of the Regulations in the United States and European Union. *Regul. Toxicol. Pharmacol.* **2016**, *76*, 199–208. [CrossRef]
13. US Food and Drug Administration. Biosimilar Development, Review, and Approval. Available online: https://www.fda.gov/drugs/biosimilars/biosimilar-development-review-and-approval (accessed on 13 August 2020).
14. Isaacs, J.; Gonçalves, J.; Strohal, R.; Castañeda-Hernández, G.; Azevedo, V.; Dörner, T.; McInnes, I. The Biosimilar Approval Process: How Different is it? *Consid. Med.* **2017**, *1*. [CrossRef]
15. European Medicines Agency. Biosimilar Medicines: Overview. Available online: https://www.ema.europa.eu/en/human-regulatory/overview/biosimilar-medicines-overview (accessed on 25 November 2020).
16. European Medicines Agency. Guideline on Similar Biological Medicinal Products Containing Biotechnology-Derived Proteins as Active Substance: Non-Clinical and Clinical Issues. Available online: https://www.ema.europa.eu/en/documents/scientific-guideline/guideline-similar-biological-medicinal-products-containing-biotechnology-derived-proteins-active_en-2.pdf (accessed on 13 August 2020).
17. US Food and Drug Administration. Development of Therapeutic Protein Biosimilars: Comparative Analytical Assessment and Other Quality-Related Considerations Guidance for Industry DRAFT GUIDANCE. Available online: https://www.fda.gov/vaccines-blood-biologics/guidance-compliance-regulatory-information-biologics/biologics-guidances (accessed on 13 August 2020).
18. Chapman, K.; Adjei, A.; Baldrick, P.; da Silva, A.; De Smet, K.; DiCicco, R.; Hong, S.S.; Jones, D.; Leach, M.W.; McBlane, J.; et al. Waiving In Vivo Studies for Monoclonal Antibody Biosimilar Development: National and Global Challenges. *MAbs* **2016**, *8*, 427–435. [CrossRef] [PubMed]
19. European Medicines Agency. Guideline on Similar Biological Medicinal Products Containing Biotechnology-Derived Proteins as Active Substance: Quality Issues (Revision 1). Available online: https://www.ema.europa.eu/en/documents/scientific-guideline/guideline-similar-biological-medicinal-products-containing-biotechnology-derived-proteins-active_en-0.pdf (accessed on 13 August 2020).
20. Cilia, M.; Ruiz, S.; Richardson, P.; Salmonson, T.; Serracino-Inglott, A.; Wirth, F.; Borg, J.J. Quality Issues Identified During the Evaluation of Biosimilars by the European Medicines Agency's Committee for Medicinal Products for Human Use. *AAPS Pharm. Sci. Tech.* **2018**, *19*, 489–511. [CrossRef] [PubMed]
21. Christl, L. FDA's Overview of the Regulatory Guidance for the Development and Approval of Biosimilar Products in the US. Available online: https://www.fda.gov/files/drugs/published/FDA%E2%80%99s-Overview-of-the-Regulatory-Guidance-for-the-Development-and-Approval-of-Biosimilar-Products-in-the-US.pdf (accessed on 13 August 2020).
22. Tesser, J.R.; Furst, D.E.; Jacobs, I. Biosimilars and the Extrapolation of Indications for Inflammatory Conditions. *Biologics* **2017**, *11*, 5–11. [CrossRef]
23. Weise, M.; Bielsky, M.C.; De Smet, K.; Ehmann, F.; Ekman, N.; Giezen, T.J.; Gravanis, I.; Heim, H.K.; Heinonen, E.; Ho, K.; et al. Biosimilars: What Clinicians Should Know. *Blood* **2012**, *120*, 5111–5117. [CrossRef] [PubMed]
24. Schellekens, H.; Lietzan, E.; Faccin, F.; Venema, J. Biosimilar Monoclonal Antibodies: The Scientific Basis for Extrapolation. *Expert Opin. Biol. Ther.* **2015**, *15*, 1633–1646. [CrossRef]
25. European Medicines Agency. Medicines. Available online: https://www.ema.europa.eu/en/search/search/field_ema_web_topics%3Aname_field/Biosimilars (accessed on 13 August 2020).

26. US Food and Drug Administration. Biosimilar Product Information: FDA-Approved Biosimilar Products. Available online: https://www.fda.gov/drugs/biosimilars/biosimilar-product-information (accessed on 13 August 2020).
27. Greene, L.; Singh, R.M.; Carden, M.J.; Pardo, C.O.; Lichtenstein, G.R. Strategies for Overcoming Barriers to Adopting Biosimilars and Achieving Goals of the Biologics Price Competition and Innovation Act: A Survey of Managed Care and Specialty Pharmacy Professionals. *J. Manag. Care. Spec. Pharm.* **2019**, *25*, 904–912. [CrossRef]
28. Halimi, V.; Daci, A.; Ancevska Netkovska, K.; Suturkova, L.; Babar, Z.U.; Grozdanova, A. Clinical and Regulatory Concerns of Biosimilars: A Review of Literature. *Int. J. Environ. Res. Public Health* **2020**, *17*, 5800. [CrossRef]
29. Cazap, E.; Jacobs, I.; McBride, A.; Popovian, R.; Sikora, K. Global Acceptance of Biosimilars: Importance of Regulatory Consistency, Education, and Trust. *Oncologist* **2018**, *23*, 1188–1198. [CrossRef]
30. World Health Organization. WHO Questions and Answers: Similar Biotherapeutic Products. Available online: http://www.who.int/biologicals/publications/trs/areas/biological_therapeutics/TRS_977_Annex_2.pdf (accessed on 13 August 2020).
31. US Food and Drug Administration. Clinical Pharmacology Data to Support a Demonstration of Biosimilarity to a Reference Product: Guidance for Industry. Available online: https://www.fda.gov/media/88622/download (accessed on 20 November 2020).
32. Cohen, S.; Emery, P.; Greenwald, M.; Yin, D.; Becker, J.C.; Melia, L.A.; Li, R.; Gumbiner, B.; Thomas, D.; Spencer-Green, G.; et al. A Phase I Pharmacokinetics Trial Comparing PF-05280586 (a Potential Biosimilar) and Rituximab in Patients with Active Rheumatoid Arthritis. *Br. J. Clin. Pharmacol.* **2016**, *82*, 129–138. [CrossRef] [PubMed]
33. Palaparthy, R.; Udata, C.; Hua, S.Y.; Yin, D.; Cai, C.H.; Salts, S.; Rehman, M.I.; McClellan, J.; Meng, X. A Randomized Study Comparing the Pharmacokinetics of the Potential Biosimilar PF-06438179/GP1111 with Remicade® (Infliximab) in Healthy Subjects (REFLECTIONS B537-01). *Expert Rev. Clin. Immunol.* **2018**, *14*, 329–336. [CrossRef]
34. Stalker, D.; Ramaiya, A.; Kumbhat, S.; Zhang, J.; Reid, S.; Martin, N. Pharmacodynamic and Pharmacokinetic Equivalences of Epoetin Hospira and Epogen® After Multiple Subcutaneous Doses to Healthy Male Subjects. *Clin. Ther.* **2016**, *38*, 1090–1101. [CrossRef] [PubMed]
35. Stalker, D.; Reid, S.; Ramaiya, A.; Wisemandle, W.A.; Martin, N.E. Pharmacokinetic and Pharmacodynamic Equivalence of Epoetin Hospira and Epogen After Single Subcutaneous Doses to Healthy Male Subjects. *Clin. Ther.* **2016**, *38*, 1778–1788. [CrossRef] [PubMed]
36. Yao, H.M.; Ottery, F.D.; Borema, T.; Harris, S.; Levy, J.; May, T.B.; Moosavi, S.; Zhang, J.; Summers, M. PF-06881893 (Nivestym), a Filgrastim Biosimilar, Versus US-Licensed Filgrastim Reference Product (US-Neupogen®): Pharmacokinetics, Pharmacodynamics, Immunogenicity, and Safety of Single or Multiple Subcutaneous Doses in Healthy Volunteers. *Biodrugs* **2019**, *33*, 207–220. [CrossRef]
37. Yin, D.; Barker, K.B.; Li, R.; Meng, X.; Reich, S.D.; Ricart, A.D.; Rudin, D.; Taylor, C.T.; Zacharchuk, C.M.; Hansson, A.G. A Randomized Phase 1 Pharmacokinetic Trial Comparing the Potential Biosimilar PF-05280014 with Trastuzumab in Healthy Volunteers (REFLECTIONS B327-01). *Br. J. Clin. Pharmacol.* **2014**, *78*, 1281–1290. [CrossRef] [PubMed]
38. Knight, B.; Rassam, D.; Liao, S.; Ewesuedo, R. A Phase I Pharmacokinetics Study Comparing PF-06439535 (a Potential Biosimilar) with Bevacizumab in Healthy Male Volunteers. *Cancer Chemother. Pharmacol.* **2016**, *77*, 839–846. [CrossRef] [PubMed]
39. Lee, A.; Shirley, M. PF-06410293: An Adalimumab Biosimilar. *Biodrugs* **2020**, *34*, 695–698. [CrossRef]
40. Moosavi, S.; Borema, T.; Ewesuedo, R.; Harris, S.; Levy, J.; May, T.B.; Summers, M.; Thomas, J.S.; Zhang, J.; Yao, H.M. PF-06881894, a Proposed Biosimilar to Pegfilgrastim, Versus US-Licensed and EU-Approved Pegfilgrastim Reference Products (Neulasta®): Pharmacodynamics, Pharmacokinetics, Immunogenicity, and Safety of Single or Multiple Subcutaneous Doses in Healthy Volunteers. *Adv. Ther.* **2020**, *37*, 3370–3391. [CrossRef]
41. European Medicines Agency. Biosimilars in the EU: Information Guide for Healthcare Professionals. Available online: https://www.ema.europa.eu/en/documents/leaflet/biosimilars-eu-information-guide-healthcare-professionals_en.pdf (accessed on 10 December 2020).
42. US Food and Drug Administration. Labeling for Biosimilar Products: Guidance for Industry. Available online: https://www.fda.gov/media/96894/download (accessed on 10 December 2020).
43. Health Canada. Guidance Document: Information and Submission Requirements for Biosimilar Biologic Drugs. Available online: www.hc-sc.gc.ca/index-eng.php (accessed on 13 August 2020).
44. Pharmaceutical and Food Safety Bureau Ministry of Health Labour and Welfare. Guideline for the Quality, Safety, and Efficacy Assurance of Follow-on Biologics. Available online: https://www.pmda.go.jp/files/000153851.pdf (accessed on 25 November 2020).

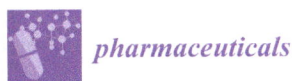

Article

Type and Extent of Information on (Potentially Critical) Quality Attributes Described in European Public Assessment Reports for Adalimumab Biosimilars

Ali M. Alsamil [1,2], Thijs J. Giezen [3,4], Toine C. Egberts [1,5], Hubert G. Leufkens [1] and Helga Gardarsdottir [1,5,6,*]

1. Division of Pharmacoepidemiology and Clinical Pharmacology, Utrecht Institute of Pharmaceutical Sciences, Faculty of Science, Utrecht University, 3584 CG Utrecht, The Netherlands; a.m.alsamil@uu.nl (A.M.A.); A.C.G.Egberts@uu.nl (T.C.E.); H.G.M.Leufkens@uu.nl (H.G.L.)
2. Pharmaceutical Product Evaluation Directorate, Drug sector, Saudi Food and Drug Authority, Riyadh 13513-7148, Saudi Arabia
3. Foundation Pharmacy for Hospitals in Haarlem, 2035 RC Haarlem, The Netherlands; tgiezen@sahz.nl
4. Department of Clinical Pharmacy, Spaarne Gasthuis, 2035 RC Haarlem, The Netherlands
5. Department of Clinical Pharmacy, University Medical Center Utrecht, 3584 CX Utrecht, The Netherlands
6. Department of Pharmaceutical Sciences, University of Iceland, 107 Reykjavik, Iceland
* Correspondence: h.gardarsdottir@uu.nl; Tel.: +31-30-2537324

Abstract: Regulatory approval of biosimilars predominantly relies on biosimilarity assessments of quality attributes (QAs), particularly the potentially critical QAs (pCQAs) that may affect the clinical profile. However, a limited understanding exists concerning how EU regulators reflect the biosimilarity assessments of (pC)QAs in European public assessment reports (EPARs) by different stakeholders. The type and extent of information on QAs and pCQAs in EPARs were evaluated for seven adalimumab biosimilars. Seventy-seven QAs, including 31 pCQAs, were classified and assessed for type (structural and functional attributes) and extent (biosimilarity interpretation and/or test results) of information in EPARs. Reporting on the QAs (35–75%) varied between EPARs, where the most emphasis was placed on pCQAs (65–87%). Functional attributes (54% QAs and 92% pCQAs) were reported more frequently than structural attributes (8% QAs and 22% pCQAs). About 50% (4 structural and 12 functional attributes) of pCQAs were consistently reported in all EPARs. Regulators often provided biosimilarity interpretation (QAs: 83% structural and 80% functional; pCQAs: 81% structural and 78% functional) but rarely include test results (QAs: 1% structural and 9% functional and pCQAs: 3% structural and 9% functional). Minor differences in structural attributes, commonly in glycoforms and charge variants, were often observed in adalimumab biosimilars but did not affect the functions and clinical profile. Despite the variability in reporting QAs in EPARs, the minor observed differences were largely quantitative and not essentially meaningful for the overall conclusion of biosimilarity of the seven adalimumab biosimilars.

Keywords: adalimumab; biosimilar; biosimilarity assessment; quality attributes (QAs); potentially critical quality attributes (pCQAs); European public assessment reports (EPARs)

Highlights

- Comparing adalimumab biosimilars at the level of quality attributes (QAs), as reported in EPARs, showed that the reporting frequencies of QAs vary between biosimilars compared with the same reference biological (Humira®).
- Regulators emphasized reporting of potentially critical QAs (pCQAs) in EPARs and more consistently reported functional pCQAs because they are directly related to the drug mechanisms of action and provide valuable information for clinical performance and the extrapolation of indications.
- Regulators often observed minor differences in structural attributes, most commonly in glycoforms and charge variants, between the biosimilar and reference biological,

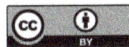

though this had no effect on the functions and clinical profiles and did not preclude biosimilarity.
- Regulators provided a biosimilarity interpretation but rarely reported test results for QAs in EPARs, impeding the interpretation by EPAR users.

1. Introduction

Biological drugs have become important treatment options for numerous diseases, including cancer and inflammatory diseases [1]. After patent expiration of the reference biologicals, biosimilars contribute to improved patient access to treatment due to competition, resulting in lower prices. Unlike small molecule drugs, biological drugs, including biosimilars, are large and complicated molecules produced through a complex process using living microorganisms. Variability within and between batches is an inherent feature of the production of biologicals [2,3]. Therefore, biosimilars are, generally, not exact replications of the reference biological but are highly similar [4].

The leading regulatory and health authorities in highly regulated markets, such as the European Medicines Agency (EMA), the United States Food and Drug Administration (US FDA), and the World Health Organization (WHO), have established frameworks and guidelines for the development, assessment, and approval of biosimilars [5–8]. Biosimilar development and regulatory approval predominantly rely on demonstrating the biosimilarity to the reference biological, which involves a stepwise comparability assessment. The comparability assessment of quality attributes (QAs) is a fundamental step, and it forms the basis for establishing biosimilarity and determining the scope and range of the in-vitro and clinical studies needed for biosimilar approval [9–12]. Minor differences in QAs between the biosimilar and reference biological may exist but should not be clinically relevant to obtaining regulatory approval.

Quality attributes are measurable molecular characteristics that describe the physical, chemical, biological, and microbiological properties of a drug molecule [13]. Some QAs are classified as potentially critical QAs (pCQAs) because they may affect the biological activity (potency) and the clinical drug profile, which includes pharmacokinetics (PK), pharmacodynamics (PD), safety, immunogenicity, and efficacy [14]. This criticality can be illustrated by a recent example where a biosimilar company discovered a drift in antibody-dependent cell-mediated cytotoxicity (ADCC) activity due to shifts in afucosylated glycans of the reference biological trastuzumab [15], which was associated with a reduced event-free survival rate [16]. Several studies have provided valuable insight into various risk assessment tools for identifying pCQAs [17–22]. Some pCQAs apply to all biologicals, but some pCQAs are specific to a biological and information about these may (d)evolve over time as more knowledge of the product and manufacturing process becomes available. The pharmaceutical industry generally defines which QAs are considered pCQAs based on the available information and the manufacturer risk assessment [23–32]. For biosimilars, the test results of all QAs must remain within the range of variability set by analyzing different batches of the reference biological. Scientific justification is needed if any deviation occurs in the QAs, especially in pCQAs. This rigorous assessment should also be followed when changes are introduced to the manufacturing processes of approved biologicals, including biosimilars [33–36].

Since the regulatory approval of the first biosimilar in Europe in 2006, 49 unique biosimilars marketed under 69 brand names for 15 reference biologicals have received a positive opinion from the EMA's Committee for Medicinal Products for Human Use (CHMP) as of November 2020 [37]. Currently, the reference biological adalimumab, sold under the brand name Humira® by AbbVie Corporation, USA, has the largest number of biosimilars approved in the EU market. Adalimumab is an anti-tumor necrosis factor-α (TNF-α) monoclonal antibody that prevents the interaction of TNF-α with its receptors and is indicated for the treatment of various immune-mediated inflammatory diseases [23,38,39].

Despite the established and stringent regulatory pathway of biosimilars in Europe, the adoption of biosimilars in clinical practice is challenged by a lack of knowledge and understanding of the scientific rationale behind their approval [40–42]. In Europe, regulators have taken actions to increase transparency for the biosimilar approval process to improve stakeholder understanding of biosimilars through various communication media. The European public assessment report (EPAR) is an unbiased source through which the EMA publishes and broadcasts information to stakeholders about regulatory assessments for all medicinal products approved by the European Commission (EC) [37]. Previous studies have provided an in-depth overview of the clinical evidence reported in EPARs that supports approval of biosimilars in general [43,44] and approval of adalimumab biosimilars in particular [45]. These studies have shown that variations exist in reporting clinical data that confirm the biosimilarity of biosimilars to a reference biological, but they have not explored the reporting of the QAs that are the basis of biosimilar approval. The biosimilarity assessment of QAs is increasingly reported in scientific publications of biosimilars [46], which needed to be systematically consulted with the corresponding EPARs to obtain comprehensive information on biosimilarity at the quality level [47]. However, a limited understanding exists concerning how EU regulators reflect the biosimilarity assessment of (pC)QAs in EPARs by different stakeholders.

Therefore, this study aims to evaluate the QAs and pCQAs reported in EPARs using adalimumab biosimilars as a case study in terms of (1) consistency of QA and pCQA reporting between biosimilars of the same reference biological (i.e., adalimumab), (2) Type of the reported QAs and pCQAs (i.e., structural or functional attributes), and (3) how biosimilarity interpretation and test results were described for the reported (pC)QAs. We hypothesized that EU regulators are more focused in the reporting of pCQAs and the biosimilar interpretation because these are more likely to be of clinical relevance.

2. Results

2.1. Characteristics of the Included European Public Assessment Reports of Adalimumab Biosimilars

As of 30 November 2020, seven unique adalimumab biosimilars (11 brand names) had received marketing authorization from the EC. Three of the seven biosimilars (i.e., ABP501, GP2017, and MSB11022) were marketed under more than one brand name. Rapporteurs from 11 member states prepared the initial EPARs of the seven adalimumab biosimilars. Rapporteurs from two (Finland and Austria) of the 11 member states were involved in more than one EPAR of adalimumab biosimilars (Table 1).

Table 1. Characteristics of the included initial European public assessment reports (EPARs) of adalimumab biosimilars [48–58].

Company Code	Date of Initial EPAR Publication (mm/yyyy)	Brand Names	EU Member State of Rapporteurs (Rapporteur and Co-Rapporteur)
ABP501	04-2017	Amgevita® Solymbic® *	Sweden and Italy
SB5	08-2017	Imraldi®	Finland and Austria
BI695501	11-2017	Cyltezo® *	Austria and Germany
GP2017	08-2018	Hefiya® Halimatoz® Hyrimoz®	Austria and Ireland
FKB327	09-2018	Hulio®	Belgium and United Kingdom
MSB11022	04-2019	Idacio® Kromeya® *	Netherlands and Lithuania
PF06410293	02-2020	Amsparity®	Finland and Romania

* Solymbic®, Cyltezo® and Kromeya® were approved by the European Medicines Agency (EMA) but voluntarily withdrawn by the applicant for commercial reasons.

2.2. Types of Reported (Potentially Critical) Quality Attributes

In general, the frequency of reported QAs (range: 27 (35%)–58 (75%)) varied between EPARs of adalimumab biosimilars, with most emphasis placed on the reporting of the pCQAs (range: 20 (65%)–27 (87%)). The proportion of reported pCQAs was comparable for all biosimilars. Overall, 16 (21%) of all QAs were reported in all EPARs of adalimumab biosimilars. Of the 31 pCQAs, 29 (94%) were reported at least in one EPAR, and 16 (52%) were consistently reported in all included EPARs (Table 2). Two (6%) pCQAs related to structural attributes were not reported in any included EPAR: post-translation modifications (PTMs) including neuraminic N-glycolyl acid and galactose alpha-1,3-galactose (Figure S1).

Table 2. Reporting of the quality attributes (QAs) and potentially critical quality attributes (pCQAs) stratified by structural and functional attributes and the company code of adalimumab biosimilars in the included European public assessment reports (EPARs).

Company Code	All QAs (n = 77, 100%)	Type of QAs		All pCQAs (n = 31, 100%)	Type of pCQAs	
		Structural (n = 53, %)	Functional (n = 24, %)		Structural (n = 18, %)	Functional (n = 13, %)
ABP501	36 (47%)	18 (34%)	18 (75%)	20 (65%)	7 (39%)	13 (100%)
SB5	49 (64%)	27 (51%)	22 (92%)	27 (87%)	14 (78%)	13 (100%)
BI695501	27 (35%)	12 (23%)	15 (63%)	20 (65%)	7 (39%)	13 (100%)
GP2017	52 (68%)	34 (64%)	18 (75%)	27 (87%)	14 (78%)	13 (100%)
FKB327	58 (75%)	39 (74%)	19 (79%)	27 (87%)	14 (78%)	13 (100%)
MSB11022	42 (55%)	20 (38%)	22 (92%)	25 (81%)	12 (67%)	13 (100%)
PF06410293	46 (60%)	27 (51%)	19 (79%)	24 (77%)	12 (67%)	12 (92%)
Consistent for all biosimilars	16 (21%)	4 (8%)	12 (54%)	16 (52%)	4 (22%)	12 (92%)

Overall, functional attributes (54% QAs and 92% pCQAs) were more often consistently reported than structural attributes (8% QAs and 22% pCQAs) in EPARs of adalimumab biosimilars (Table 2). Consistent reporting of functional pCQAs was high, with 12 (92%) out of 13 pCQAs reported in all EPARs, including binding to soluble- and transmembrane-TNFα (s-TNFα and tm-TNFα), (ADCC), and complement-dependent cytotoxicity (CDC) activity and binding to complement component 1q (C1q), neonatal Fc receptor (FcRn), and six Fcγ-receptors. Of the 18 structural pCQAs, only four (22%) were consistently reported in all EPARs, including amino acid sequence and disulfide bridges, glycosylation, and aggregates (Figure S1).

2.3. Extent of Information on Reported (Potentially Critical) Quality Attributes

In general, no differences were observed in the extent of the reported information between the QAs and pCQAs in all EPARs of adalimumab biosimilars. Regulators frequently provided biosimilarity interpretations of the reported QAs (83% structural and 80% functional) and pCQAs (81% structural and 78% functional) but rarely included test results with or without biosimilarity interpretations of the reported QAs (1% structural and 9% functional) and pCQAs (3% structural and 9% functional) (Figure 1).

The total number of reported QAs included with a biosimilarity interpretation in EPARs was 69 QAs and the number varied (range: 10–58 QAs) for adalimumab biosimilars. The interpretation of the biosimilarity of the reported QAs was most frequently reported as being similar (range: 7–44 QAs) than having minor differences (range: 1–18 QAs) (Table S1). Thirty-one QAs, including fifteen pCQAs, were observed with minor differences in at least one adalimumab biosimilar. The most common structural pCQAs with minor differences were the four glycoforms (galactosylated glycans, high mannose glycans, afucosylated glycans, and sialylated glycans) and the charge variants (acidic and basic variants). While functional pCQAs were more often similar between the biosimilar and reference biological, minor differences were observed for the functional pCQAs tm-TNFα binding, ADCC activity, and C1q binding in two adalimumab biosimilars: GP2017 and PF-06410293 (Figure S1).

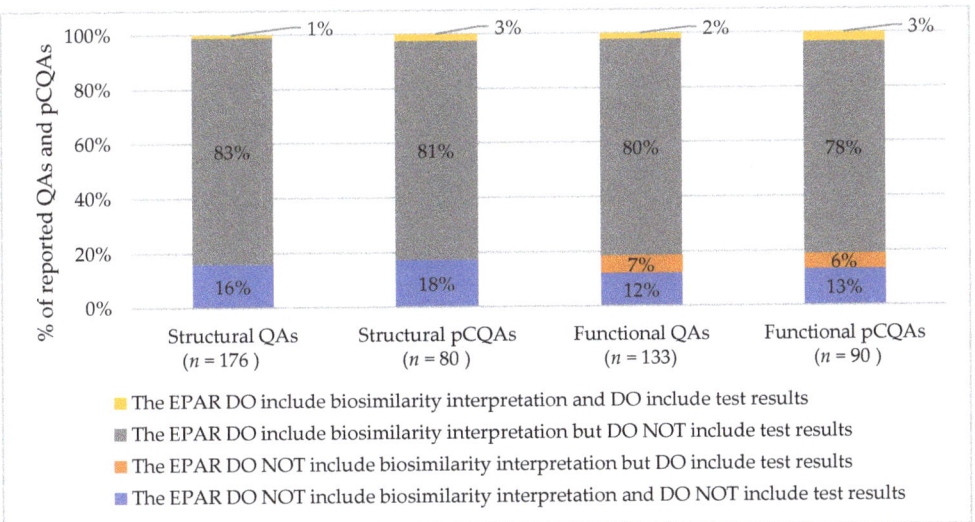

Figure 1. Comparison of the extent of reported information on quality attributes (QAs) and potentially critical quality attributes (pCQAs) stratified by the types of QAs and pCQAs (structural and functional) reported in all EPARs of adalimumab biosimilars included.

Regulators provided both biosimilarity interpretations and test results in EPARs for only five pCQAs, including the protein concentration and binding to FcγRIIIa for ABP501 and the high mannose glycans, ADCC activity, and binding to FcγRIIIa for MSB11022 (Table S2). Of those five pCQAs, only the test results of high mannose glycans, which were slightly lower in the MSB11022 biosimilar (range = 1.9–2.5%) compared to the reference biological (range = 5.3–12.0%), were interpreted by the regulators as minor difference. Figure S1 shows reporting of the type and extent of information on QAs and pCQAs described in the EPARs of adalimumab biosimilars included.

3. Discussion

The present study evaluated the type and extent of information on QAs and pCQAs reported in EPARs by EU regulators for seven adalimumab biosimilars approved in Europe as of November 2020. In general, reporting of QAs (ranging from 27 (35%) to 58 (75%)) varied between EPARs of adalimumab biosimilars, where the most emphasis was on reporting pCQAs (ranging from 20 (65%) to 27 (87%)). About 50% (4 structural and 12 functional attributes) of pCQAs were consistently reported in all EPARs. Functional attributes (54% QAs and 92% pCQAs) were more frequently and consistently reported than structural attributes (8% QAs and 22% pCQAs). Minor differences between adalimumab biosimilars and the reference biological in certain structural attributes, most commonly in glycoforms and charge variants, were often observed by regulators. Regulators reported on the biosimilarity interpretation but rarely presented the test results underlying their interpretation in EPARs. However, QA and pCQA data not reported in the EPARs do not necessarily indicate that they were neither submitted by companies nor assessed by regulators during the stringent regulatory process.

This study highlights some variations in reporting biosimilarity assessments at the quality level in EPARs. Despite this variability in QA reporting, pCQAs were most frequently and consistently reported by EU regulators in EPARs. The variation in QA reporting between EPARs is consistent with the variability in reporting clinical data, which was explained by the flexibility in regulatory requirements (i.e., a case-by-case basis) [43,44]. However, such flexibility cannot explain the variability in reporting of QAs and pCQAs for biosimilars, particularly those containing the same active substance and compared to the same reference biological (e.g., Humira® in the case of adalimumab), that were assessed based on the same regulatory standards for establishing biosimilarity. The variability in QA reporting may be explained by the fact that the EPARs are prepared by various rapporteurs (i.e., regulators) from different member states. Nevertheless, regulators diligently reported the pCQAs, which are all considered to be of relevance because these may potentially affect functions (biological and immunochemical activity) and the clinical profile, including the pharmacokinetics, pharmacodynamics, safety, immunogenicity and efficacy of the drug. It is, however, important to note that learning on pCQAs is an ongoing process, which will likely result in changes to the current list over time.

The direct or indirect relationship between structural and functional QAs and the clinical profile influences the determination of pCQAs [19]. This relationship can be illustrated by the four structural pCQAs, including the amino acid sequence, disulfide bridges, aggregates, and glycosylation, which were consistently reported in EPARs. A mismatch in amino acid sequence and disulfide bridges can change the structural conformation affecting the biological activity and clinical performance, which were identical to the reference biological for all adalimumab biosimilars. Aggregates can elicit immunogenic responses by inducing neutralizing antibodies, hypersensitivity reactions, and infusion-related reactions in vivo. The propensity of aggregation may increase with some structural attributes (e.g., disulfide bridges, oxidation, and deamidation) if these are inadequately controlled. For all adalimumab biosimilars, aggregate levels were similar to the reference biological. Glycosylation is a PTM that occurs through an enzymatic process at specific sites in a protein drug and can influence the biological activity (potency and efficacy), serum half-life clearance (pharmacokinetics), and immunogenicity (safety). Minor differences in glycosylation were observed in adalimumab biosimilars, which are the most frequent notable differences in biosimilars and reference biologicals in general [9–12].

In practice, minor differences in QAs and pCQAs are expected for biosimilars due to the use of various manufacturing processes, cell lines, and materials [35]. These minor differences have also been observed between batches of a reference biological, primarily when a company introduces manufacturing changes [2,3,23]. The galactosylated glycans, high mannose glycans, afucosylated glycans, and sialylated glycans are types of glycoforms where minor differences have most commonly been reported (Figure S1). Galactosylated glycans may influence C1q binding and CDC activity, whereas high mannose glycans may influence pharmacokinetics parameters. However, structure-activity relationship studies and pivotal pharmacokinetics trials indicate that these are not affected by minor differences in galactosylated and high mannose glycans [48,49,51–57]. The same applies to afucosylated and sialylated glycans, which may influence Fcγ-receptors and ADCC activity [51–58]. These examples demonstrate the importance of structure-activity relationship studies and pharmacokinetics and pharmacodynamics trials in assessing the potential effect of minor differences in pCQAs in biosimilarity assessments. Minor differences in acidic and basic variants in several adalimumab biosimilars were attributed to changes in c-terminal lysin [48,49,51–54,58], which is generally cleaved in human serum with no effect on clinical profiles, and were thus considered noncritical QAs. Minor differences for certain functional pCQAs were attributed to minor differences in certain structural QAs and pCQAs, which were observed and reported by EU regulators in EPARs for GP2017 and PF06410293. For both biosimilars, the minor differences in ADCC activity disappeared when using an in-vitro assay with more physiological conditions in peripheral blood mononuclear cells. For GP2017, the aggregate levels were slightly higher using size-exclusion chromatography and slightly lower using analytical ultracentrifugation than the reference biological, which was considered a minor and clinically irrelevant difference by regulators. This ADCC and aggregate example indicates the importance of using orthogonal methods to assess the (dis)similarity of QAs. Based on these observations, minor differences in these pCQAs seem to be quantitative (i.e., numerical values) but do not preclude the overall conclusion for biosimilarity and are considered clinically irrelevant.

The underlying reason functional pCQAs are more frequently and consistently reported in EPARs could relate to their direct relationship with the mechanisms of action (MoAs). The primary MoA of adalimumab involves binding to, and neutralizing TNF-α. Adalimumab also mediates effector functions, such as ADCC and CDC activity, by binding to tm-TNF-α, C1q (for CDC), and Fcγ-receptors. The relevance of ADCC or CDC activity to the primary MoA and efficacy of adalimumab is not well established but may be important, particularly in inflammatory bowel disease [45]. Binding to tm-TNFα can trigger potential biological functions known as "referred signaling," which may play a role in some therapeutic indications (e.g., inflammatory bowel disease). For GP2017, regulators reported minor differences in the binding to tm-TNFα, for which the scientific justifications provided by the company were not available in the EPAR for GP2017. However, the developer company of GP2017 reported functional and pharmacological characterizations demonstrating indistinguishable binding profiles and subsequent induction of reverse signaling to support the rationale for extrapolation across indications [28]. Therefore, functional pCQAs provide the final insight into the (dis)similarity at the quality level and useful information in predicting the outcomes of clinical studies [9–11], forming the basis for supporting the extrapolation of biosimilars across all indications authorized for the reference biological [59–62].

Regulators frequently describe the biosimilarity interpretation of reported QAs and pCQAs but rarely present the test result data, impeding the interpretation by EPAR users. For example, in EPARs, minor differences are frequently expressed subjectively as "slightly lower" or "slightly higher," but the exact extent to which the difference is minor remains unclear for most reported QAs and pCQAs. A more appropriate method would be in line with what was reported in the EPAR of MSB11022, in which the ranges of high mannose glycans (ranging from 1.9% to 2.5%) and the reference adalimumab (ranging from 5.3% to 12.0%) were reported. Such information on the test results allows for a better understanding of the regulatory interpretation and scientific justification behind the regulatory approval of biosimilars.

The present study used a classification scheme to investigate in a standardized manner how EU regulators present information on the biosimilarity of QAs and pCQAs in EPARs. The focus on the pCQAs to be considered in biosimilarity assessment, which may affect the clinical profiles of adalimumab products, was a strength of this investigation. The selection of adalimumab pCQAs was based on the literature review, providing an overview concerning which QAs are considered pCQAs with the current knowledge. This study stresses the importance of EPARs as a source of information that provides insight into the scientific evidence underpinning the regulatory approval of biosimilars.

Our study does have some limitations, which are noted as follows. First, these study findings are restricted to adalimumab biosimilars, which may hamper the generalizability to biosimilars of other biological molecules. Nevertheless, even if a biosimilarity assessment of another molecule is conducted with a different set of QAs and pCQAs, the findings, especially the focus on reporting the pCQAs, are expected to be comparable to other types of biosimilars because all EPARs are published by the same regulatory agency (i.e., EMA). Second, the generalizability of our findings to the regulatory reports from various jurisdictions, such as in the US FDA review reports, is unknown and beyond the scope of this study. Third, the QA classification scheme may not have captured all pCQAs of adalimumab because no consensus list is currently available. However, a literature search for publications on comparability and biosimilarity studies of adalimumab products was performed, and no pCQAs were identified that were not included in our classification.

Our observations reveal that minor differences in certain QAs between biosimilars and reference biological can occur at the same level of variability between pre- and post-manufacturing change batches of the reference biological [23,35,63], which reassures the biosimilar regulation system. Although EU regulators have focused on describing pCQAs, these critical attributes were not explicitly defined in EPARs. Because biosimilar companies have conducted extensive analyses to define pCQAs based on their risk assessments, it would be preferable if regulators clearly define which QAs are identified as pCQAs by the companies. A clear definition of pCQAs in EPARs would enable stakeholders to better understand the links between QAs and the clinical profile and the meaning of the QAs concerning patient safety and product efficacy. The pCQAs may also (d)evolve over the drug life cycle based on the knowledge gained regarding the product and process. Standardized reporting of pCQAs in EPARs would benefit regulatory learning by allowing future researches to track pCQAs over time. Learning of pCQAs over time might result in reducing the need for comparative clinical trials and streamlining biosimilar approvals [9–12].

Although the EMA quality guidance of biosimilars provides high-level information on QAs, the guidance was last updated in 2014 and may not reflect the current state of knowledge and regulatory experience regarding QAs for biosimilars [5]. The lack of information on pCQAs in the guidance is understandable because these were not entirely known in the early years of biosimilar regulation. Nevertheless, the accumulated and long experience of EU biosimilar regulation as reflected in EPARs would fuel regulatory guidance with product-specific pCQAs, making the regulatory standard more visible and predictable.

As EPARs are considered an unbiased information source, there is great value in providing insight into the biosimilarity assessment of QAs for various stakeholders involved in biosimilar development, adoption, and regulation. The pharmaceutical industry can use EPARs to learn from past successes and failures and predict the regulatory process, and EPARs as such may contribute to reducing the time and cost of biosimilar development [64]. Healthcare professionals (HCPs) can use EPARs to understand the QA assessment's crucial role during the regulatory approval of biosimilars [65,66]. Reporting more extensive information about pCQAs in EPARs could help HCPs understand the predominant role of QAs and the reduced weight of evidence from comparative clinical trials in biosimilar approval. Among HCPs, pharmacists are uniquely positioned to take a leading role in informing other HCPs and patients about the scientific evidence underpinning biosimilar approval. Such efforts could increase confidence in and acceptance of using biosimilars in medical practice to fully capture the societal and patients benefits offered by biosimilars. Non-European regulatory authorities can use EPARs to support their own decision-making process, relying on the regulatory assessment undertaken by competent authorities in the world [67–72]. Therefore, EPARs could contribute to accelerating the regulatory review process and patients access to biosimilars in non-European jurisdictions.

For a comprehensive understanding of biosimilarity concepts and the predominant role of QAs in the approval of biosimilars, continued improvement in presenting biosimilarity assessments of QAs in EPARs is recommended. One method could include applying a structured uniform approach to QA reporting in EPARs. Such an approach may enhance the completeness and consistency of QA data and avoid missing crucial regulatory reflection on clinically relevant pCQAs. Greater consistency in QA reporting could make the EPAR a valuable and reliable tool for stakeholders to support evidence-based education to address the lack of knowledge and understanding of the scientific rationale behind biosimilar approval. Biosimilarity assessments of QAs in EPARs could be summarized in a standardized format that includes the type of evaluated QAs, explicit definition of the pCQAs, the test methods used and their results, the biosimilarity interpretation and scientific justification of the differences, if applicable. This summary could be achieved through adopting the International Pharmaceutical Regulators Program's regulatory review templates to optimize the current content with respect to biosimilarity assessment of QAs in EPARs [73]. Alternatively, initiating a project similar to the collaborative study between the EMA and European network for health technology assessment [74], which has resulted in a template to improve the contribution of EPARs in health technology assessments of relative drug effectiveness.

4. Methods

4.1. Study Cohort

In this study, the initial EPARs of all adalimumab biosimilars approved by the EMA before 30 November 2020 were included. The initial EPARs of adalimumab biosimilars were retrieved from the official EMA website (http://www.ema.europa.eu (accessed on 1 June 2020)) [37]. The EPAR contains a summary of the submitted registration dossier and the scientific assessment undertaken by the CHMP, a body that advises the EC on marketing authorization of medicines for human use. Only the initial EPAR of each adalimumab biosimilar released following the final EC decision was included in this study because biosimilarity assessments of QAs and pCQAs between biosimilar and reference biological are presented only in the initial EPARs.

The initial EPARs were used to extract baseline characteristics for each adalimumab biosimilar, including the company code(s), brand name(s), date of the initial EPAR publication, and member states of the rapporteurs responsible for the assessment. Some adalimumab biosimilars are produced by the same manufacturer but marketed under different brand names (e.g., the company code for Hefiya®, Halimatoz®, and Hyrimoz® is GP2017) for which the registration dossier and initial EPARs are identical. In such cases, only the EPAR of one brand name (e.g., Hefiya® for GP2017) was included in the study for subsequent analysis. The date of the initial EPAR publication was defined as the month and year when the EPAR was published by the EMA, which is generally the same date as the EC decision on marketing authorization. The member state was defined as the rapporteurs' European country of origin. The rapporteurs are the two CHMP members who led the regulatory assessment of a marketing authorization application.

4.2. Information on (Potentially Critical) Quality Attributes in EPARs

The study outcome was the determination of how EU regulators report information on the biosimilarity assessment of QAs and pCQAs in the EPARs. Two aspects were studied: the type and extent of information on the reported QAs and pCQAs.

4.2.1. Types of Reported (Potentially Critical) Quality Attributes

The types of QAs and pCQAs reported in the biosimilarity assessment were identified from the quality, non-clinical, and clinical sections of the initial EPARs. A general classification scheme of QAs was used to extract information from the EPARs. Information about the development of the classification scheme has been described elsewhere [46]. In short, the first draft was developed by the authors based on information from the EMA and US FDA biosimilar guidelines [5–7] and publicly available information relevant to the molecular characterization of a biological drug. The classification scheme was validated by regulators involved in the quality assessment of biosimilars at the Dutch Medicines Evaluation Board (MEB) to ensure that no critical and relevant QAs were missed. The classification scheme divides the QAs into seven types with additional subtypes of structural (physiochemical properties, primary structure, higher-order structure, PTMs and purity and impurities) and functional attributes (biological and immunochemical activity), resulting in the classification of 77 (53 structural and 24 functional) QAs of biologicals considered in the biosimilarity assessment (Figure 2) [46,47].

Subsequently, a list of pCQAs was defined in a two-step process. First, the pCQAs of adalimumab were identified from scientific publications presenting comparability or biosimilarity studies of adalimumab products, including the reference biological (Humira®) and corresponding biosimilars [23–32]. The publications were selected from an updated search of our previous systematic review [46]. From this search, an initial list of 29 pCQAs of adalimumab was constructed based on the pCQAs proposed by the authors. Second, the initial list was compared with the pCQAs identified for monoclonal antibodies, in general, in the previous literature [17–22] to verify and broaden the initial selection of pCQAs. If a new pCQA was identified in this second step, the authors (A.M.A., T.J.G., and H.G.) discussed its relevancy to adalimumab and reached a consensus on the inclusion of the attribute. In this way, two pCQAs were added to the initial list, resulting in a final list of 31 (18 structural and 13 functional) pCQAs considered relevant to adalimumab products. These pCQAs were classified according to the previously described scheme (Figure 2).

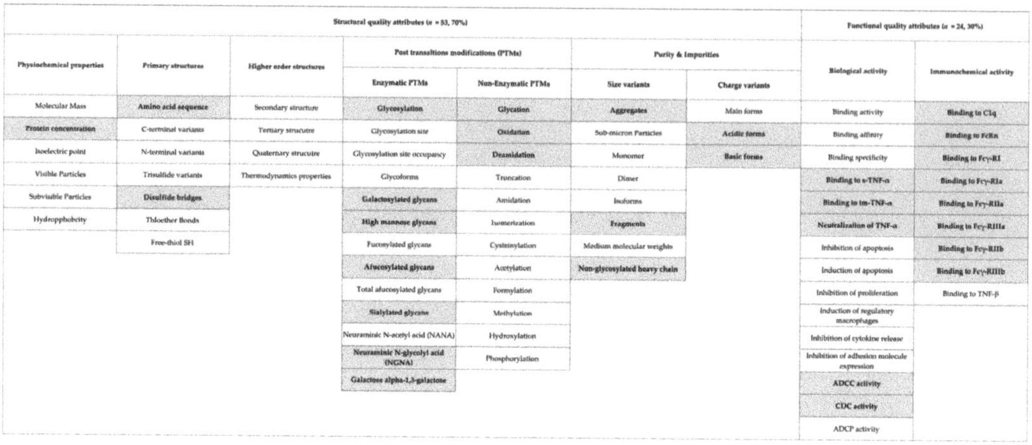

Figure 2. Classification scheme for 77 common quality attributes (QAs) of biologicals including 31 potentially critical quality attributes (pCQAs) relevant to adalimumab. The pCQAs are presented in gray boxes. Definitions: ADCC: antibody-dependent cellular cytotoxicity, ADCP: antibody-dependent cellular phagocytosis, CDC: complement-dependent cytotoxicity, C1q: complement component 1q, TNFα: tumor necrosis factor-alpha, s-TNFα: surface tumor necrosis factor-alpha, tm-TNFα: transmembrane tumor necrosis factor-alpha, Fc: fragment crystallizable, FcR: Fc receptor.

4.2.2. Extent of Reported Information on (Potentially Critical) Quality Attributes

The extent of the information on QAs and pCQAs provided in the EPARs was categorized by whether a biosimilarity interpretation was reported (yes/no) and whether test results were reported (yes/no) for a given QA or pCQA. The four possible combinations of answers resulted in four categories for each reported QA and pCQA (Table 3) [47].

Biosimilarity interpretation was defined as reported (yes) if the EPAR contained keywords demarcating the regulatory interpretation of the biosimilarity of a QA and pCQA as identical, similar, or having minor differences. The interpretation of *similar* included wording such as "same," "match," "(highly) similar," "comparable," and "consistent".

Test results were defined as reported (yes) if the EPAR included the quantitative or qualitative acceptance criteria of a given QA and pCQA, which included the numerical limits, range, and distribution, as shown in the examples in Table 3, or other suitable visual assessment measures, such as the spectra for higher-order structures and chromatograms for purity and impurities.

4.3. *Data Analysis*

The frequency of the reported QAs and pCQAs stratified by structural and functional attributes was used to express the consistency in reporting the QAs and pCQAs of adalimumab biosimilars by EU regulators in EPARs. A QA and pCQA was considered to be consistently reported if EU regulators describe it in all included EPARs. The proportion of reported QAs and pCQAs for the four reporting categories (see Table 3) was calculated and stratified by structural and functional attributes to compare the extent of information on reported QAs and pCQAs in EPARs. If the regulatory interpretation of the biosimilarity or test results were presented for a given QA or pCQA in the EPARs, the type of interpretation (identical, similar, or minor differences) and the acceptance biosimilarity criteria were identified.

Table 3. Definitions of the four reporting categories for the quality attributes (QAs) and potentially critical quality attributes (pCQAs) reported in biosimilarity assessments in the initial European public assessment reports (EPARs) [47].

Reporting Categories		Biosimilarity Interpretation	
		No	Yes
Test results	No	Reported QAs and pCQAs include no biosimilarity interpretation and no test results, for example: - The amino acid sequence and N-glycosylation site were compared. - The protein concentration was determined. - Binding to FcRn and Fcγ-RIIIa was studied, and a comparison of ADCC activity was performed. - Neutralization of TNFα, binding to s-TNFα, and binding to tm-TNFα were addressed.	Reported QAs and pCQAs include the biosimilarity interpretation but not test results, for example: - The amino acid sequence and N-glycosylation site of the biosimilar were identical to those of the reference. - The protein concentration was similar to that of the reference. - Minor differences with no clinical relevance were observed in glycation, galactosylated N-glycans, high mannose N-glycans, fucosylated N-glycans, and sialylated glycans. - The FcRn, C1q binding, CDC, ADCC, and neutralization of TNFα were comparable with those of the reference.
	Yes	Reported QAs and pCQAs include the test results but not the biosimilarity interpretation, for example: - The levels of high mannose N-glycans (biosimilar: 1.9–2.5%; reference: 5.3–12.0%). - The K_D ranges for Fcγ-RIIIa binding (biosimilar: 6.2–10.1 nM; reference: 3.8–8.0 nM) - The EC_{50} values for inhibiting cytokine release (204 pM, 294 pM and 200 pM for the three batches of tested biosimilars and 177 pM, 168 pM and 222 pM for the three batches of tested reference biological). - ADCC activity (biosimilar: 89–107%; reference: 84–115%)	Reported QAs and pCQAs include the biosimilarity interpretation and test results, for example: - Minor differences with no clinical relevance were observed in the levels of high mannose N-glycans (biosimilar: 1.9–2.5%; reference: 5.3–12.0%). - ADCC activity (biosimilar: 89–107%; reference: 84–115%) was comparable/similar between the two products.

ADCC: antibody-dependent cellular cytotoxicity, CDC: complement-dependent cytotoxicity, EC_{50}: half-maximal effective concentration, TNFα: tumor necrosis factor-alpha, s-TNFα: surface tumor necrosis factor-alpha, tm-TNFα: transmembrane tumor necrosis factor-alpha, Fc: fragment crystallizable, FcR: Fc receptor, K_D: equilibrium dissociation constant, nM: nanomoles, pM: picomoles.

5. Conclusions

In conclusion, we found variations in the frequency of reported QAs between EPARs of adalimumab biosimilars. The minor differences in the identified QAs did not affect functions and clinical performance and seem to be largely quantitative differences and not essentially meaningful for the overall conclusion of biosimilarity.

In line with our hypothesis, the pCQAs, specifically functional pCQAs, were reported most frequently and consistently in EPARs, as these reflect the MoA and can potentially affect the clinical profile. Greater consistency could be applied in reporting of QAs with more emphasis on pCQAs in EPARs, which could improve the understanding of the relationship between QAs and the clinical profile, which may positively contribute to adopting biosimilars in clinical practice.

Supplementary Materials: The following are available online at https://www.mdpi.com/1424-8247/14/3/189/s1, Figure S1: The types of and extent of information on quality attributes (QAs) and potentially critical QAs (pCQAs, in bold and gray boxes) as part of biosimilarity assessment reported by regulators in the initial European public assessment reports (EPARs) of seven adalimumab biosimilars; Table S1: Types of biosimilarity interpretation of reported quality attributes (QAs) stratified by the company code of adalimumab biosimilars in the European public assessment reports

(EPARs); Table S2: Comparison of potentially critical quality attributes (pCQAs) where test results and interpretation were reported for ABP501 and MSB11022 biosimilar.

Author Contributions: Conceptualization, A.M.A., T.J.G., T.C.E., H.G.L., and H.G.; methodology, A.M.A., T.J.G., T.C.E., H.G.L., and H.G.; validation, A.M.A., T.J.G., and H.G.; formal analysis, A.M.A.; investigation, A.M.A., T.J.G., T.C.E., H.G.L., and H.G.; resources, T.J.G., T.C.E., H.G.L., and H.G.; data curation, A.M.A.; writing—original draft preparation, A.M.A.; writing—review and editing, A.M.A., T.J.G., T.C.E., H.G.L., and H.G.; visualization, A.M.A.; supervision, T.J.G., T.C.E., H.G.L., and H.G.; project administration, T.J.G., T.C.E., H.G.L., and H.G.; funding acquisition, A.M.A.; All authors have read and agreed to the published version of the manuscript.

Funding: This study was funded by the Saudi Food and Drug Authority (SFDA) as a part of a Doctor of Philosophy (Ph.D.) project for A.M.A. The SFDA has no role in any aspect of the study, including the preparation, review, the approval of the manuscript, nor the decision to publish the manuscript.

Institutional Review Board Statement: Not applicable.

Informed Consent Statement: Not applicable.

Data Availability Statement: The datasets during and/or analyzed during the current study are available from the corresponding author on reasonable request.

Acknowledgments: The authors acknowledge the contribution of Lotte A. Minnema for constructive suggestion on the search strategy and Magdalena A. Gamba for kind advice on the process of data collection.

Conflicts of Interest: A.M.A., T.J.G., T.C.E., H.G.L., and H.G. declare that they have no conflict of interest.

References

1. Walsh, G. Biopharmaceutical benchmarks 2018. *Nat. Biotechnol.* **2018**, *36*, 1136–1145. [CrossRef] [PubMed]
2. Schiestl, M.; Stangler, T.; Torella, C.; Cepeljnik, T.; Toll, H.; Grau, R. Acceptable changes in quality attributes of glycosylated biopharmaceuticals. *Nat. Biotechnol.* **2011**, *29*, 310–312. [CrossRef] [PubMed]
3. Planinc, A.; Dejaegher, B.; Vander Heyden, Y.; Viaene, J.; Van Praet, S.; Rappez, F.; Van Antwerpen, P.; Delporte, C. Batch-to-batch N-glycosylation study of infliximab, trastuzumab and bevacizumab, and stability study of bevacizumab. *Eur. J. Hosp. Pharm.* **2017**, *24*, 286–292. [CrossRef] [PubMed]
4. Moorkens, E.; Vulto, A.G.; Huys, I. Biosimilars: Regulatory Frameworks for Marketing Authorization of Biosimilars: Where Do We Go from Here. *EPLR* **2018**, *2*, 31. [CrossRef]
5. EMA. *Similar Biological Medicinal Products Containing Biotechnology-Derived Proteins as Active Substance: Quality Issues*; European Medicines Agency (EMA)-Publications: Amsterdam, The Netherlands, 2014.
6. EMA. *Guideline on Similar Biological Medicinal Products*; European Medicines Agency (EMA)-Publications: Amsterdam, The Netherlands, 2015.
7. USFDA. *Development of Therapeutic Protein Biosimilars: Comparative Analytical Assessment and Other Quality-Related Considerations*; US Food and Drug Adminstration (USFDA)-Publications: Silver Spring, MD, USA, 2019.
8. WHO. *Guidelines on Evaluation of Similar Biotherapeutic Products (SBPs)*; World Health Orgnization (WHO)-Publications: Geneva, Switzerland, 2009.
9. Schiestl, M.; Ranganna, G.; Watson, K.; Jung, B.; Roth, K.; Capsius, B.; Trieb, M.; Bias, P.; Marechal-Jamil, J. The Path Towards a Tailored Clinical Biosimilar Development. *BioDrugs* **2020**, *34*, 297–306. [CrossRef]
10. Webster, C.J.; Wong, A.C.; Woollett, G.R. An Efficient Development Paradigm for Biosimilars. *BioDrugs* **2019**, *33*, 603–611. [CrossRef]
11. Wolff-Holz, E.; Tiitso, K.; Vleminckx, C.; Weise, M. Evolution of the EU Biosimilar Framework: Past and Future. *BioDrugs* **2019**, *33*, 621–634. [CrossRef]
12. Bielsky, M.C.; Cook, A.; Wallington, A.; Exley, A.; Kauser, S.; Hay, J.L.; Both, L.; Brown, D. Streamlined approval of biosimilars: Moving on from the confirmatory efficacy trial. *Drug Discov. Today* **2020**, *25*, 1910–1918. [CrossRef] [PubMed]
13. EMA. *ICH Guideline Q8 (R2) on Pharmaceutical Development Step 5*; International Conference on Harmonization (ICH)-Publications: Geneva, Switzerland, 2015.
14. Walsh, G.; Jefferis, R. Post-translational modifications in the context of therapeutic proteins. *Nat. Biotechnol.* **2006**, *24*, 1241–1252. [CrossRef]
15. Kim, S.; Song, J.; Park, S.; Ham, S.; Paek, K.; Kang, M.; Chae, Y.; Seo, H.; Kim, H.C.; Flores, M. Drifts in ADCC-related quality attributes of Herceptin®: Impact on development of a trastuzumab biosimilar. *MAbs* **2017**, *9*, 704–714. [CrossRef]
16. Pivot, X.; Pegram, M.; Cortes, J.; Lüftner, D.; Lyman, G.H.; Curigliano, G.; Bondarenko, I.; Yoon, Y.C.; Kim, Y.; Kim, C. Three-year follow-up from a phase 3 study of SB3 (a trastuzumab biosimilar) versus reference trastuzumab in the neoadjuvant setting for human epidermal growth factor receptor 2-positive breast cancer. *Eur. J. Cancer* **2019**, *120*, 1–9. [CrossRef]

17. Vulto, A.G.; Jaquez, O.A. The process defines the product: What really matters in biosimilar design and production? *Rheumatology* **2017**, *56*, iv14–iv29. [CrossRef]
18. Eon-Duval, A.; Broly, H.; Gleixner, R. Quality attributes of recombinant therapeutic proteins: An assessment of impact on safety and efficacy as part of a quality by design development approach. *Biotechnol. Prog* **2012**, *28*, 608–622. [CrossRef]
19. Kwon, O.; Joung, J.; Park, Y.; Kim, C.W.; Hong, S.H. Considerations of critical quality attributes in the analytical comparability assessment of biosimilar products. *Biologicals* **2017**, *48*, 101–108. [CrossRef] [PubMed]
20. Vandekerckhove, K.; Seidl, A.; Gutka, H.; Kumar, M.; Gratzl, G.; Keire, D.; Coffey, T.; Kuehne, H. Rational Selection, Criticality Assessment, and Tiering of Quality Attributes and Test Methods for Analytical Similarity Evaluation of Biosimilars. *AAPS J.* **2018**, *20*, 68. [CrossRef] [PubMed]
21. Berridge, J.; Seamon, K.; Venugopal, S. *A-MAb: A Case Study in Bioprocess Development*; CASSS and ISPE, CMC Biotech Working Group: Emeryville, CA, USA, 2009; pp. 1–278.
22. Vessely, C.; Bussineau, C. QbD in biopharmaceutical manufacturing and biosimilar development. In *Biosimilars*; Springer: Berlin/Heidelberg, Germany, 2018; pp. 187–219.
23. Tebbey, P.W.; Varga, A.; Naill, M.; Clewell, J.; Venema, J. Consistency of quality attributes for the glycosylated monoclonal antibody Humira® (adalimumab). *MAbs* **2015**, *7*, 805–811. [CrossRef]
24. Liu, J.; Eris, T.; Li, C.; Cao, S.; Kuhns, S. Assessing Analytical Similarity of Proposed Amgen Biosimilar ABP 501 to Adalimumab. *BioDrugs* **2016**, *30*, 321–338. [CrossRef] [PubMed]
25. Velayudhan, J.; Chen, Y.F.; Rohrbach, A.; Pastula, C.; Maher, G.; Thomas, H.; Brown, R.; Born, T.L. Demonstration of Functional Similarity of Proposed Biosimilar ABP 501 to Adalimumab. *BioDrugs* **2016**, *30*, 339–351. [CrossRef]
26. Lee, J.J.; Yang, J.; Lee, C.; Moon, Y.; Ahn, S.; Yang, J. Demonstration of functional similarity of a biosimilar adalimumab SB5 to Humira(®). *Biologicals* **2019**, *58*, 7–15. [CrossRef]
27. Lee, N.; Lee, J.J.; Yang, H.; Baek, S.; Kim, S.; Kim, S.; Lee, T.; Song, D.; Park, G. Evaluation of similar quality attribute characteristics in SB5 and reference product of adalimumab. *MAbs* **2019**, *11*, 129–144. [CrossRef] [PubMed]
28. Kronthaler, U.; Fritsch, C.; Hainzl, O.; Seidl, A.; da Silva, A. Comparative functional and pharmacological characterization of Sandoz proposed biosimilar adalimumab (GP2017): Rationale for extrapolation across indications. *Expert Opin. Biol. Ther.* **2018**, *18*, 921–930. [CrossRef]
29. Schreiber, S.; Yamamoto, K.; Muniz, R.; Iwura, T. Physicochemical analysis and biological characterization of FKB327 as a biosimilar to adalimumab. *Pharmacol. Res. Perspect.* **2020**, *8*, e00604. [CrossRef] [PubMed]
30. Magnenat, L.; Palmese, A.; Fremaux, C.; D'Amici, F.; Terlizzese, M.; Rossi, M.; Chevalet, L. Demonstration of physicochemical and functional similarity between the proposed biosimilar adalimumab MSB11022 and Humira®. *MAbs* **2017**, *9*, 127–139. [CrossRef]
31. Derzi, M.; Shoieb, A.M.; Ripp, S.L.; Finch, G.L.; Lorello, L.G.; O'Neil, S.P.; Radi, Z.; Syed, J.; Thompson, M.S.; Leach, M.W. Comparative nonclinical assessments of the biosimilar PF-06410293 and originator adalimumab. *Regul. Toxicol. Pharmacol.* **2020**, *112*, 104587. [CrossRef]
32. Zhang, E.; Xie, L.; Qin, P.; Lu, L.; Xu, Y.; Gao, W.; Wang, L.; Xie, M.H.; Jiang, W.; Liu, S. Quality by Design-Based Assessment for Analytical Similarity of Adalimumab Biosimilar HLX03 to Humira®. *AAPS J.* **2020**, *22*, 69. [CrossRef]
33. Lee, J.F.; Litten, J.B.; Grampp, G. Comparability and biosimilarity: Considerations for the healthcare provider. *Curr. Med. Res. Opin.* **2012**, *28*, 1053–1058. [CrossRef] [PubMed]
34. Raghavan, R.R.; McCombie, R. ICH Q5E Comparability of Biotechnological/Biological Products Subject to Changes in Their Manufacturing Processes. In *ICH Quality Guidelines*; Wiley: Hoboken, NJ, USA, 2018; Volume 409.
35. Ramanan, S.; Grampp, G. Drift, evolution, and divergence in biologics and biosimilars manufacturing. *BioDrugs* **2014**, *28*, 363–372. [CrossRef]
36. van der Plas, R.M.; Hoefnagel, M.H.N.; Hillege, H.L.; Roes, K.C.B. Pragmatic rules for comparability of biological medicinal products. *Biologicals* **2020**, *63*, 97–100. [CrossRef]
37. EMA. *Human Medicines*; European Medicines Agency (EMA): Amsterdam, The Netherlands, 2020.
38. AbbVie. *HUMIRA (Adalimumab) Injection, Full Prescribing Information*; AbbVie Inc.: North Chicago, IL, USA, 2009.
39. Tracey, D.; Klareskog, L.; Sasso, E.H.; Salfeld, J.G.; Tak, P.P. Tumor necrosis factor antagonist mechanisms of action: A comprehensive review. *Pharmacol. Ther.* **2008**, *117*, 244–279. [CrossRef] [PubMed]
40. Barbier, L.; Simoens, S.; Vulto, A.G.; Huys, I. European Stakeholder Learnings Regarding Biosimilars: Part II-Improving Biosimilar Use in Clinical Practice. *BioDrugs* **2020**, *34*, 797–808. [CrossRef] [PubMed]
41. Barbier, L.; Simoens, S.; Vulto, A.G.; Huys, I. European Stakeholder Learnings Regarding Biosimilars: Part I-Improving Biosimilar Understanding and Adoption. *BioDrugs* **2020**, *34*, 783–796. [CrossRef]
42. Moorkens, E.; Jonker-Exler, C.; Huys, I.; Declerck, P.; Simoens, S.; Vulto, A.G. Overcoming Barriers to the Market Access of Biosimilars in the European Union: The Case of Biosimilar Monoclonal Antibodies. *Front. Pharmacol.* **2016**, *7*, 193. [CrossRef] [PubMed]
43. Mielke, J.; Jilma, B.; Jones, B.; Koenig, F. An update on the clinical evidence that supports biosimilar approvals in Europe. *Br. J. Clin. Pharmacol.* **2018**, *84*, 1415–1431. [CrossRef]
44. Mielke, J.; Jilma, B.; Koenig, F.; Jones, B. Clinical trials for authorized biosimilars in the European Union: A systematic review. *Br. J. Clin. Pharmacol.* **2016**, *82*, 1444–1457. [CrossRef] [PubMed]
45. Bellinvia, S.; Cummings, J.R.F.; Ardern-Jones, M.R.; Edwards, C.J. Adalimumab Biosimilars in Europe: An Overview of the Clinical Evidence. *BioDrugs* **2019**, *33*, 241–253. [CrossRef] [PubMed]

46. Alsamil, A.M.; Giezen, T.J.; Egberts, T.C.; Leufkens, H.G.; Vulto, A.G.; van der Plas, M.R.; Gardarsdottir, H. Reporting of quality attributes in scientific publications presenting biosimilarity assessments of (intended) biosimilars: A systematic literature review. *Eur. J. Pharm. Sci.* **2020**, *154*, 105501. [CrossRef] [PubMed]
47. Alsamil, A.M.; Giezen, T.J.; Egberts, T.C.; Leufkens, H.G.; Gardarsdottir, H. Comparison of consistency and complementarity of reporting biosimilar quality attributes between regulatory and scientific communities: An adalimumab case study. *Biologicals* **2021**, *69*, 30–37. [CrossRef]
48. EMA. *EPAR Amgevita, EMA/CHMP/106922/2017*; European Medicines Agency (EMA): Amsterdam, The Netherlands, 2017.
49. EMA. *EPAR Solymbic, EMA/CHMP/106921*; European Medicines Agency (EMA): Amsterdam, The Netherlands, 2017.
50. EMA. *EPAR Cyltezo, EMA/CHMP/750187*; European Medicines Agency (EMA): Amsterdam, The Netherlands, 2017.
51. EMA. *EPAR Hefiya, EMA/CHMP/520007*; European Medicines Agency (EMA): Amsterdam, The Netherlands, 2018.
52. EMA. *EPAR Halimatoz, EMA/CHMP/519681*; European Medicines Agency (EMA): Amsterdam, The Netherlands, 2018.
53. EMA. *EPAR Hyrimoz, EMA/CHMP 404076*; European Medicines Agency (EMA): Amsterdam, The Netherlands, 2018.
54. EMA. *EPAR Hulio, EMA/CHMP/541826*; European Medicines Agency (EMA): Amsterdam, The Netherlands, 2019.
55. EMA. *EPAR Idacio, EMA/CHMP/124342*; European Medicines Agency (EMA): Amsterdam, The Netherlands, 2019.
56. EMA. *EPAR Kromeya, EMA/CHMP/214726*; European Medicines Agency (EMA): Amsterdam, The Netherlands, 2019.
57. EMA. *EPAR Amsparity, EMA/CHMP/2756*; European Medicines Agency (EMA): Amsterdam, The Netherlands, 2020.
58. EMA. *EPAR Imraldi, EMA/CHMP/559383*; European Medicines Agency (EMA): Amsterdam, The Netherlands, 2017.
59. Weise, M.; Kurki, P.; Wolff-Holz, E.; Bielsky, M.C.; Schneider, C.K. Biosimilars: The science of extrapolation. *Blood* **2014**, *124*, 3191–3196. [CrossRef]
60. Ebbers, H.C.; Chamberlain, P. Controversies in Establishing Biosimilarity: Extrapolation of Indications and Global Labeling Practices. *BioDrugs* **2016**, *30*, 1–8. [CrossRef] [PubMed]
61. Declerck, P.; Danesi, R.; Petersel, D.; Jacobs, I. The Language of Biosimilars: Clarification, Definitions, and Regulatory Aspects. *Drugs* **2017**, *77*, 671–677. [CrossRef]
62. Tesser, J.R.; Furst, D.E.; Jacobs, I. Biosimilars and the extrapolation of indications for inflammatory conditions. *Biologics* **2017**, *11*, 5–11. [CrossRef]
63. Ebbers, H.C.; Fehrmann, B.; Ottosen, M.; Hvorslev, N.; Høier, P.; Hwang, J.W.; Chung, J.; Lim, H.T.; Lee, S.; Hong, J.; et al. Batch-to-Batch Consistency of SB4 and SB2, Etanercept and Infliximab Biosimilars. *BioDrugs* **2020**, *34*, 225–233. [CrossRef]
64. Papathanasiou, P.; Brassart, L.; Blake, P.; Hart, A.; Whitbread, L.; Pembrey, R.; Kieffer, J. Transparency in drug regulation: Public assessment reports in Europe and Australia. *Drug Discov. Today* **2016**, *21*, 1806–1813. [CrossRef]
65. Cohen, H.; Beydoun, D.; Chien, D.; Lessor, T.; McCabe, D.; Muenzberg, M.; Popovian, R.; Uy, J. Awareness, knowledge, and perceptions of biosimilars among specialty physicians. *Adv. Ther.* **2016**, *33*, 2160–2172. [CrossRef]
66. Hallersten, A.; Fürst, W.; Mezzasalma, R. Physicians prefer greater detail in the biosimilar label (SmPC)–results of a survey across seven European countries. *Regul. Toxicol. Pharmacol.* **2016**, *77*, 275–281. [CrossRef] [PubMed]
67. Liberti, L.; Breckenridge, A.; Hoekman, J.; Leufkens, H.; Lumpkin, M.; McAuslane, N.; Stolk, P.; Zhi, K.; Rägo, L. Accelerating access to new medicines: Current status of facilitated regulatory pathways used by emerging regulatory authorities. *J. Public Health Policy* **2016**, *37*, 315–333. [CrossRef]
68. Liberti, L.; Stolk, P.; McAuslane, N.; Somauroo, A.; Breckenridge, A.; Leufkens, H. Adaptive licensing and facilitated regulatory pathways: A survey of stakeholder perceptions. *Clin. Pharmacol. Ther.* **2015**, *98*, 477–479. [CrossRef]
69. Luigetti, R.; Bachmann, P.; Cooke, E.; Salmonson, T. Collaboration, not competition: Developing new reliance models. *WHO Drug Inf.* **2016**, *30*, 558.
70. WHO. *Good Regulatory Practices: Guidelines for National Regulatory Authorities for Medical Products*; Working Document QAS/16.686. Draft for comment Prepared by EMP/RSS; WHO: Geneva, Switzerland, 2016.
71. Roth, L.; Bempong, D.; Babigumira, J.B.; Banoo, S.; Cooke, E.; Jeffreys, D.; Kasonde, L.; Leufkens, H.G.; Lim, J.C.; Lumpkin, M. Expanding global access to essential medicines: Investment priorities for sustainably strengthening medical product regulatory systems. *Glob. Health* **2018**, *14*, 102. [CrossRef]
72. Kang, H.N.; Thorpe, R.; Knezevic, I.; Casas Levano, M.; Chilufya, M.B.; Chirachanakul, P.; Chua, H.M.; Dalili, D.; Foo, F.; Gao, K.; et al. Regulatory challenges with biosimilars: An update from 20 countries. *Ann. N. Y. Acad. Sci.* **2020**. [CrossRef]
73. IPRP. *The Basics of Analytical Comparability of Biosimilar Monoclonal Antibody for Regulatory Reviewers*; The International Pharmaceutical Regulators Programme (IPRP)-Publications: Valparaiso, IN, USA, 2018.
74. Berntgen, M.; Gourvil, A.; Pavlovic, M.; Goettsch, W.; Eichler, H.-G.; Kristensen, F.B. Improving the contribution of regulatory assessment reports to health technology assessments—A collaboration between the European Medicines Agency and the European network for Health Technology Assessment. *Value Health* **2014**, *17*, 634–641. [CrossRef] [PubMed]

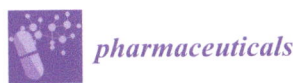

Review

Informing Patients about Biosimilar Medicines: The Role of European Patient Associations

Yannick Vandenplas [1,*], Steven Simoens [1], Philippe Van Wilder [2], Arnold G. Vulto [1,3] and Isabelle Huys [1]

1. Department of Pharmaceutical and Pharmacological Sciences, KU Leuven, 3000 Leuven, Belgium; steven.simoens@kuleuven.be (S.S.); a.vulto@gmail.com (A.G.V.); Isabelle.huys@kuleuven.be (I.H.)
2. Ecole de Santé Publique, Université Libre de Bruxelles (ULB), 1050 Brussels, Belgium; Philippe.Van.Wilder@ulb.be
3. Hospital Pharmacy, Erasmus University Medical Center, 3015 GD Rotterdam, The Netherlands
* Correspondence: yannick.vandenplas@kuleuven.be; Tel.: +32-1632-5629

Abstract: Biosimilar medicines support the sustainability of national healthcare systems, by reducing costs of biological therapies through increased competition. However, their adoption into clinical practice largely depends on the acceptance of healthcare providers and patients. Patients are different from health care professionals (HCPs), who are informing themselves professionally. For patients, the biosimilar debate only becomes actual when they are confronted with disease and drug choices. This paper provides a literature review on how patients are and should be informed about biosimilars, searching in scientific databases (i.e., Medline, Embase). Several large surveys have shown a lack of knowledge and trust in biosimilars among European patients in recent years. This review identified five main strategies to inform patients about biosimilars: (1) provide understandable information, (2) in a positive and transparent way, (3) tailored to the individual's needs, (4) with one voice, and (5) supported by audiovisual material. Moreover, the importance of a multistakeholder approach was underlined by describing the role of each stakeholder. Patients are a large and diffuse target group to be reached by educational programs. Therefore, patient associations have become increasingly important in correctly informing patients about biosimilar medicines. This has led to widespread biosimilar information for patients among European patient associations. Therefore, a web-based screening of European Patients' Forum (EPF) and International Alliance of Patients' Organizations (IAPO) member organizations on publicly available information about biosimilars was performed. We found that the level of detail, correctness, and the tone of the provided information varied. In conclusion, it is paramount to set up a close collaboration between all stakeholders to communicate, develop, and disseminate factual information about biosimilars for patients.

Keywords: biosimilar; biological; information; education; communication; patient; Europe

Citation: Vandenplas, Y.; Simoens, S.; Van Wilder, P.; Vulto, A.G.; Huys, I. Informing Patients about Biosimilar Medicines: The Role of European Patient Associations. *Pharmaceuticals* 2021, 14, 117. https://doi.org/10.3390/ph14020117

Academic Editor: Jean Jacques Vanden Eynde
Received: 31 December 2020
Accepted: 1 February 2021
Published: 4 February 2021

Publisher's Note: MDPI stays neutral with regard to jurisdictional claims in published maps and institutional affiliations.

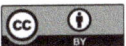

Copyright: © 2021 by the authors. Licensee MDPI, Basel, Switzerland. This article is an open access article distributed under the terms and conditions of the Creative Commons Attribution (CC BY) license (https://creativecommons.org/licenses/by/4.0/).

1. Introduction

Since their introduction to the European market in 2006, biosimilar medicines have contributed to a more sustainable healthcare system in several European markets [1]. Biosimilars are biological medicines that contain a version of the active substance of an already authorized biological medicine in the European Economic Area (EEA) [2]. They are allowed to enter the market when market exclusivities of the original biological product have expired, and market authorization has been granted by the European Commission (EC). Market authorization is achieved after a rigorous regulatory evaluation process by the European Medicines Agency (EMA) and subsequent approval of the EC. This guarantees that biosimilars are as effective and safe as their reference product, making them equal treatment options for patients [2,3]. Several benefits have been identified following the increased competition induced by biosimilar market entry [4]. Due to the decreased costs of biological medicines, generated savings could be allocated to providing patients with more access to biological therapies. In addition, these savings can be utilized to finance high-cost innovative treatments [1,5,6].

However, the extent to which these benefits are being captured in Europe largely depends on the adoption of biosimilars by European Union (EU) member states. Adoption into clinical practice might be hampered by limited healthcare provider (HCP) and patient acceptance of biosimilars. Often, besides other factors such as the absence of tangible incentives, a lack of acceptance among HCPs and patients comes down to shortcomings in knowledge and understanding about biosimilars [7–9]. Patients' access to information and education about biosimilar medicines is therefore considered as one of the key elements for a sustainable market [10]. Hence, policy initiatives aiming to increase understanding among clinicians and patients have been implemented in most European countries in past years [11,12].

Several studies have brought an inadequate understanding and acceptance among European patients about biosimilars to light, underlining the need for information and education of patients [13–19]. Especially when transitioning or *switching* current original (or innovator) biological therapy to its biosimilar, the value of adequate patients' understanding about biosimilars cannot be underestimated [20]. Clinical studies have proven the positive effect on patient outcomes when patients with rheumatological disorders were properly informed before transitioning to a biosimilar [21,22]. The authors attributed the improvement in patient outcomes after a structured communication strategy to a reduction in the risk of *nocebo effects*. The nocebo effect is described as the worsening of symptoms associated or an increase in side effects with a negative attitude towards a given therapy, in this case the biosimilar medicine. A lack of patient knowledge is the main underlying reason for negative attitudes towards biosimilars, contributing to nocebo effects and possible treatment failure [20,23].

Educating patients about biosimilars is crucial to provide clarity and prevent misinformation [9,20,24]. Patients need access to understandable and evidence-based information that allows them to make informed decisions about their treatment. Regulatory authorities, medical scientific associations, and patient organizations have therefore been active in developing and disseminating educational material on biosimilars for European patients during past years. However, information and educational material are widespread, requiring a mapping of the available material [8,9]. Mapping the available information or material for patients makes it possible to have an overview of what material exists, and to verify the information found for its scientific correctness. In addition, a proper inventory will facilitate the dissemination of information through collaboration between stakeholders.

This review aimed to provide an overview of existing scientific literature on how to inform patients about biosimilars and compile available information about biosimilars for patients, developed or disseminated by European patient associations. Based on this review, an overview of the important aspects when talking to patients about biosimilars is provided for policymakers, healthcare providers, patient organizations, and other relevant stakeholders, in support of a sustainable market for off-patent biological and biosimilar medicines in Europe.

2. Methods
2.1. Literature Review

This comprehensive structured literature review identified articles on what information patients need about biosimilars and how this information can be communicated, by looking into scientific databases (Embase, Medline) using a structured search strategy (Cfr. Supplementary Table S1). Relevant English-language scientific publications published between 2006 and 2020 were included. This period was chosen since biosimilars have been introduced in Europe in 2006, thereby encompassing the whole period of time when biosimilars were available on the European market. Search terms were related to patient communication about biosimilars and included the following terms: 'biosimilar', 'information', 'education', 'communication', 'knowledge', and 'patient'. All terms were modified according to the respective scientific database. Both abstracts and full texts were included in the analysis. Only articles relevant to the European landscape were within the scope of this analysis. Articles were searched up to the 21st of October 2020.

All identified records were imported from Embase or Pubmed into Mendeley software to remove duplicates. Next, all articles were screened on title and abstract for relevance in the Rayyan (Qatar Computing Research Institute, Doha, Qatar) software. In a third step, articles were carefully reviewed based on their full text. Lastly, reference lists of included articles were searched for additional relevant articles. The articles included in the final analysis were analyzed qualitatively according to the thematic framework method [25]. A combination of inductive and deductive coding was used, since some aspects were already identified as relevant for this research question. During the initial coding step, general themes were identified prior to the literature review. Similar codes were grouped together to form the coding tree. Second, the identified literature was coded deductively. Meanwhile, additional codes were created inductively and added to the coding tree.

2.2. Mapping of Patient Information

A web-based screening on relevant patient information (i.e., general information not intended for educational purposes) or educational material (i.e., brochures, toolboxes, position papers, audiovisual material, etc.) was performed to provide an overview of the educational material disseminated by European patient organizations. This screening included all public websites of European Patients' Forum (EPF) and European International Alliance of Patients' Organizations (IAPO) members. EPF and IAPO are two major umbrella associations, uniting a large number of European patient organizations in a variety of disease areas. Websites were screened on available information about biosimilars by searching for 'biosimilar' or related terms in the search bar. In addition, the name of the respective patient association was combined with the term 'biosimilar' via Google to make sure no information was missed.

After all identified information was analyzed and mapped together, the tone in which each association reports about biosimilars was evaluated on a five-point Likert scale. This was done by scoring the overall attitude towards biosimilar medicines on the following scale: "− −" (negative), "−" (somewhat negative), "0" (neutral), "+" (somewhat positive), "+ +" (positive). Neutral information was taken as a starting point. Neutral information refers to factually correct information about biosimilars, without any additional positive or negative undertone. The initial scoring was done by one researcher (Y.V.), and afterwards reviewed by four other researchers (S.S., A.G.V., P.V.W., I.H.).

The purpose of the web-based screening was (1) to examine to what extent patient information about biosimilars is provided on their public websites, (2) to have a closer look at the actual content of these materials, and (3) to evaluate the tone in which they report about biosimilars. All different types of information found was schematically listed per patient association (Table 1).

Table 1. European Patients' Forum (EPF) and International Alliance of Patients' Organizations (IAPO) members providing biosimilar information for patients.

Patient Association	Disease Area	Country/Region of Origin	Available Information	Attitude towards Biosimilars [1]
Association for the Protection of Patients' Rights (Asociácia na Ochranu Práv Pacientov, AOPP)	N/A	Slovak Republic	**Short article** about biosimilar medicines (i.e., What are they, how are they produced, the difference with original biologicals) [26]. Lastly, **a link to the EC brochure** (questions and answers about biosimilars for patients) in Slovakian is provided [26].	+
Digestive Cancers Europe (DiCE)	Colorectal cancer	Europe	**Position paper** of DiCE about the use of biosimilar medicines in colorectal cancer (including general information on originator biologicals and biosimilars, biologicals in CRC, access and availability of biologicals, safety and effectiveness of biosimilars). The position paper will be extended to educational materials (video, educational leaflet, checklist to support HCPs) [27]. **General information** on biosimilar and biological medicines, including a frequently asked questions (FAQ) document [28].	+ +
European Federation of Crohn's and Ulcerative Colitis Associations (EFCCA)	Ulcerative colitis and Crohn's disease	Europe	**Link to the EC brochure** is provided [29]. **Summary of a workshop** on biosimilars (and biologicals in general) organized by EFCCA [30]. **Short article** on biosimilars in the EFCCA magazine, focusing also on the potential benefits of biosimilar medicines [31].	0
European Multiple Sclerosis Platform (EMSP)	Multiple sclerosis	Europe	**Link to the EC brochure** is provided [32].	+
European Parkinson's Disease Association (EPDA)	Parkinson's disease	Europe	**Brief information** on what biological medicines are, with a section on biosimilars. No detailed information is provided [33].	−
International Diabetes Federation European Region (IDF Europe)	Diabetes	International	**Position paper** on biosimilars for the treatment of people with diabetes. This document includes information on the difference with generics (focusing the difference between biosimilars and their reference products), the regulatory framework, impact of biosimilars on healthcare systems, and recommendations for clinical practice [34].	− −
Malta Health Network (MHN)	N/A	Malta	**Link to the EUPATI toolbox** on biosimilar medicines, directed at patients [35].	0
Platform for Patient Organizations (Plataforma de Organizaciones de Pacientes)	N/A	Spain	**Specific web page** about biological medicines in general and biosimilars, including information on their definitions, interchangeability, substitution, and position statements [36].	−
European Federation of Neurological Associations (EFNA)	Neurological disorders	Europe	**Link to the EC brochure** is provided [37].	+

Table 1. Cont.

Patient Association	Disease Area	Country/Region of Origin	Available Information	Attitude towards Biosimilars [1]
European Institute of Women's Health (EIWH)	N/A	Europe	Link to the EC brochure is provided [38].	+
National Coalition of Dutch Patients (Patiëntenfederatie Nederland)	N/A	Netherlands	Brief information on key concepts of biosimilars [39]. Link to a brochure (question and answer) about biosimilars developed by the Dutch competent authority, including general information, their position on interchangeability and switching, and infographics about biosimilar medicines [40].	+ +
Flemish Patient Platform (Vlaams Patiëntenplatform) (FPP)	N/A	Belgium	Very brief information on biological and biosimilar medicines ('copy of original biological, equal to generics') [41]. Link to specific information from the Belgian regulatory authority is provided. This information includes: definition, general information, pharmacovigilance, available biosimilars (not up to date), and links to several other brochures (EC, EMA, etc.) [42].	−
European Patients' Forum (EPF)	N/A	Europe	A link to the EC brochure is provided. Several EPF members collaborated with EC and EMA on the EC brochure about biosimilar medicines for patients [43]. A summary of the yearly biosimilar stakeholder event by the EC [44].	0
International Federation of Psoriasis Associations (IFPA)	Psoriasis	International	Position statement on the use of biosimilar medicines for the treatment of psoriasis, including the definition, general information, switching, regulatory requirements [45].	−
Psoriasis Action (Acción Psoriasis)	Psoriasis	Spain	Link to a video where biosimilars are explained by an expert [46]. Short article about biosimilar medicines, explaining general information about them [47,48].	0
International Alliance of Patients' Organizations (IAPO)	N/A	International	Biosimilars toolkit, developed in collaboration with IFPMA, is publicly available on the IAPO website. The toolkit contains information on several aspects of biologicals in general, and biosimilar medicines specifically: general information, regulatory requirements, pharmacovigilance, how to talk to patients about biosimilars, biologicals in low- and middle-income countries, key recommendations (as mentioned by WHO), and FAQs about biosimilars [49].	0

[1] The evaluation of the overall attitude towards biosimilars for each patient organization is done on a five-point Likert scale. The scale is as follows: "− −" (negative), "−" (somewhat negative), 0 (neutral), "+" (somewhat positive), and "+ +" (positive).

3. Results

3.1. Literature Review

After a screening of 1319 records, a total of 51 articles were included in this literature review. Although conference abstracts ($n = 6$) were also eligible for inclusion, most identified records were full-text articles ($n = 45$). Most articles were identified through the structured literature search after title and abstract screening ($n = 38$). Nonetheless, the screening of reference lists resulted in 13 additional records. A complete overview of the literature search process is included in Supplementary Table S1 and Figure S1.

3.1.1. Points to Consider When Talking to Patients about Biosimilars

In the vast body of literature, we can conclude that several specific aspects are essential when informing patients about biosimilars. An overview of these aspects is provided below.

Provide Understandable and Up-to-Date Information

Biosimilars are a relatively new and difficult concept for patients. It is therefore important that the given information to patients is easy to understand and not overly complicated. The message must be concise, using simple language, avoiding redundant medical jargon [50–52]. When informing the patient face-to-face, make sure they understand all information by asking questions and involving them in the discussion [52]. In this way, the patient will feel more involved and can participate in the discussion as well. In addition, the information must be up-to-date and adapted to the most recent insights [53]. It should not contain outdated concepts or outdated data.

Communicate Positively

Several studies have already shown that it is crucial to positively formulate the message about biosimilars towards patients. An empathic and positive communication (including positive framing) or attitude increase the acceptance to switch and reduce the development of nocebo effects after transitioning to a biosimilar [54–58]. An open and positive communication, emphasizing the equalities and not the differences between the reference product and its biosimilar, should be the norm when talking to patients. Information or communication should avoid messages such as: "biosimilars have no meaningful differences with their reference product". Instead, the similarities must be underlined in any communication to reassure patients that biosimilars are equal treatment alternatives [20,58,59]. When transitioning to a biosimilar, it is unnecessary to mention all possible side effects. It is rather recommended to provide patients with the opportunity to contact their physicians or nurse when any unexpected side effect would occur [60]. Moreover, a positive communication about biosimilars should be adopted for information towards HCPs as well, thereby supporting overall acceptance of biosimilars in clinical practice [9,50].

Patients generally feel that their physician's opinion and attitude on biosimilars strongly influences their decision to use a biosimilar [61]. Yet, an open and positive attitude should be adopted by all healthcare providers (i.e., physicians, nurses, and pharmacists) who communicate with patients. This involves empathy, reassurance, and nonverbal elements in their communication towards patients when discussing medicines in general [51,62]. It will be essential to educate HCPs using these communication techniques or 'soft skills' in the future.

Provide Information Tailored to the Individual Patients' Needs

A one-size-fits-all approach to communicate or inform patients about biosimilars does not exist, nor would it be appropriate [8,63]. Some patients will naturally be more concerned about their treatment and ask for more information. While other patients trust their physician completely and will express no further concerns about biosimilars [55,60,64]. However, many patients will be somewhere between these two extremes of the spectrum, highlighting the importance of tailored communication. Providing too much information could lead to unnecessary concerns of patients, while giving too little information could leave patients with remaining concerns [65]. It is the task of all HCPs to assess the individual patients' needs and find the right balance. Specific tools or questionnaires exist to assess prior beliefs or concerns of patients about their medicine, such as the Beliefs about Medicine Questionnaire (BMQ) [63]. The BMQ might help HCPs stratify patients based on their prior thoughts about biosimilars before transitioning.

In addition, information should be tailored to the individual patient's demographics and health literacy as well [66]. For example, patients affiliated to a patient association or previously treated with a biological medicine generally have a better knowledge about biosimilars [16]. Some patients might have already looked for information about biosimilars elsewhere, given the broad access to information on the internet [64,67]. It is therefore advised to account for this and assess whether their prior knowledge is factual. Furthermore, in order to make sure that the information is accessible for all patients, educational material should be translated into local languages.

Communicate with One Voice

As already touched upon in the above, communication towards patients must be consistent across resources, so confusion among patients is avoided. Homogenous information leads to higher acceptance and better treatment outcomes after transitioning to a biosimilar [54,57]. Stakeholders should therefore deliver the same message or speak with *one voice* to patients about biosimilars [7,20]. Such an approach means that all healthcare providers are involved and educated about biosimilars, ensuring a coherent and unified message to patients. Not only the information itself, but also the way it is explained to patients should be coherent (i.e., positive and open communication, tailored information) [68].

Make Use of Supportive Material

Several ways exist to inform patients in addition to oral communication of the HCP with the patient. In the context of transitioning or switching to biosimilars, written informed consent before transitioning could be considered. Such information must be in the patient's native language, include only key information on biosimilars, the reasons why transitioning is considered, and who to contact if they have any issues or concerns [50,54,57,69].

For general information accessible to patients, a variety of audiovisual aids can be used, such as videos, infographics, podcasts, and pictures [50,52]. All these ways may contribute to the understandability and confidence in the key biosimilar concepts. Moreover, for subcutaneous biosimilars, instructional leaflets or videos about the injection device might be useful as well. Since patients are increasingly seeking health-related information on the internet, such audiovisual material can be made broadly accessible online [67]. For example, the European Medicines Agency (EMA) and European Commission (EC) developed an animated video explaining the general concepts of biosimilar medicines [70].

3.1.2. Information Needs of Patients about Biosimilar Medicines

A multitude of studies has been performed in past years assessing the level of knowledge about or attitudes towards biosimilar medicines among European patients. In general, most of these studies concluded that the level of knowledge of patients is limited, as well as that confidence in biosimilars is rather low. In particular, limited knowledge about the general concepts of biological and biosimilar medicines is reported [13–17,19,54,56,71–73]. Doubts around efficacy, safety, and extrapolation of indications were revealed among most patient populations (i.e., oncology, psoriasis, rheumatology, IBD). It goes without saying that correct information and education can resolve these concerns and lack of knowledge.

A tailored approach was already pointed out earlier in this review in the context of direct communication of HCPs towards patients. The specific biosimilar concepts that should be explained by HCPs will therefore vary from patient to patient, depending on the individual needs and level of understanding. It used to be common practice that the basic concepts about biological medicines, and biosimilars in particular (e.g., definitions, safety, efficacy, regulatory approval, etc.), have to be clearly explained to patients when transitioning to a biosimilar [20,60,74]. However, nowadays current practice has evolved towards providing the message that another brand of the same medicine will be used, with the same efficacy and safety outcomes at a lower cost.

There is still a lack of clarity about which aspects of biosimilars should be included when developing educational material for patients [8]. It should be borne in mind that patients themselves look for information about biosimilars on the internet, potentially finding incorrect information. The purpose of providing information is to counter such negative reports as well [9,74,75]. Therefore, publicly available information or educational material about biosimilars for patients should address the general definitions of biological and biosimilar medicines in an understandable way. This should include the thorough regulatory evaluation process of EMA that assures the same clinical efficacy and safety between the original and biosimilar product. The potential benefits of biosimilars can also be considered, albeit in understandable language and as direct benefits (i.e., increase in access to necessary medicines or access to treatments at an earlier disease stage) [8,54,76]. However, it should be avoided that the impression is created that the patient is treated with biosimilars only for the sake of cost savings. Other essential concepts such as extrapolation of indication may be explained as well, although overly detailed information should always be avoided [8,20].

3.1.3. Reaching the Patient

All stakeholders, particularly healthcare providers, play a role in informing patients about biosimilars. It must be stressed that communicating with patients should be a multistakeholder effort [8,20,77]. This includes physicians, nurses, pharmacists, scientific associations, regulatory bodies, and patient associations. In the following, we summarize the role of each stakeholder in informing patients about biosimilars (Figure 1).

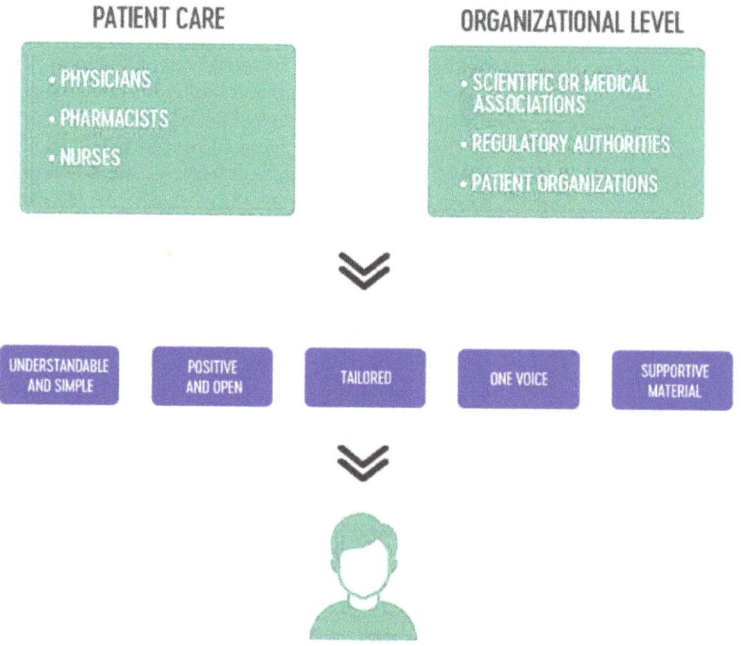

Figure 1. The multistakeholder approach using five main strategies for informing patients about biosimilars.

Role of Physicians

Treatment decisions must be based on shared decision-making between patients and their physician. In most European countries, physicians have the ultimate responsibility in making treatment choices. Physicians will often be the first point of contact for patients when treatment decisions are being made, and they should therefore ensure a trusted relationship with the patient. Good communication, based on informed discussions and shared decision-making with the physician, is known to benefit adherence to a prescribed medicine, and thus the adoption of biosimilars [5,20,21,74]. However, shared-decision making about medical therapy in general is not yet established to the same extent in every European country [78,79].

Previous research involving patient surveys has shown that physicians are the most trusted source of information about biosimilars [17,19,80]. However, several surveys among European physicians have concluded that physicians' knowledge on biosimilar medicines could be improved [50]. As a result, it is clear that physicians should be properly trained about biosimilars and be able to communicate adequately about them to the patient. As mentioned earlier, physicians must therefore be trained in communication techniques as well [65].

Role of Nurses

Nurses play a key role in the daily care for patients and are ideally placed to inform patients by addressing questions or concerns about their medicine. Usually, nurses administer the medication and spend the most time with patients, which allows them to have a closer relationship with the patient [81]. When transitioning from a reference product to its biosimilar, the important role of nurses has been pointed out in several publications during past years [7,8,52,81,82]. Building further on their profound experience with educating patients, nurses can guide patients in the process when transitioning to a biosimilar and manage nocebo effects. Additionally, following the transition or initiation with a biosimilar, patients may have further questions or concerns at home. To prevent any additional concerns or even discontinuation of their treatment, nurses should serve as a contact point to patients [58,83]. For subcutaneously administered biologicals, where injection devices may differ, nurses provide the necessary explanation and guidance to use the new injection device [52].

The above reasons make it clear that nurses are a critical link in the multidisciplinary team, particularly when making the transition to a biosimilar. This has been recognized by the European Specialist Nurses Organization (ESNO), by developing an elaborate communication guide for nurses when transitioning to a biosimilar in 2017 [84]. This document has been translated into eight languages and can serve as a reference document for nurses.

Role of Pharmacists

The main task of a pharmacist is often simplified to the delivery of medicines. However, pharmacists also have an important task of providing information to patients, although regional differences exist among European countries in their role in direct patient counseling. Especially community pharmacists serve as a first-line contact for patients for any questions about their medicine, including biosimilar medicines [58,66]. Pharmacists thereby contribute to medication adherence by increasing confidence in biosimilar medicines among patients. They may also have to explain differences in injection devices, since subcutaneously administered biosimilars are often dispensed in community or outpatient pharmacies.

For biosimilars delivered in the hospital setting, pharmacists have an increasing role in educating the medical staff about biosimilars [85,86]. The Dutch association of hospital pharmacists (NVZA) has developed a practical guidance document (i.e., toolbox) on how to implement biosimilars in the hospital setting, thereby emphasizing the role of hospital pharmacists in this process [87]. As medicine experts, clinical pharmacists can serve as a coordinator of the medical team to address patients' concerns about biosimilars when preparing the switch to a biosimilar. Their role should be further explored in the future, particularly in the context of transitioning to biosimilars in the hospital setting.

Role of Scientific or Medical Associations

Several European scientific associations have developed educational material for patients in past years about biosimilars. Due to their extensive scientific expertise and background, they are an important source of unbiased information about the use of biosimilars [62,66,71]. The European Society for Medical Oncology (ESMO) developed educational leaflets about biosimilars for patients [88]. ESMO uses infographics to explain the key concepts and potential advantages of biosimilars in understandable language. The European League Against Rheumatism (EULAR) has developed a document with general information about biosimilars as well. The main questions or concerns patients may have are addressed in this question and answer brochure [89,90]. Additionally, the need for more patient educational material is highlighted in this document.

Role of Regulatory Authorities

European regulatory agencies and national competent authorities have a supporting role in disseminating unbiased information about biosimilars in general [55,66,91]. However, room for improvement was recently pointed out for European national competent authorities to disseminate biosimilar information to the public [92]. The widespread patient brochure developed by the European Commission (EC) and European Medicines Agency (EMA) has become a reference document for patients, and is being referred to by many national authorities [93]. This brochure was developed in cooperation with the European Patients' Forum (EPF) in 2016, explaining the key concepts about biological and biosimilar medicines in lay language. It is also publicly available in a more concise video format [70]. In recent years, this material has been translated into all European languages [93]. National authorities should continue facilitating the dissemination of this document, as it provides coherent and factual information about biosimilars in understandable language and graphical format [92].

Role of Patient Associations

Patient organizations are a trusted source of information for patients about biosimilars. Patients rely on their respective associations or advocacy groups to clarify complex concepts such as biosimilars [16,19]. Patient associations can also serve as a discussion board to discuss complex matters such as biosimilars and share experiences among patients [17]. If patient associations are committed to developing educational material themselves, they should join forces with medical and scientific associations. In this way, it can be ensured that the information is evidence-based and up-to-date [13,71].

A schematic overview of the multistakeholder approach, using the five identified strategies, is provided in Figure 1. The section below takes a closer look at the role of patient associations in developing and disseminating information about biosimilars to patients.

3.2. Information Provided by European Patient Organizations

In total, public websites of 75 European Patients' Forum (EPF) members and 95 members of the International Alliance of Patients' Organizations (IAPO) were consulted. As some organizations were part of both EPF and IAPO, 159 unique members were screened. Of these 159 patient organizations, 16 were actively disseminating information on biosimilars via their website. An overview summarizing all patient organizations, along with the type of information, is provided in Table 1.

Patient associations active in providing information about biosimilars are representing patients with a variety of diseases or regions. The main disease areas are those where biosimilars are marketed today, such as rheumatology, diabetes, oncology, inflammatory bowel diseases, and psoriasis. The majority of these associations only provide brief information on biosimilars, by explaining key concepts or merely providing a link to the patient brochure developed by the European Commission (EC) [93]. Nonetheless, some patient organizations have developed their own educational material or even produced position statements on the use of biosimilar medicines within their specific disease area. All identified information or educational material on biosimilars intended for patients is summarized below (Table 1).

The Slovakian Association for the Protection of Patients' Rights (AOPP) provides a short article briefly explaining the main characteristics of originator biological and biosimilar medicines. For more information, they refer patients to the EC brochure [26].

One of the larger patient associations discussed in this review is Digestive Cancers Europe (DiCE). It is the umbrella organization of a larger group or national associations representing patients with colorectal, gastric, and pancreatic cancers. DiCE has committed itself in recent years to several educational initiatives. In 2019, they developed a position paper on biosimilars for the treatment of colorectal cancer [27]. In this well-structured paper, they touch on the definitions of biologicals, with specific information about biosimilar medicines. They also draw attention to the benefits of biosimilar usage, in particular the increase in access to biological medicines. Problems regarding unequal access to biologicals among European countries are mentioned, including the possible role of biosimilars to overcome these to a certain extent. More recently, in the context of the licensing of bevacizumab biosimilars in Europe, DiCE started a larger project to provide educational material about biosimilars for patients and HCPs [28].

Similar to DiCE, the European Federation of Crohn's and Ulcerative Colitis Associations (EFCCA) is the umbrella organization representing national Crohn's and ulcerative colitis patient associations. Like most patient associations discussed in this review, they mention the EC brochure about biosimilars for patients. EFCCA also wrote an article about biosimilars, mentioning specific information on biosimilars and their benefits for healthcare systems in their monthly magazine. In this article, EFCCA emphasizes the importance of generics and biosimilars for a competitive market and a more sustainable healthcare system. In addition, they state that physicians should not be obliged to prescribe a biosimilar purely on the grounds of cost, but should be allowed to exercise appropriate clinical judgment and always involve patients in the decision making process [31].

Even though no biosimilars have been marketed yet for the treatment of Parkinson's Disease, the European Parkinson's Disease Association (EPDA) provides a brief explanation of biologicals in general, as well as of biosimilar medicines. They emphasize that all biological medicines are prone to structural variability and the possible consequences on clinical outcomes. Due to the varying composition of biologicals, patient safety may be a concern. The only specific information given on biosimilars is that they aim for the same mechanism of action as the original, even though different cells are used during the production process [33].

The International Diabetes Federation Europe or IDF Europe is the umbrella organization of European national associations for patients with diabetes. IDF Europe has developed a position paper on the use of biosimilars among patients with diabetes in 2017 [34]. In this extensive position document, several topics are highlighted such as the difference between biosimilars and generics, the European legal framework, and the potential impact of biosimilars on healthcare systems. The paper ends with a set of recommendations for the use of biosimilars in clinical practice. Under the list of recommendations, IDF Europe states that stable patients on insulin treatment should not be switched to a biosimilar without good clinical reasons and evidence of interchangeability. Furthermore, patients should always be informed and involved in the decision-making process, based on an informed discussion with their physician. They demand more information for patients from national regulatory authorities, specifically about biosimilar medicines. Routine education for patients with diabetes, facilitated by national authorities, should include a section on biosimilars. However, the position paper emphasizes possible clinical differences between insulin biosimilars and reference products. According to the authors, not enough clinical evidence exists to ensure biosimilars are equally safe and effective as their reference product. Possible immunogenicity risks are pointed out, especially when switching the reference biological with its biosimilar. To support this statement, they refer to an epoetin biosimilar (HX-575) that showed an increased occurrence of adverse events linked to a higher immunogenicity of the biosimilar. However, the article they refer to does not mention a possible difference between the biosimilar and originator of epoetin due to increased immunogenicity [94]. Instead, the article describes several cases of pure red cell aplasia (PRCA) with epoetin treatment, among which a trial with a biosimilar of epoetin. The particular clinical study being referred to reported two cases of neutralizing antibodies with the epoetin biosimilar [95]. An extensive analysis revealed that contamination during primary packaging of the prefilled syringes explained the increase in neutralizing antibodies [96]. The manufacturing process was therefore improved, followed by the completion of new open-label study without any patients developing neutralizing antibodies. Subsequently, the respective biosimilar HX-575 was authorized on the European market in 2016. This type of information is an example of a false narrative, by supporting incorrect conclusions with references from published scientific articles. Such kind of incorrect and negatively framed information should be avoided, since it may harm the trust in biosimilar medicines among patients with diabetes and potentially lead to a slower adoption of biosimilars [9].

Malta Health Network (MHN), the national association for Maltese patients, provides a link to the EUPATI toolbox on biosimilar medicines [35]. Although this information is rather difficult to find on the MHN website, the EUPATI toolbox provides understandable information on biological medicines, including biosimilars, for patients [97].

The Spanish Platform for Patient Organizations published an article for patients about biological and biosimilar medicines in 2017 [36]. Definitions about biologicals, biosimilars, and the difference with generic medicines are highlighted. They underline the importance of therapeutic freedom of physicians when prescribing biosimilars, and switching must always be in close dialogue with the patient. While they are not opposed to switching the original product with the biosimilar, they state that there is insufficient evidence to support switching.

Another national patient association is the National Coalition of Dutch Patients, which provides simple and understandable information about biosimilars on its website [39]. Like many other patient associations discussed in this review, the importance of involving the patient in the decision to prescribe a biosimilar is mentioned. For further information, they refer patients to a brochure developed by the Dutch competent authority [40]. This is a structured document providing information about biological and biosimilar medicines in understandable language for patients. Moreover, the question and answer structure of the document might increase the understandability of the brochure. In contrast to other informational material discussed in this article, the same effect of the biosimilar and the reference product is emphasized instead of no expected differences. In general, a more favorable position towards switching to a biosimilar is noted. Yet, switching must remain the physician's responsibility, and the necessary consultation with the patient is required.

The Flemish Patient Platform (FPP) unites Dutch-speaking Belgian patient associations. FPP mentions very limited information on biosimilars, merely explaining that they are biological medicines. FPP refers to biosimilars as copies, similar to generic medicines, which is too simplistic and incorrect. Furthermore, they advise patients to look at the Belgian national competent authority's information on biosimilars [42]. Here, general information about biosimilars is provided, including definitions, approved biosimilars, and guidance when switching to biosimilars. However, this web page is not up to date and only contains information of approved biosimilars until 2016.

The European Multiple Sclerosis Platform (EMSP), European Federation of Neurological Associations (EFNA), European Institute of Women's Health (EIWH), and European

Patients' Forum (EPF) only posted the link to the EC brochure for patients on their website [32,37,38,43].

Three additional patient organization members of IAPO were identified that provide educational material for patients on their website. The International Federation of Psoriasis Associations (IFPA) is the overarching organization of national patient associations representing patients with psoriasis. IFPA recently developed a position paper about the use of biosimilars for the treatment of psoriasis [45]. They acknowledge that biosimilars do not lead to different clinical outcomes compared with their reference product. Again, the patient–physician dialogue is underlined when making treatment decisions in general, which includes decisions to switch to a biosimilar. However, they mention transitioning to a biosimilar should not be done for patients with stable disease control. This shows some hesitance to use biosimilars among patients with psoriasis already treated by biological medicines.

Psoriasis Action, the Spanish patient association for patients with psoriasis, provides several sources of biosimilar information. They share a short video in which a professor explains what biosimilars are to Spanish patients [47]. A video with a more extensive explanation is also provided, intended for patients who prefer more detailed information on biosimilars [48]. Psoriasis Action also published a more general piece of information for patients, where generalities of biological and biosimilar medicines are explained in a specific article [46].

Last but not least, IAPO also developed educational material for patients about biosimilars in collaboration with the International Federation of Pharmaceutical Manufacturers and Associations (IFPMA). On their website, extensive documentation on biological and biosimilar medicines can be found in their toolkit for patients, from which they developed a second version in 2017 [49]. The toolkit includes fact sheets, infographics, frequently asked questions, and a decision guide for patients when choosing between an original biological or biosimilar product. Their educational material includes general information on biological and biosimilar medicines, regulatory requirements, pharmacovigilance, and a communication guide for HCPs. The toolkit is intended for patient organizations worldwide for distribution to their patients. In contrast to the initial version of this toolkit of 2013, which was made available in English, Spanish, and Portuguese, the second version is only available in English [98].

4. Discussion

This article looked at the relevant elements to consider when informing patients about biosimilars. In addition, an overview of the information and educational material by the major European patient associations was provided. Based on this overview, all available material was evaluated on its tone and correctness.

4.1. Communication Strategies to Inform Patients about Biosimilars

Five main points of attention were identified when informing patients about biosimilars. **First** of all, information has to be provided in an understandable way. Patients generally have no scientific background, so one must make sure not to overly complicate the given message [50–53]. **Second**, a positive attitude when talking to patients about medicines in general is paramount [20,51,58,62]. Emphasis must be put on the similarities between biosimilars and their reference product, rather than the possible differences. This can be done by conveying the message that the biosimilar has similar clinical outcomes, instead of no expected differences [59]. An open and positive way of communicating has shown to generate trust, and subsequently improve treatment outcomes and adherence [56,57]. HCPs should therefore be trained on the proper use of such communication strategies with patients. **Third**, a one-size-fits-all approach is not desirable when communicating directly to patients since each patient's individual needs and level of understanding might differ [8,60,63,64,66]. A tailored approach is therefore preferred. It is the task of each member of the multidisciplinary team to assess these needs and to adapt their communication strategy accordingly. This brings us to the **fourth** point of attention, the *one voice* principle. In essence, this means that everyone informing patients about biosimilars has to provide a coherent message. Communication towards patients must be consistent across channels, thereby avoiding suspicion by generating trust between healthcare providers and patients [7,20,54,58,68]. **Fifth**, the use of supportive audiovisual material (i.e., videos, infographics, brochures) may help bringing the information across in a clear and understandable way [9,50,52,67]. Such supportive material closes the gap between the complexity of the biosimilar concepts and the need for understandable information.

A series of studies pointed to a lack of knowledge and trust in biosimilars in various relevant patient populations, making clear the necessity of education [13–17,19,54,56,71–73]. However, the purpose of informing patients should not be to create a high level of knowledge among the whole patient population. This would not be feasible, nor desirable. After all, it is not intended to inform all patients about a treatment the vast majority will not need. Instead, information about biosimilars should be reaching those patients who require such information. In other words, patients who may or will be treated with biosimilars in the near future. This approach differs from informing HCPs about biosimilars, as they all need to have a good understanding of biosimilars.

Educating patients about medicines in general, but in particular biosimilars, should always be a multistakeholder effort [8,20,60,77]. Each stakeholder has its own role to fulfill in order to provide correct, unbiased, understandable, and coherent information. Physicians, nurses, and pharmacists have a coordinating role and are key partners to remove doubts and generate trust in biosimilars, as for any kind of medicine [52,60,85,86]. In addition, other parties such as regulatory authorities, medical societies, and patient associations have a supporting role in informing patients. They are all regarded by patients as reliable sources of information. However, the identified list of stakeholders is not exhaustive, since other stakeholders that were not mentioned in the literature may also play a role. For example, academia might support the development of evidence-based information as a trusted and unbiased source of information. Other national authorities, such as payers and health technology assessment (HTA) bodies, could also disseminate information about biosimilars to patients. Some stakeholders may be of particular importance in the creation of information or educational material (e.g., scientific associations, professional associations, academia), whereas others (e.g., healthcare providers, patient associations, regulatory authorities) in the dissemination of information to patients. Moreover, pharmaceutical companies also play a role in informing the wider public about biosimilar medicines. One must acknowledge that many informational campaigns are supported by pharmaceutical industry, thereby facilitating the development of factual information as well.

4.2. The Role of European Patient Organizations

A variety of information and educational material for patients about biosimilar medicines is made public by European patient organizations. Yet, the quality and level of detail vary among different associations, and it is not clear whether the identified information is effectively reaching the patient. This overview of information was based on a web-based screening. However, one should be aware that information made accessible via the internet will not reach every patient who needs such information. After all, not every citizen across Europe has the opportunity to consult the internet. That is why it remains important that healthcare providers fulfill their role to reach patients, and that patient associations themselves do not limit themselves to disseminating information via their websites.

Patient associations often refer to the biosimilar brochure of the European Commission, which was translated in all European languages in recent years. Some patient organizations have developed educational brochures or position statements about the use of biosimilars by themselves. They generally all agree on the fact that biosimilars are equal treatment options ensuring a sustainable healthcare system and underline that the decision to prescribe a biosimilar should be a shared decision involving the patient. Nonetheless, some patient associations should be cautious not to fall prey to negatively framed, incorrect, or outdated information about biosimilars. Several patient associations provide detailed information on biosimilars, but express a rather negative attitude in particular towards transitioning from the reference product to a biosimilar (e.g., IDF Europe, Spanish Platform for Patient Organizations, and IFPA). Others provide or refer to incorrect or outdated information, such as EPDA, IDF Europe, and Flemish Patient Platform. The most pronounced example of this is IDF Europe, where they support their concerns about switching to biosimilar insulins by information that was incorrectly interpreted and taken out of context. Generally, national patient associations adopt the position on biosimilars of their European umbrella organization. However, this does not prevent national associations from formulating their own positions that differ from incorrect European ones. For example, the recommendations of the Dutch Diabetes Association about insulin biosimilars are in line with current scientific evidence and do therefore not correspond to those from IDF Europe [99]. A clear contrast was observed when looking at biosimilar information or educational material of DiCE and National Coalition of Dutch Patients. In particular, DiCE puts emphasis on the fact that if biosimilars are implemented on a wider scale, they could help closing the gap in gaining access to the highest standards of care for the treatment of colorectal cancer. The National Coalition of Dutch Patients repeatedly states that biosimilar medicines have the same efficacy, safety, and quality as their reference products. This is an example of positive framing since most information on biosimilars mentions that no meaningful differences are expected with originator biologicals, which is correct, yet framed more neutrally.

Information should always be evidence-based and therefore in line with the most recent scientific developments. As for all stakeholders, patient associations should distance themselves from positions or opinions about biosimilars that are not scientifically or incorrectly substantiated. Clear collaboration with independent and knowledgeable experts to develop such material is necessary to avoid incorrect information. With this overview, we have taken a critical look at the available information about biosimilars for patients developed by major European patient associations.

4.3. Future Perspectives

During past years, the way that most treatment decisions are made has evolved towards shared decision-making [100]. The choice for an originator biological or a biosimilar must therefore be based on a coherent information stream to the patient. Several communication strategies have been identified in this review, guaranteeing correct information is provided adequately to patients. However, not all communication strategies have proven effective in actually increasing patient knowledge and confidence in biosimilars. Moreover, they have not proven to meet the appropriate behavioral objectives among patients. Future research assessing the actual impact of communication strategies based on a behavioral model could help clarify these unmet needs.

Most recommendations identified during this literature review are based on empirical grounds. Communication strategies emerging from theoretical concepts could be explored as well in the future. This would contribute to the overall picture on how to inform patients about biosimilar medicines and increase the robustness of the conclusions.

4.4. Strengths and Limitations of the Study

The main conclusions of this study are based on a structured literature review and a web-based mapping of available information by European patient organizations. This study provides an overview of existing scientific literature on how to effectively inform patients about biosimilar medicines. The structured approach allows for reliable conclusions regarding information strategies for patients about biosimilars. This article is the first of its kind to compile the provided information of the major European patient organizations (i.e., EPF and IAPO members), with the purpose to have an overview of available information or educational material.

Although the literature review was conducted in a structured way, no systematic review was conducted and thus the selection of articles was not based on an agreement between two independent researchers. As a consequence, selection bias might have occurred during the title and abstract screening phase. Furthermore, the web-based mapping only allows for the collection of information that is publicly available on the websites of the patient associations of interest. Educational efforts that were not made available on their websites were therefore not included in this review. The researchers chose to include members of EPF and IAPO in the mapping of information, hence some available information on biosimilars by other European patient associations that are not members of these umbrella organizations might have been missed. Although the assessment of the tone in which patient associations report about biosimilars can be seen as subjective, it does provide an interesting picture of the overall attitude of each individual organization and the differences between them.

5. Conclusions

It is important to set up a close collaboration between all stakeholders to develop and effectively disseminate correct information about biosimilars to patients, bringing together scientific associations, professional associations (including physicians, nurses, and pharmacists), regulatory authorities, and patient associations. Informing and educating patients on biosimilars should be part of a wider approach to support the adoption of biosimilars in Europe. European member states should consider informing patients on biosimilars in their policy frameworks more actively. It is imperative that European national authorities support biosimilar medicines to safeguard an affordable and sustainable healthcare system within their country.

Supplementary Materials: The following are available online at https://www.mdpi.com/1424-8247/14/2/117/s1, Table S1: Structured literature search methodology, and Figure S1: PRISMA flow diagram of the literature review.

Author Contributions: I.H., A.G.V., and Y.V. developed the idea for and were involved in the design of the study. Y.V. was involved in the data collection and drafted the initial version of the manuscript. I.H., A.G.V., S.S., and P.V.W. critically reviewed the manuscript. All authors have read and agreed to the published version of the manuscript.

Funding: This manuscript is supported by KU Leuven and the Belgian National Institute for Health and Disability Insurance (NIHDI).

Institutional Review Board Statement: Not applicable.

Informed Consent Statement: Not applicable.

Data Availability Statement: The data presented in this study are available on request from the corresponding author.

Acknowledgments: This article is based on the preparatory work of master students' projects by Julie Brown, Ben Janssens, Seppe Lenaerts, Marie Pardon, and Olivia Wagman. The authors would like to thank all five master students for their efforts. The authors also express their appreciation towards the Pharmaceutical Policy Department of NIHDI for their support in this research project.

Conflicts of Interest: This research project is funded by the Belgian National Institute for Health and Disability Insurance (NIHDI). S.S., I.H. and A.G.V. have founded the KU Leuven Fund on Market Analysis of Biologics and Biosimilars following Loss of Exclusivity (MABEL). S.S. was involved in a stakeholder roundtable on biologics and biosimilars sponsored by Amgen, Pfizer and MSD; he has participated in advisory board meetings for Sandoz, Pfizer and Amgen; he has contributed to studies on biologics and biosimilars for Hospira (together with A.G.V. and I.H.), Celltrion, Mundipharma and Pfizer, and he has had speaking engagements for Amgen, Celltrion and Sandoz. A.G.V. is involved in consulting, advisory work and speaking engagements for a number of companies, a.o. AbbVie, Accord, Amgen, Biogen, EGA, Pfizer/Hospira, Mundipharma, Roche, Sandoz. P.V.W. acted as health care consultant to public and private organizations, including pharmaceutical companies and their professional associations. All other authors declare that the research was conducted in the absence of any commercial or financial relationships that could be construed as a potential conflict of interest.

References

1. IQVIA. Advancing Biosimilar Sustainability in Europe. Available online: https://www.biosimilars-nederland.nl/wp-content/uploads/2018/10/okt_2018_IQVIA_Pfizer_Advancing-Biosimilar-Sustainability-in-Europe.pdf (accessed on 2 February 2020).
2. European Medicines Agency (EMA). *Guideline on Similar Biological Medicinal Products*; European Medicines Agency: Amsterdam, The Netherland, 2014; pp. 1–7.
3. Wolff-Holz, E.; Tiitso, K.; Vleminckx, C.; Weise, M. Evolution of the EU Biosimilar Framework: Past and Future. *BioDrugs* 2019, 33, 621–634. [CrossRef] [PubMed]
4. Dutta, B.; Huys, I.; Vulto, A.G.; Simoens, S. Identifying Key Benefits in European Off-Patent Biologics and Biosimilar Markets: It is Not Only about Price! *BioDrugs* 2020, 34, 159–170. [CrossRef]
5. Razanskaite, V.; Bettey, M.; Downey, L.; Wright, J.; Callaghan, J.; Rush, M.; Whiteoak, S.; Ker, S.; Perry, K.; Underhill, C.; et al. Biosimilar Infliximab in Inflammatory Bowel Disease: Outcomes of a Managed Switching Programme. *J. Crohn's Colitis* 2017, 11, 690–696. [CrossRef] [PubMed]
6. IQVIA. *The Impact of Biosimilar Competition in Europe*; European Medicines Agency (EMA): Amsterdam, The Netherland, 2020.
7. Peyrin-Biroulet, L.; Danese, S.; Cummings, F.; Atreya, R.; Greveson, K.; Pieper, B.; Kang, T. Anti-TNF biosimilars in Crohn's Disease: A patient-centric interdisciplinary approach. *Expert Rev. Gastroenterol. Hepatol.* 2019, 13, 731–738. [CrossRef]
8. Barbier, L.; Simoens, S.; Vulto, A.G.; Huys, I. European Stakeholder Learnings Regarding Biosimilars: Part II—Improving Biosimilar Use in Clinical Practice. *BioDrugs* 2020, 34, 797–808. [CrossRef] [PubMed]
9. Cohen, H.P.; McCabe, D. The Importance of Countering Biosimilar Disparagement and Misinformation. *BioDrugs* 2020, 34, 407–414. [CrossRef] [PubMed]
10. Vulto, A.G.; Vanderpuye-Orgle, J.; Van Der Graaff, M.; Simoens, S.; Dagna, L.; Macaulay, R.; Majeed, B.; Lemay, J.; Hippenmeyer, J.; Gonzalez-McQuire, S. Sustainability of Biosimilars in Europe: A Delphi Panel Consensus with Systematic Literature Review. *Pharmaceuticals* 2020, 13, 400. [CrossRef] [PubMed]
11. Rémuzat, C.; Kapuśniak, A.; Caban, A.; Ionescu, D.; Radière, G.; Mendoza, C.; Toumi, M. Supply-side and demand-side policies for biosimilars: An overview in 10 European member states. *J. Mark. Access Health Policy* 2017, 5, 1307315. [CrossRef] [PubMed]
12. Moorkens, E.; Vulto, A.G.; Huys, I.; Dylst, P.; Godman, B.; Keuerleber, S.; Claus, B.; Dimitrova, M.; Petrova, G.; Sović-Brkičić, L.; et al. Policies for biosimilar uptake in Europe: An overview. *PLoS ONE* 2017, 12, e0190147. [CrossRef]
13. Jacobs, I.; Singh, E.; Sewell, K.L.; Al-Sabbagh, A.; Shane, L.G. Patient attitudes and understanding about biosimilars: An international cross-sectional survey. *Patient Prefer. Adherence* 2016, 10, 937–948. [CrossRef]
14. Aladul, M.I.; Fitzpatrick, R.W.; Chapman, S.R. Patients' Understanding and Attitudes towards Infliximab and Etanercept Biosimilars: Result of a UK Web-Based Survey. *BioDrugs* 2017, 31, 439–446. [CrossRef] [PubMed]
15. Azevedo, A.; Bettencourt, A.; Selores, M.; Torres, T. Biosimilar Agents for Psoriasis Treatment: The Perspective of Portuguese Patients. *Acta Med. Port.* 2018, 31, 496–500. [CrossRef] [PubMed]
16. Frantzen, L.; Cohen, J.-D.; Tropé, S.; Beck, M.; Munos, A.; Sittler, M.-A.; Diebolt, R.; Metzler, I.; Sordet, C.; Sordet, I.C. Patients' information and perspectives on biosimilars in rheumatology: A French nation-wide survey. *Jt. Bone Spine* 2019, 86, 491–496. [CrossRef] [PubMed]
17. Peyrin-Biroulet, L.; Lönnfors, S.; Roblin, X.; Danese, S.; Avedano, L. Patient Perspectives on Biosimilars: A Survey by the European Federation of Crohn's and Ulcerative Colitis Associations: Table 1. *J. Crohn's Colitis* 2017, 11, 128–133. [CrossRef] [PubMed]
18. Waller, J.; Sullivan, E.; Piercy, J.; Black, C.M.; Kachroo, S. Assessing physician and patient acceptance of infliximab biosimilars in rheumatoid arthritis, ankylosing spondyloarthritis and psoriatic arthritis across Germany. *Patient Prefer. Adherence* 2017, 11, 519–530. [CrossRef] [PubMed]
19. Van Overbeeke, E.; De Beleyr, B.; De Hoon, J.; Westhovens, R.; Huys, I. Perception of Originator Biologics and Biosimilars: A Survey Among Belgian Rheumatoid Arthritis Patients and Rheumatologists. *BioDrugs* 2017, 31, 447–459. [CrossRef] [PubMed]
20. Kristensen, L.E.; Alten, R.; Puig, L.; Philipp, S.; Kvien, T.K.; Mangues, M.A.; Hoogen, F.V.D.; Pavelka, K.; Vulto, A.G. Non-pharmacological Effects in Switching Medication: The Nocebo Effect in Switching from Originator to Biosimilar Agent. *BioDrugs* 2018, 32, 397–404. [CrossRef] [PubMed]
21. Tweehuysen, L.; Huiskes, V.J.B.; Bemt, B.J.F.V.D.; Vriezekolk, J.E.; Teerenstra, S.; Hoogen, F.H.J.V.D.; Ende, C.H.V.D.; Broeder, A.A.D. Open-Label, Non-Mandatory Transitioning from Originator Etanercept to Biosimilar SB4. *Arthritis Rheumatol.* 2018, 70, 1408–1418. [CrossRef] [PubMed]
22. Tweehuysen, L.; Bemt, B.J.F.V.D.; Van Ingen, I.L.; De Jong, A.J.L.; Van Der Laan, W.H.; Hoogen, F.H.J.V.D.; Broeder, A.A.D. Subjective Complaints as the Main Reason for Biosimilar Discontinuation After Open-Label Transition From Reference Infliximab to Biosimilar Infliximab. *Arthritis Rheumatol.* 2018, 70, 60–68. [CrossRef] [PubMed]
23. Pouillon, L.; Socha, M.; Demoré, B.; Thilly, N.; Abitbol, V.; Danese, S.; Peyrin-Biroulet, L. The nocebo effect: A clinical challenge in the era of biosimilars. *Expert Rev. Clin. Immunol.* 2018, 14, 739–749. [CrossRef] [PubMed]
24. Kravvariti, E.; Kitas, G.D.; Mitsikostas, D.D.; Sfikakis, P.P. Nocebos in rheumatology: Emerging concepts and their implications for clinical practice. *Nat. Rev. Rheumatol.* 2018, 14, 727–740. [CrossRef]

25. Gale, N.K.; Heath, G.; Cameron, E.; Rashid, S.; Redwood, S. Using the framework method for the analysis of qualitative data in multi-disciplinary health research. *BMC Med. Res. Methodol.* **2013**, *13*, 117. [CrossRef]
26. Assocation for the Protection of Patients' Rights (AOPP). Biosimilary Alebo Biologicky Podobné Lieky—Čo by Ste O Nich Mali Vedie? Available online: https://www.aopp.sk/clanok/biosimilary-alebo-biologicky-podobne-lieky-co-ste-o-nich-mali-vediet (accessed on 18 November 2020).
27. Digestive Cancers Europe. Position Paper on the Use of Biosimilar Medicines in Colorectal Cancer. Available online: https://digestivecancers.eu/digestive-cancers-europe-has-developed-a-position-paper-on-the-use-of-biosimilars-medicine-in-colorectal-cancer/ (accessed on 20 November 2020).
28. Digestive Cancers Europe. Biosimilar Education in Metastatic Colorectal Cancer. Available online: https://www.digestivecancers.eu/campaigning-and-education/biosimilar-education-in-metastatic-colorectal-cancer/ (accessed on 18 November 2020).
29. European Federation of Crohn's and Ulcerative Colitis Assocations. European Commission Publication on Biosimilars. Available online: https://www.efcca.org/en/european-commission-publication-biosimilars (accessed on 19 November 2020).
30. European Federation of Crohn's and Ulcerative Colitis Assocations. Biologics and Biosimilars: Advocacy Workshop on Patient Safety. Available online: https://www.efcca.org/sites/default/files/Biologics-Biosimilars-Exec-Summary-WEB_0.pdf (accessed on 23 November 2020).
31. European Federation of Crohn's and Ulcerative Colitis Assocations. EFCCA Magazine. Available online: https://www.efcca.org/sites/default/files/EFCCA_Magazine_%23_10_May_2014.pdf (accessed on 20 November 2020).
32. European Multiple Sclerosis Platform (EMSP). European Commission Publishes Guide on Biosimilar Medicines. Available online: http://www.emsp.org/news-messages/european-commission-publishes-guide-biosimilar-medicines/ (accessed on 23 November 2020).
33. European Parkinson's Disease Association. Managing Your Parkinson's Medication. Available online: https://www.epda.eu.com/about-parkinsons/treatments/managing-your-medication/ (accessed on 20 November 2020).
34. International Diabetes Federation Europe. IDF Europe Position on Biosimilars in the Treatment of People with Diabetes. Available online: https://idf.org/images/IDF_Europe_Position_on_Biosimilars.pdf (accessed on 20 November 2020).
35. Malta Health Network. European Patients' Academy (EUPATI) Patient Education Toolbox. Available online: https://www.maltahealthnetwork.org/projects/european-patients-academy-eupati-patient-education-toolbox-english/ (accessed on 20 November 2020).
36. Plataforma de Organizaciones de Patientes. Los Pacientes Ante Los Medicamentos Biológicos. Available online: https://www.plataformadepacientes.org/actualidad/los-pacientes-ante-los-medicamentos-biologicos (accessed on 20 November 2020).
37. European Federation of Neurological Associations (EFNA). EMA Publishes Educational Material on Biosimilar Medicines. Available online: https://www.efna.net/ema-publish-educational-material-on-biosimilar-medicines/ (accessed on 23 November 2020).
38. European Institute of Women's Health (EIWH). Guide on Biosimilars for Healthcare Professionals. Available online: https://eurohealth.ie/2019/11/12/guide-on-biosimilars-for-healthcare_professionals/?highlight=biosimilar (accessed on 23 November 2020).
39. Patiëntenfederatie Nederland. Biosimilar Medicijn. Available online: https://kennisbank.patientenfederatie.nl/app/answers/detail/a_id/2177/~{}/biosimilar-medicijn/ (accessed on 20 November 2020).
40. College ter Beoordeling van Geneesmiddelen. Antwoorden op Vragen over Biologische Medicijnen. Available online: https://www.cbg-meb.nl/onderwerpen/medicijninformatie-originele-biologische-medicijnen-en-biosimilars/documenten/brochures/2020/01/01/biologische-medicijnen (accessed on 20 October 2020).
41. Vlaams Patiëntenplatform. Wat Zijn Biosimilairen? Available online: http://vlaamspatientenplatform.be/themas/medicatie-1 (accessed on 23 November 2020).
42. Federaal Agentschap voor Geneesmiddelen en Gezondheidsproducten. Biosimilars. Available online: https://www.fagg.be/nl/MENSELIJK_gebruik/geneesmiddelen/geneesmiddelen/procedures_vhb/Registratie_procedures/Biosimilars (accessed on 20 November 2020).
43. European Patients' Forum (EPF). A Sustainable Framework for Biosimilar Medicines in Europe. Available online: https://www.eu-patient.eu/news/latest-epf-news/2018/a-sustainable-framework-for-biosimilars-medicines-in-europe/ (accessed on 23 November 2020).
44. European Patients' Forum (EPF). Recent News on EU Developments on Biosimilars. Available online: https://www.eu-patient.eu/news/latest-epf-news/2016/a-couple-of-initiatives-from-the-european-commission-on-biosimilar-medicines/ (accessed on 23 November 2020).
45. International Federation of Psoriasis Associations. The International Federation of Posriasis Associations' Statement on Biosimilars. Available online: https://ifpa-pso.com/wp-content/uploads/2020/03/IFPA-statement-on-biosimilars1.pdf (accessed on 20 November 2020).
46. Acción Psoriasis. Biosimilares: Una Nueva Revolución. Available online: https://www.accionpsoriasis.org/investigacion/innovacion/441-biosimilares-una-nueva-revolucion.html (accessed on 20 November 2020).
47. Acción Psoriasis. Que Son Los Medicamentos Biosimilares? Available online: https://www.accionpsoriasis.org/component/allvideoshare/video/que-son-los-medicamentos-biosimilares.html?Itemid=590 (accessed on 20 November 2020).
48. Acción Psoriasis. Conferencia Sobre Medicamentos Biosimilares. Available online: https://www.accionpsoriasis.org/component/allvideoshare/video/conferencia-sobre-medicamentos-biosimilares.html?Itemid=590 (accessed on 20 November 2020).

49. International Alliance of Patients' Organizations. Biosimilars Toolkit. Available online: https://www.iapo.org.uk/biosimilars-toolkit (accessed on 20 November 2020).
50. Barbier, L.; Simoens, S.; Vulto, A.G.; Huys, I. European Stakeholder Learnings Regarding Biosimilars: Part I—Improving Biosimilar Understanding and Adoption. *BioDrugs* **2020**, *34*, 783–796. [CrossRef] [PubMed]
51. Drossman, D.A. 2012 David Sun Lecture: Helping Your Patient by Helping Yourself—How to Improve the Patient–Physician Relationship by Optimizing Communication Skills. *Am. J. Gastroenterol.* **2013**, *108*, 521–528. [CrossRef] [PubMed]
52. Armuzzi, A.; Avedano, L.; Greveson, K.; Kang, T. Nurses are Critical in Aiding Patients Transitioning to Biosimilars in Inflammatory Bowel Disease: Education and Communication Strategies. *J. Crohn's Colitis* **2019**, *13*, 259–266. [CrossRef] [PubMed]
53. Fiorino, G.; Caprioli, F.; Daperno, M.; Mocciaro, F.; Principi, M.; Armuzzi, A.; Fantini, M.C.; Orlando, A.; Papi, C.; Annese, V.; et al. Use of biosimilars in inflammatory bowel disease: A position update of the Italian Group for the Study of Inflammatory Bowel Disease (IG-IBD). *Dig. Liver Dis.* **2019**, *51*, 632–639. [CrossRef] [PubMed]
54. Scherlinger, M.; Langlois, E.; Germain, V.; Schaeverbeke, T. Acceptance rate and sociological factors involved in the switch from originator to biosimilar etanercept (SB4). *Semin. Arthritis Rheum.* **2019**, *48*, 927–932. [CrossRef] [PubMed]
55. Colloca, L.; Panaccione, R.; Murphy, T.K. The Clinical Implications of Nocebo Effects for Biosimilar Therapy. *Front. Pharmacol.* **2019**, *10*, 1372. [CrossRef] [PubMed]
56. Gasteiger, C.; Jones, A.S.K.; Kleinstäuber, M.; Lobo, M.; Horne, R.; Dalbeth, N.; Petrie, K.J. Effects of Message Framing on Patients' Perceptions and Willingness to Change to a Biosimilar in a Hypothetical Drug Switch. *Arthritis Rheum.* **2020**, *72*, 1323–1330. [CrossRef] [PubMed]
57. Tweehuysen, L.; Huiskes, V.; Bemt, B.V.D.; Hoogen, F.V.D.; Broeder, A.D. FRI0200 Higher acceptance and persistence rates after biosimilar transitioning in patients with a rheumatic disease after employing an enhanced communication strategy. *Poster Present.* **2017**, *76*, 557. [CrossRef]
58. Gecse, K.B.; Cumming, F.; D'Haens, G. Biosimilars for inflammatory bowel disease: How can healthcare professionals help address patients' concerns? *Expert Rev. Gastroenterol. Hepatol.* **2019**, *13*, 143–155. [CrossRef] [PubMed]
59. Nabhan, C.; Feinberg, B.A. Behavioral Economics and the Future of Biosimilars. *J. Natl. Compr. Cancer Netw.* **2017**, *15*, 1449–1451. [CrossRef]
60. Pouillon, L.; Danese, S.; Hart, A.; Fiorino, G.; Argollo, M.; Selmi, C.; Carlo-Stella, C.; Loeuille, D.; Costanzo, A.; Lopez, A.; et al. Consensus Report: Clinical Recommendations for the Prevention and Management of the Nocebo Effect in Biosimilar-Treated IBD Patients. *Aliment. Pharmacol. Ther.* **2019**, *49*, 1181–1187. [CrossRef] [PubMed]
61. Azevedo, V.F.; Kos, I.A.; Ariello, L. The Experience with Biosimilars of Infliximab in Rheumatic Diseases. *Curr. Pharm. Des.* **2017**, *23*, 6752–6758. [CrossRef] [PubMed]
62. Janjigian, Y.Y.; Bissig, M.; Curigliano, G.; Coppola, J.; Latymer, M. Talking to patients about biosimilars. *Futur. Oncol.* **2018**, *14*, 2403–2414. [CrossRef] [PubMed]
63. Edwards, C.J.; Hercogová, J.; Albrand, H.; Amiot, A. Switching to biosimilars: Current perspectives in immune-mediated inflammatory diseases. *Expert Opin. Biol. Ther.* **2019**, *19*, 1001–1014. [CrossRef] [PubMed]
64. Colloca, L.; Finniss, D. Nocebo Effects, Patient-Clinician Communication, and Therapeutic Outcomes. *JAMA* **2012**, *307*, 567–568. [CrossRef] [PubMed]
65. Rezk, M.F.; Pieper, B. Treatment Outcomes with Biosimilars: Be Aware of the Nocebo Effect. *Rheumatol. Ther.* **2017**, *4*, 209–218. [CrossRef]
66. Frazer, M.B.; Bubalo, J.; Patel, H.; Siderov, J.; Cubilla, M.; De Lemos, M.L.; Dhillon, H.; Harchowal, J.; Kuchonthara, N.; Livinalli, A.; et al. International Society of Oncology Pharmacy Practitioners global position on the use of biosimilars in cancer treatment and supportive care. *J. Oncol. Pharm. Pr.* **2020**, *26*, 3–10. [CrossRef] [PubMed]
67. Tan, S.S.-L.; Goonawardene, N. Internet Health Information Seeking and the Patient-Physician Relationship: A Systematic Review. *J. Med. Internet Res.* **2017**, *19*, e9. [CrossRef]
68. Voorneveld-Nieuwenhuis, J.; Moortgat, L.; Pavic Nikolic, M.; Crombez, P.; Oomen, B. Switch Management between Similar Biological Medicines, a Communication Information Guide for Nurses. *Ann. Rheum. Dis.* **2018**, *77*, 1812–1813. [CrossRef]
69. Haghnejad, V.; Le Berre, C.; Dominique, Y.; Zallot, C.; Guillemin, F.; Peyrin-Biroulet, L. Impact of a medical interview on the decision to switch from originator infliximab to its biosimilar in patients with inflammatory bowel disease. *Dig. Liver Dis.* **2020**, *52*, 281–288. [CrossRef]
70. European Medicines Agency. Biosimilar Medicines: Overview. Available online: https://www.ema.europa.eu/en/human-regulatory/overview/biosimilar-medicines-overview (accessed on 30 December 2020).
71. Macaluso, F.S.; Leone, S.; Previtali, E.; Ventimiglia, M.; Armuzzi, A.; Orlando, A. Biosimilars: The viewpoint of Italian patients with inflammatory bowel disease. *Dig. Liver Dis.* **2020**, *52*, 1304–1309. [CrossRef] [PubMed]
72. Peyrin-Biroulet, L.; Lönnfors, S.; Avedano, L.; Danese, S. Changes in inflammatory bowel disease patients' perspectives on biosimilars: A follow-up survey. *United Eur. Gastroenterol. J.* **2019**, *7*, 1345–1352. [CrossRef] [PubMed]
73. Sullivan, E.; Piercy, J.; Waller, J.; Black, C.M.; Kachroo, S. Assessing gastroenterologist and patient acceptance of biosimilars in ulcerative colitis and Crohn's disease across Germany. *PLoS ONE* **2017**, *12*, e0175826. [CrossRef] [PubMed]
74. Kay, J.; Schoels, M.M.; Dörner, T.; Emery, P.; Kvien, T.K.; Ramiro, S.; Breedveld, F.C. Consensus-based recommendations for the use of biosimilars to treat rheumatological diseases. *Ann. Rheum. Dis.* **2018**, *77*, 165–174. [CrossRef] [PubMed]

75. Gasteiger, C.; Lobo, M.; Dalbeth, N.; Petrie, K.J. Patients' Beliefs and Behaviours Are Associated with Perceptions of Safety and Concerns in a Hypothetical Biosimilar Switch. *Rheumatol. Int.* **2020**. [CrossRef]
76. Armuzzi, A.; Bouhnik, Y.; Cummings, F.; Bettey, M.; Pieper, B.; Kang, T. Enhancing Treatment Success in Inflammatory Bowel Disease: Optimising the Use of Anti-TNF Agents and Utilising Their Biosimilars in Clinical Practice. *Dig. Liver Dis.* **2020**. [CrossRef] [PubMed]
77. D'Amico, F.; Pouillon, L.; Argollo, M.; Hart, A.; Fiorino, G.; Vegni, E.; Radice, S.; Gilardi, D.; Fazio, M.; Leone, S.; et al. Multidisciplinary Management of the Nocebo Effect in Biosimilar-Treated IBD Patients: Results of a Workshop from the NOCE-BIO Consensus Group. *Dig. Liver Dis.* **2020**, *52*, 138–142. [CrossRef] [PubMed]
78. Härter, M.; Moumjid, N.; Cornuz, J.; Elwyn, G.; van der Weijden, T. Shared Decision Making in 2017: International Accomplishments in Policy, Research and Implementation. *Z. Evidenz Fortbild. Qual. Gesundh.* **2017**, 1–5. [CrossRef]
79. Boland, L.; Graham, I.D.; Légaré, F.; Lewis, K.; Jull, J.; Shephard, A.; Lawson, M.L.; Davis, A.; Yameogo, A.; Stacey, D. Barriers and Facilitators of Pediatric Shared Decision-Making: A Systematic Review. *Implement. Sci.* **2019**, *14*, 7. [CrossRef] [PubMed]
80. Cobilinschi, C.; Opris-Belinski, D.; Codreanu, C.; Ionescu, R.; Mihailov, C.; Parvu, M.; Popoviciu, H.; Rezus, E.; Ionescu, R. Patient State of Knowledge on Biosimilars-Do Physicians Need to Improve Education Skills? *Ann. Rheum. Dis.* **2019**, *78*, 1446–1447. [CrossRef]
81. Waller, C.F.; Friganović, A. Biosimilars in Oncology: Key Role of Nurses in Patient Education. *Future Oncol.* **2020**. [CrossRef] [PubMed]
82. Wilson, P.; Wood, C. Biosimilar ESAs: A Comparative Review. *J. Ren. Care* **2015**, *41*, 53–61. [CrossRef] [PubMed]
83. Hawkins, T.; Emery, P. Biosimilar Medicines in Rheumatology. *Clin. Pharm.* **2015**, 7. [CrossRef]
84. European Specialist Nurses Organisation. Switch Management between Similar Biological Medicines: A Communication and Information Guide for Nurses. Available online: http://www.esno.org/assets/files/biosimilar-nurses-guideline-final_EN-lo.pdf (accessed on 2 December 2020).
85. Coget, E.; Laffont-Lozes, P.; Gonzalvo, V.V.; Huc, D.; De Chambrun, G.P.; Altwegg, R.; Blanc, P.; Pageaux, G.; Rosant, D.; Breuker, C. 4CPS-144 Establishment of a pharmaceutical standardised interview concerning biosimilars of infliximab in the daycare clinic of a gastroenterology department for patients affected by inflammatory bowel disease. *Sect. 4 Clin. Pharm. Serv.* **2019**, *26*, A136. [CrossRef]
86. Szlumper, C.; Topping, K.; Blackler, L.; Kirkham, B.; Ng, N.; Cope, A.; Agarwal, S.; Garrood, T.; Mercer, S. Switching to Biosimilar Etanercept in Clinical Practice. *Rheumatology* **2017**, *56*, ii139. [CrossRef]
87. Nederlandse Vereniging van Ziekenhuisapothekers. NVZA Toolbox Biosimilars: Een praktische handleiding voor succesvolle implementatie van biosimilars in de medisch specialistische zorg. Available online: https://nvza.nl/wp-content/uploads/2017/04/NVZA-Toolbox-biosimilars_7-april-2017.pdf (accessed on 15 November 2020).
88. European Society for Medical Oncology. Understanding Biosimilars for Cancer Patients. Available online: https://www.esmo.org/content/download/158275/2892910/1/ESMO-Understanding-Biosimilars-for-Cancer-Patients.pdf (accessed on 2 December 2020).
89. European League against Rheumatism. Biosimilars: What Do Patients Need to Consider? Available online: https://www.eular.org/myUploadData/files/Biosimilars_2015.pdf (accessed on 2 December 2020).
90. Skingle, D. Biosimilars: What Do Patients Need to Consider? *RMD Open* **2015**, *1*, e000141. [CrossRef] [PubMed]
91. Cazap, E.; Jacobs, I.; McBride, A.; Popovian, R.; Sikora, K. Global Acceptance of Biosimilars: Importance of Regulatory Consistency, Education, and Trust. *Oncologist* **2018**, *23*, 1188–1198. [CrossRef] [PubMed]
92. Barbier, L.; Mbuaki, A.; Simoens, S.; Vulto, A.; Huys, I. The Role of Regulatory Guidance and Information Dissemination for Biosimilars Medicines—The Perspective of Healthcare Professrionals and Industry. *Value Health* **2019**, *22*, S786–S787. [CrossRef]
93. European Commission. Information for Patients: What I Need to Know about Biosimilar Medicines? Available online: https://ec.europa.eu/growth/content/information-patients-what-i-need-know-about-biosimilar-medicines_en (accessed on 12 October 2020).
94. Bennett, C.L.; Starko, K.M.; Thomsen, H.S.; Cowper, S.; Sartor, O.; Macdougall, I.C.; Qureshi, Z.P.; Bookstaver, P.B.; Miller, A.D.; Norris, L.B.; et al. Linking Drugs to Obscure Illnesses: Lessons from Pure Red Cell Aplasia, Nephrogenic Systemic Fibrosis, and Reye's Syndrome. A Report from the Southern Network on Adverse Reactions (SONAR). *J. Gen. Intern. Med.* **2012**, *27*, 1697–1703. [CrossRef] [PubMed]
95. Haag-Weber, M.; Eckardt, K.-U.; Hörl, W.H.; Roger, S.D.; Vetter, A.; Roth, K. Safety, Immunogenicity and Efficacy of Subcutaneous Biosimilar Epoetin-α (HX575) in Non-Dialysis Patients with Renal Anemia: A Multi-Center, Randomized, Double-Blind Study. *Clin. Nephrol.* **2012**, *77*, 8–17. [CrossRef] [PubMed]
96. Seidl, A.; Hainzl, O.; Richter, M.; Fischer, R.; Böhm, S.; Deutel, B.; Hartinger, T.; Windisch, J.; Casadevall, N.; London, G.M.; et al. Tungsten-Induced Denaturation and Aggregation of Epoetin Alfa during Primary Packaging as a Cause of Immunogenicity. *Pharm. Res.* **2012**, *29*, 1454–1467. [CrossRef] [PubMed]
97. EUPATI. EUPATI Toolbox: Biosimilars. Available online: https://toolbox.eupati.eu/resources/biosimilars/ (accessed on 20 November 2020).
98. International Alliance of Patients' Organizations. Biological and Biosimilar Medicines. Available online: https://www.iapo.org.uk/biological-and-biosimilar-medicines-2013 (accessed on 1 December 2020).

99. Nederlandse Diabetes Federatie. Nederlandse Diabetes Federatie over Biosimilar Insulines: NDF Standpunt. Available online: https://diabetesfederatie.nl/images/downloads/overig/NDF_over_biosimilars_insulines-standpunt.pdf (accessed on 20 January 2021).
100. Makoul, G.; Clayman, M.L. An Integrative Model of Shared Decision Making in Medical Encounters. *Patient Educ. Couns.* **2006**, *60*, 301–312. [CrossRef] [PubMed]

MDPI
St. Alban-Anlage 66
4052 Basel
Switzerland
Tel. +41 61 683 77 34
Fax +41 61 302 89 18
www.mdpi.com

Pharmaceuticals Editorial Office
E-mail: pharmaceuticals@mdpi.com
www.mdpi.com/journal/pharmaceuticals

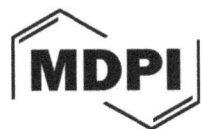

www.ingramcontent.com/pod-product-compliance
Lightning Source LLC
LaVergne TN
LVHW070703100526
838202LV00013B/1017